# New Insight into Cerebrovascular Diseases - An Updated Comprehensive Review

*Edited by Patricia Bozzetto Ambrosi, Rufai Ahmad, Auwal Abdullahi and Amit Agrawal*

Published in London, United Kingdom

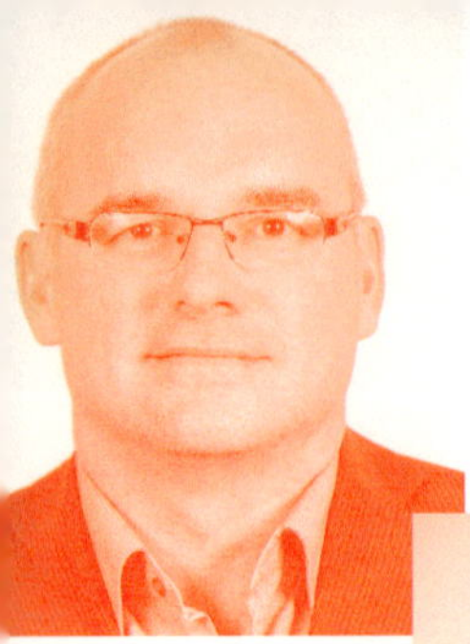
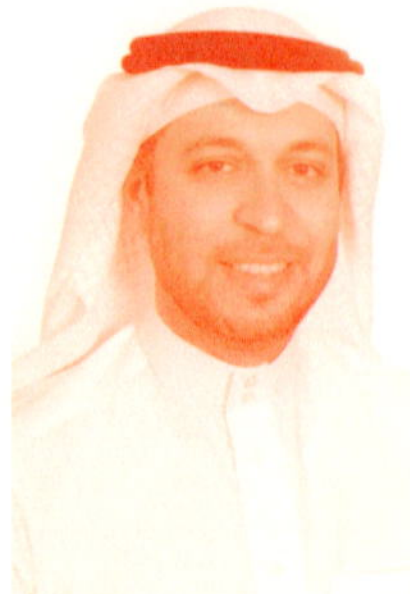
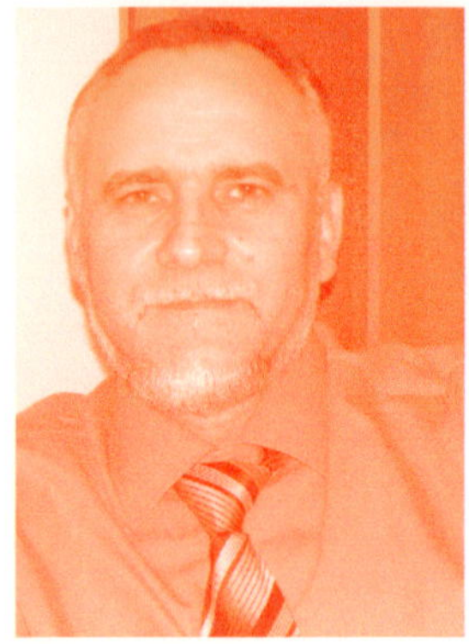
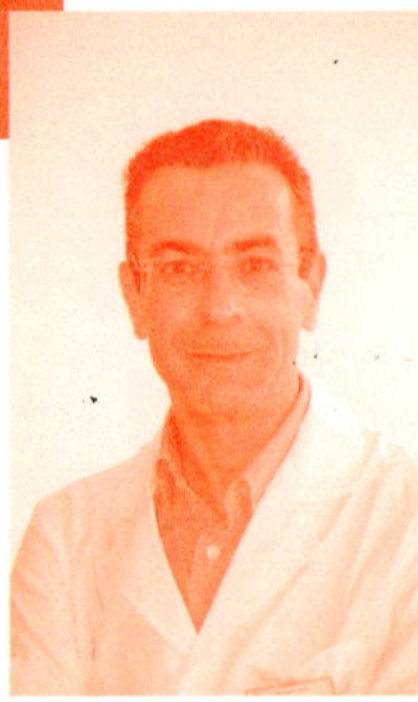
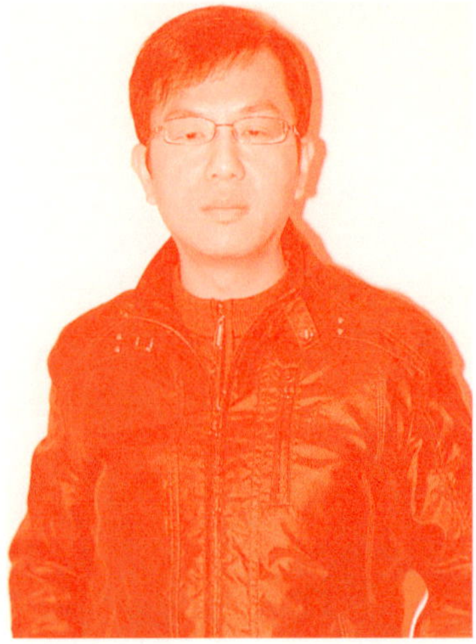
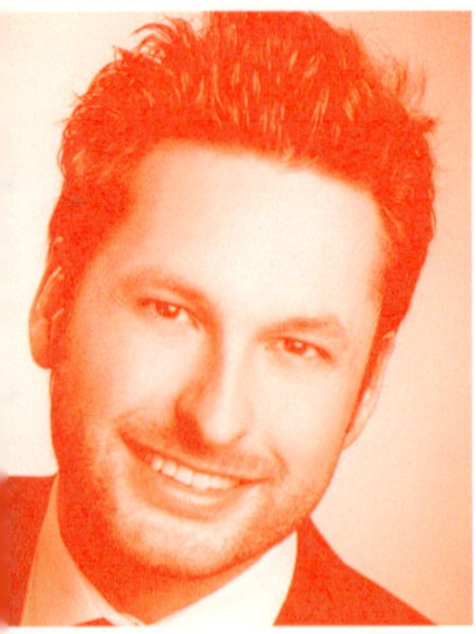
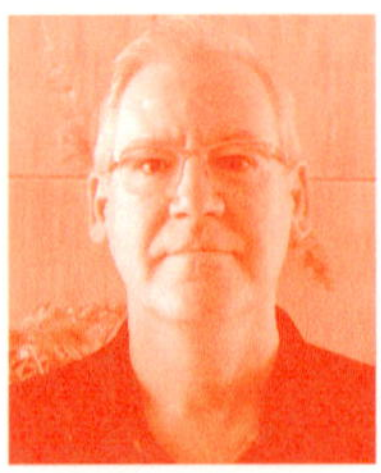

IntechOpen

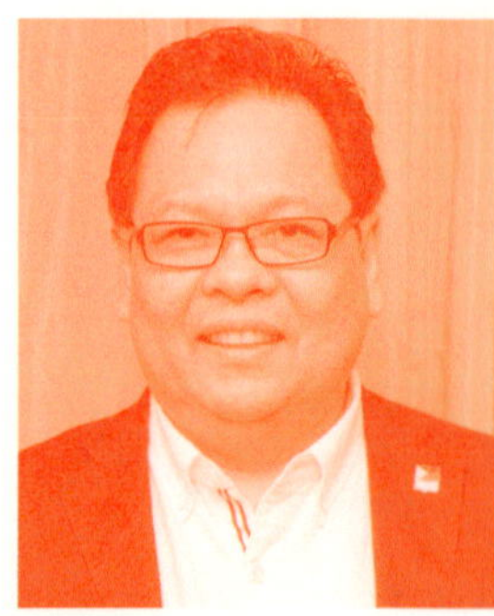
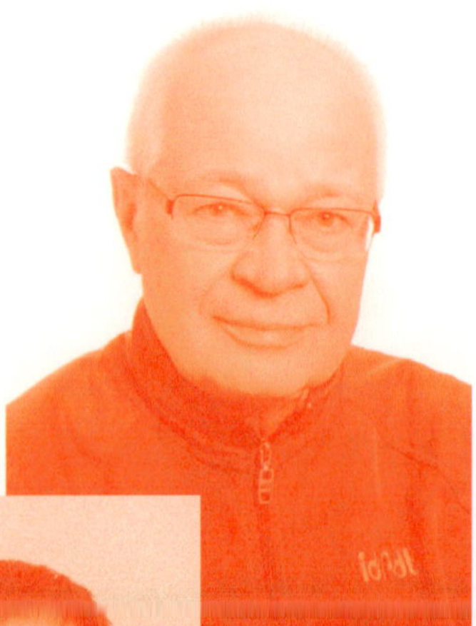
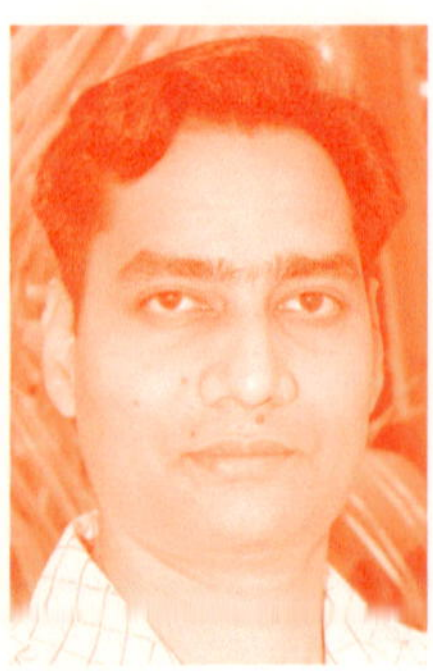
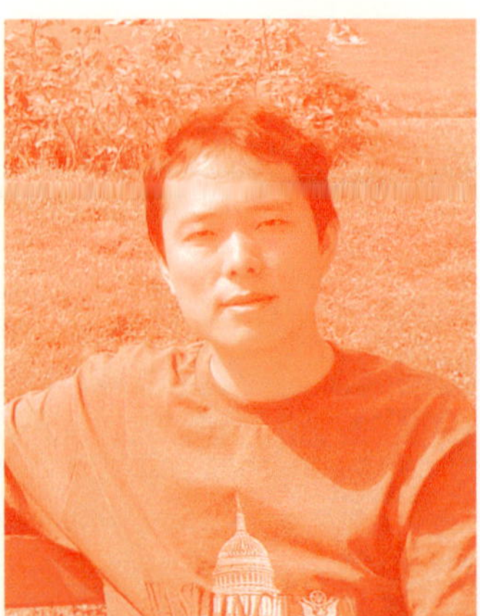
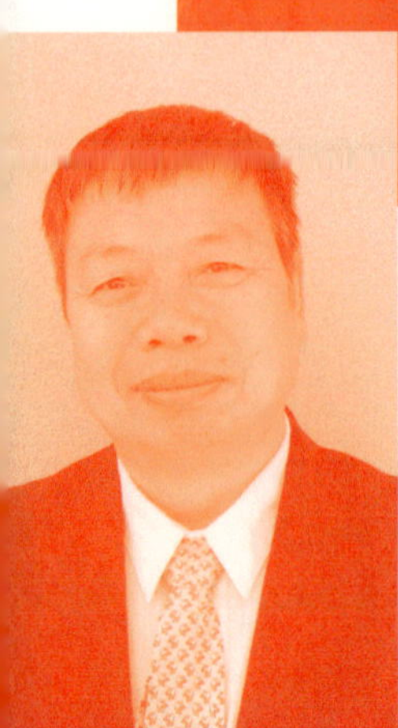
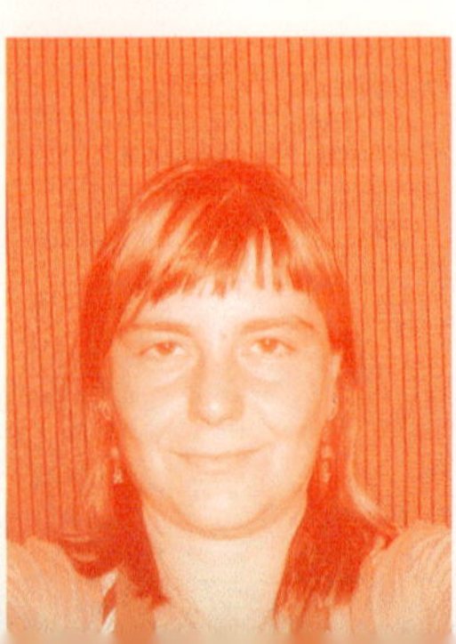

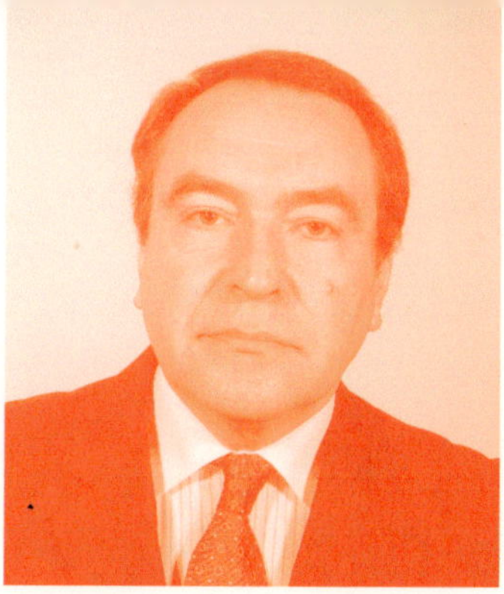
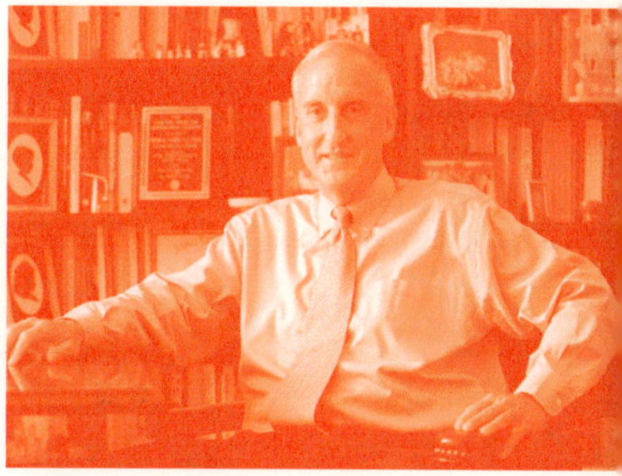
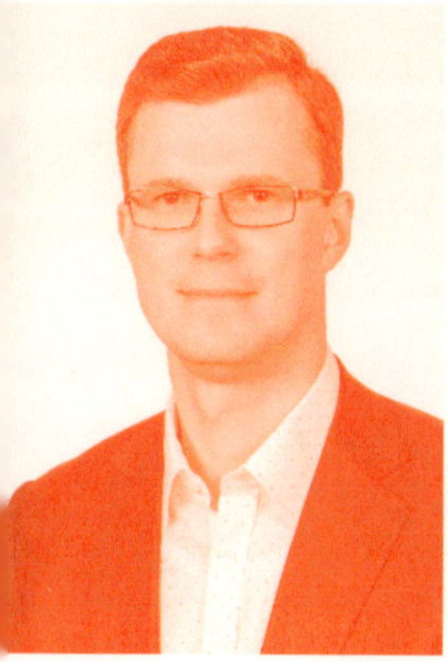
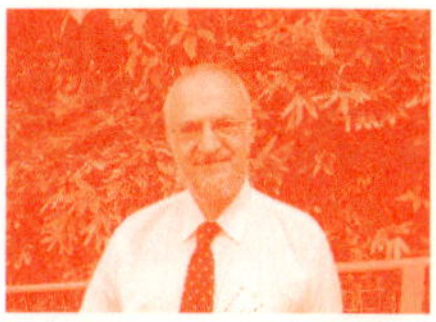
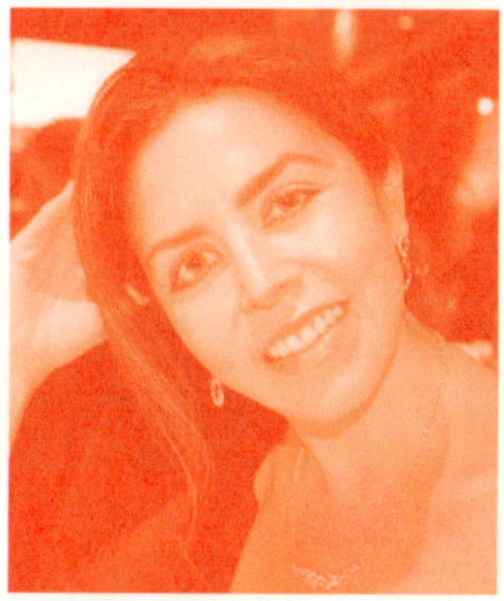

*Supporting open minds since 2005*

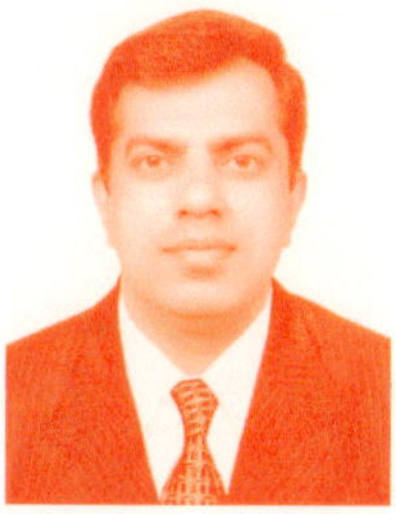
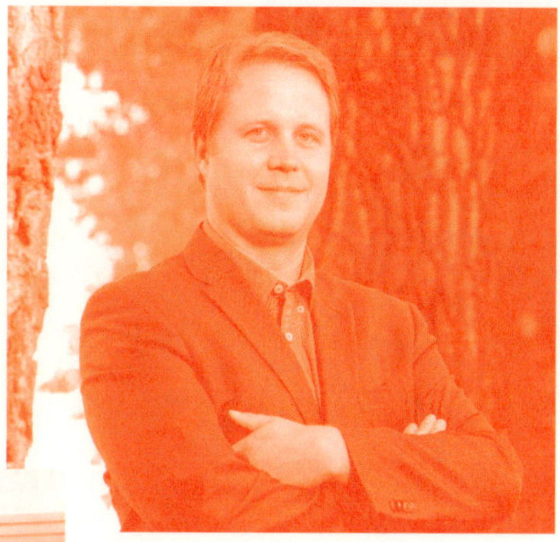
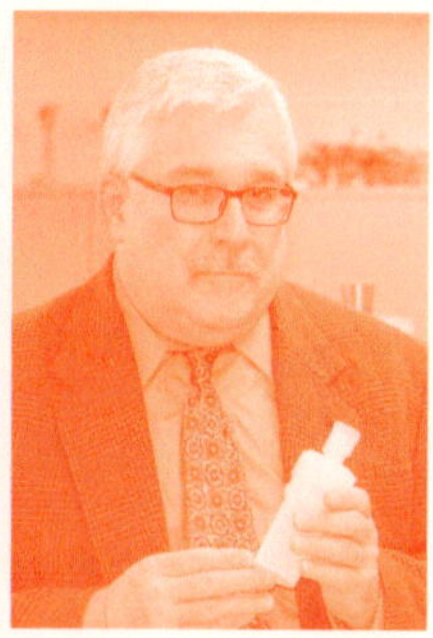
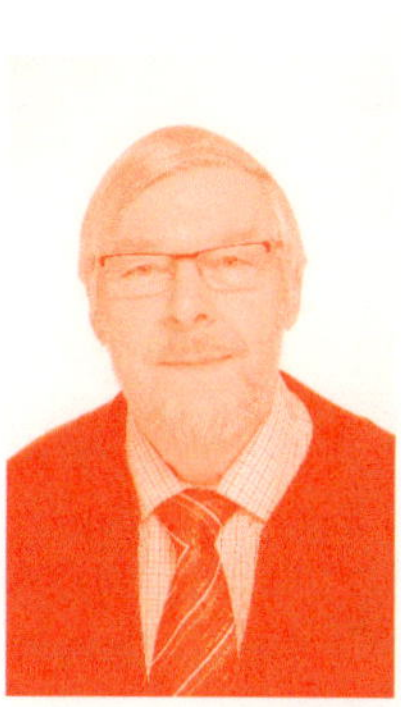
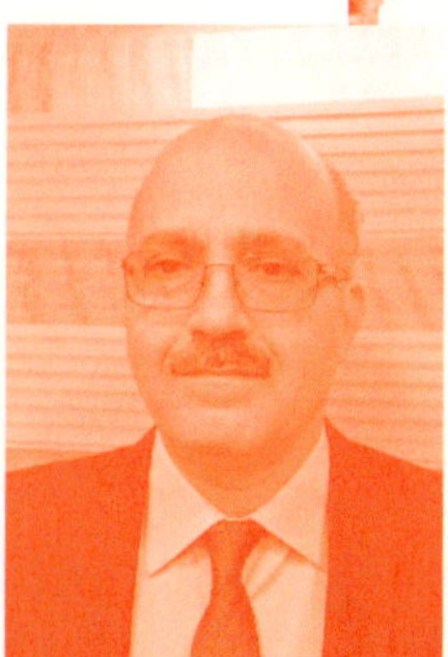
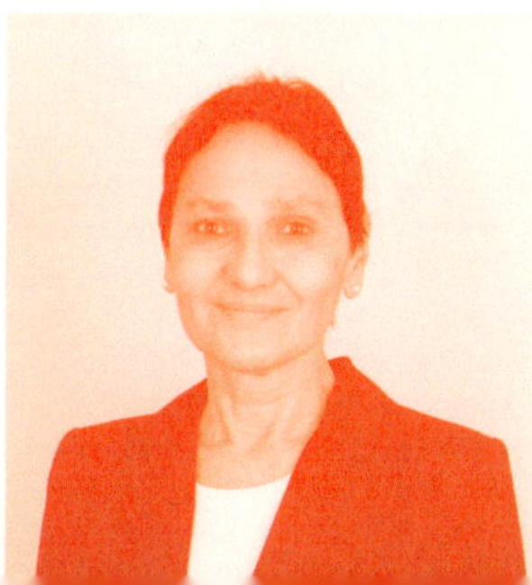
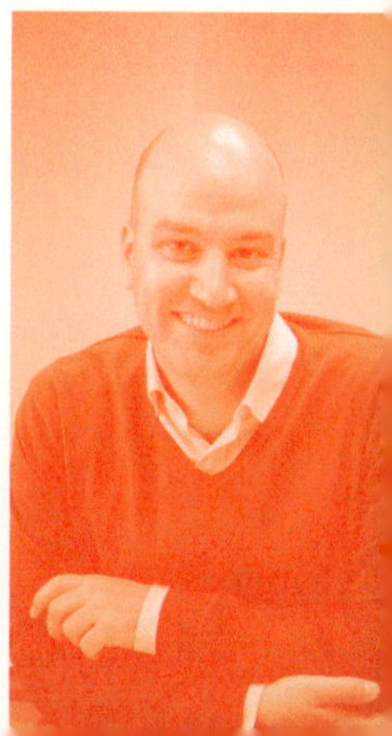

New Insight into Cerebrovascular Diseases - An Updated Comprehensive Review
http://dx.doi.org/10.5772/intechopen.84327
Edited by Patricia Bozzetto Ambrosi, Rufai Ahmad, Auwal Abdullahi and Amit Agrawal

Contributors
Ioan Alexandru Florian, Ioan Stefan Florian, Teodora Larisa Timis, Cristina Caterina Aldea, Bing Zhao, Haixia Xing, Shenghao Ding, Yaohua Pan, Jieqing Wan, Farayi Kaseke, Tecla Mlambo, Aimee Stewart, Lovemore Gwanzura, James Hakim, Rena D. Sukhdeo Singh, Abhi Pandhi, Andrei V. Alexandrov, Mehmet Erin Tüysüz, Mehmet Dedemoğlu, Mei-Ling Sharon Tai, Kuo Ghee Ong, Tsun Haw Toh, Hafez Hussain, David Altschul, Santiago Unda, Tarini Vats, Aleš Hejčl, Alena Sejkorová, Helena Švihlová, Martin Sameš, Mária Stratilová, Josef Zámečník, Jaroslav Hron, Tomáš Radovnický, Alberto Feletti, Miroslav Koblížek, Vladimír Beneš, Dan Dragomir-Daescu, Rodrigo Zapata, Geisi Saito, Kyoungjoo Cho, Dragoş Cătălin Jianu, Georgiana Munteanu, Silviana Nina Jianu, Traian Flavius Dan, Claudia Birsan, Karla Alejandra Cantú Saldaña, María Yolanda Cruz Martínez, José Juan Antonio Ibarra Arias, Hideki Nakano, Iype Cherian, Hira Burhan, Antonios El Helou, Sarah Wilson, Michael Crozier, Yaser Alahamd, Hisham Ab Ib Swehli, Sundus Sardar, Alaa Rahhal, Mawahib Ali Mohammed Elhassan, Salma Alsamel, Osama Ali Ibrahim, Ahmed Shawky Elserafy, Tarek Abdelsalam, Amit Agrawal, Ravish Rajiv Keni, Harsh Deora



First published in London, United Kingdom, 2020 by IntechOpen
IntechOpen is the global imprint of INTECHOPEN LIMITED, registered in England and Wales, registration number: 11086078, 7th floor, 10 Lower Thames Street, London, EC3R 6AF, United Kingdom
Printed in Croatia

British Library Cataloguing-in-Publication Data
A catalogue record for this book is available from the British Library

Additional hard and PDF copies can be obtained from orders@intechopen.com

New Insight into Cerebrovascular Diseases - An Updated Comprehensive Review
Edited by Patricia Bozzetto Ambrosi, Rufai Ahmad, Auwal Abdullahi and Amit Agrawal
p. cm.
Print ISBN 978-1-78985-359-9
Online ISBN 978-1-78985-360-5
eBook (PDF) ISBN 978-1-78985-099-4

For EU product safety concerns:
IN TECH d.o.o., Prolaz Marije Krucifikse Kozulić 3, 51000 Rijeka, Croatia, info@intechopen.com or visit our website at intechopen.com.

# Meet the editors

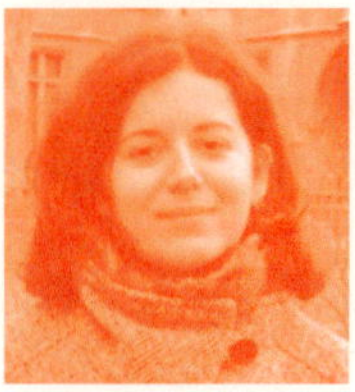

Dr. Patricia Bozzetto Ambrosi graduated in medicine from the University of Caxias do Sul, Brazil, and University of Rome Tor Vergata, Italy. She is a former researcher in morphophysiology at the University of Córdoba/Reina Sofia Hospital, Córdoba, Spain. She graduated in Neurology/ Neurosurgery at the Hospital of Restauração, SES, in Brazil and Neuroradiology/Radiodiagnostics at Paris Marie Curie University. She holds a master's degree in Medicine from the University of Nova Lisboa in Portugal and in Behavioral Sciences and Neuropsychiatry from the University of Pernambuco. She also has a PhD in Biological Sciences from the University of Pernambuco/Paris Diderot University. She is a former Fellow in Interventional Neuroradiology in France at the Ophthalmological Foundation Adolphe de Rothschild, Beaujon Hospital and Hospices Civils de Strasbourg. She was Praticien Associé in Interventional Neuroradiology at Neurologique Hospital Pierre Wertheimer, University of Lyon Claude Bernard in Lyon, France, and Visiting Professor of the University of Paris Diderot-Neuri Beaujon. She is actually an independent consultant/supervisor in neuroradiology, neuroendovascular, and imaging. She is also an academic collaborator researcher in the Cardiovascular Department at the University of Leicester. She has experience in innovative research for the development of new technologies and is also an academic editor and reviewer of several scientific publications.

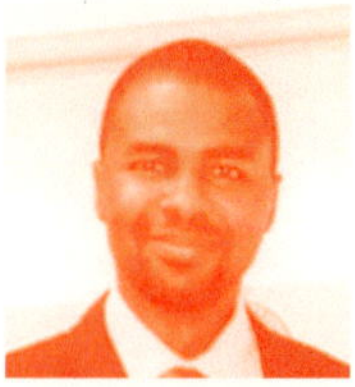

Dr. Rufai Ahmad graduated with a BSc in Physiotherapy from Bayero University, Kano, Nigeria, in 2001. He obtained his MSc and PhD in Health and Rehabilitation from the University of Southampton, UK, in 2008 and 2012, respectively. He also received his Doctor of Physiotherapy degree from the Michigan-Flint University, USA, in 2015. Dr. Ahmad is Associate Professor and Deputy Director (Procurement and Training), Directorate of Laboratory Management at Bayero University, Kano, and an Honorary Consultant Physiotherapist at Aminu Kano Teaching Hospital, Kano. He is a former Head of Department of Physiotherapy, Deputy Dean, Faculty of Allied Health Sciences, Bayero University, and editor-in-chief of the *Bayero Journal of Evidence-Based Physiotherapy*. He is currently the National President of the Nigeria Society of Physiotherapy and a member of the Medical Rehabilitation Therapists Board of Nigeria.

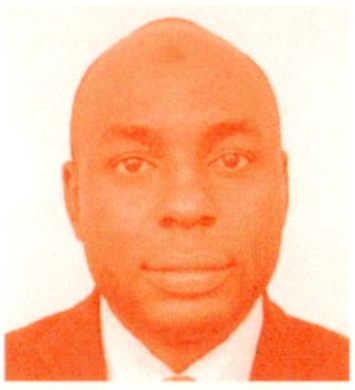

Dr. Auwal Abdullahi is a specialist neurological rehabilitation therapist at Bayero University, Kano, where he teaches and supervises both undergraduate and postgraduate students. He is a Fellow of the London of Academy of Sports and Health Sciences in Clinical Neurology Sciences. His most recent publications are on neurobiology of recovery of motor function and clinical decision making. He enjoys reading, research, teaching, and writing.

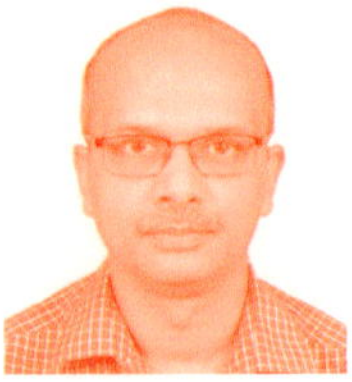

Dr. Amit Agrawal completed his neurosurgery training from the National Institute of Mental Health and Neurosciences, Bangalore, India, in 2003. Dr. Agrawal is a self-motivated, enthusiastic, and results-oriented professional with more than 16 years of rich experience in research and development, as well as teaching and mentoring in the field of neurosurgery. He is proficient in managing and leading teams for running successful process operations and has experience in developing procedures and service standards of excellence. He has attended and participated in many international- and national-level symposiums and conferences and delivered lectures on vivid topics. He has published more than 750 articles in the medical field covering various topics in several national and international journals. His expertise is in identifying training needs, designing training modules, and executing the same while working with limited resources. He has excellent communication, presentation, and interpersonal skills with proven abilities in teaching and training for various academic and professional courses. Presently, he is working at the All India Institute of Medical Sciences, Bhopal, Madhya Pradesh (India).

# Contents

# Preface

Important recent discoveries in the field of medical sciences and related disciplines have increased our understanding of cerebrovascular diseases. Cerebrovascular diseases are called by a variety of medical conditions that affect blood vessels in the brain and their hemodynamic state. The most common presentations are stroke, transient ischemic attack, vascular malformations (brain aneurysms), and arterial stenosis. Blood flows through the vessels that supply oxygen and nutrients to the brain, which are usually damaged or deformed in these disorders. If its flow is obstructed, by a blood clot that moves to the brain or by a narrowing or rupturing of blood vessels, the brain loses its energy supply, causing damage to brain tissues, causing sequelae of stroke. This spectrum of conditions involving brain vessels is of immense importance to public health, being the most common cause of disability and the second most frequent cause of death in Western society. Annually, more than 15 million people worldwide suffer a stroke, out of which five million die and another five million are permanently disabled. Technological advances in new medical therapies (calcium therapies in target vessels), advances in neurointerventionist treatment (endovascular therapies and new surgical approaches), and innovative approaches in the treatment of neurorehabilitation have strongly revolutionized the neurobiological basis of neurovascular diseases by a measure of results. The adequate correlation between central nervous system injuries and their clinical characteristics with management and results directed at neurorehabilitation represents the basis of personalized medicine, a promising perspective to explain the different individual responses to treatment and improve the current quality of care.

This book provides a comprehensive and up-to-date review of cerebrovascular diseases, as well as new information on each important related topic. This edition of the book was divided into seven sections, covering all the main aspects of cerebrovascular diseases, including Introduction (stroke load), Pathophysiology, Hemodynamics, Diagnosis, Management, Repair, and Healing. These are distributed in 18 chapters designed to assist the reader in self-examination to complete each topic. Each chapter simply represents the opinion of the authors through a particular effort to identify and separate the best of their knowledge. Although generally accepted concepts of new or controversial material have been developed, this book has been designed as a comprehensive review of cerebrovascular diseases, providing a reference source for professionals or trainees, doctors, and clinicians, all interested in cerebrovascular diseases.

Finally, I would very much like to acknowledge our achievements and to thank first of all the authors without whom this edition would not be possible. Also, I would like to thank to Dr. Ahmad, Dr. Abdullahi, and Dr. Agrawal for co-editing this project, and to Ms. Ivana Spajic, Petra Svob, Sara Bacvarova, and Sandra Maljavac who did a superb job in developing this volume to its current standard.

**Patricia Bozzetto Ambrosi**
Academic Research Collaborator with the Department of Cardiovascular Sciences,
University of Leicester,
United Kingdom

Independent Consultant in Neuroradiology, PhD
University Paris Diderot and Neuri Beaujon,
France

**Rufai Ahmad and Auwal Abdullahi**
Bayero University,
Nigeria

**Amit Agrawal**
Narayana Medical College and Hospital,
India

Section 1

# Introduction

Chapter 1

# Aging, Cerebrovascular Burden, and Cognitive Decline

*Kyoungjoo Cho*

## Abstract

Brain function is supported by the cerebrovascular system, and changes in vascular phenotype and function through aging process make the brain more susceptible to neurodegenerative diseases, particularly cognitive decline. Correspondingly, the incidence of dementia and the prevalence of neurodegenerative diseases have also increased. In aging, the vessels have been exposed to the inflammatory state by harmful factors referred to as the senescence-associated secretory phenotype (SASP). Aging is a complex process that is associated with accumulated cellular stresses and an increased stress response. The aging in the brain includes structural and functional changes, which cause brain pathologies in the elderly. Particularly, damaged neurovascular event can be a consequent trigger in the pathology of vascular cognitive impairment. This chapter introduces the current knowledge on cognitive decline according to cerebrovascular aging relevant to endothelial senescence and the changes in the SASPs.

**Keywords:** aging, cerebrovascular, cognitive impairment, senescence-associated secretory phenotype, endothelial cells

## 1. Introduction

Aging is a complex process that is associated with an accumulation of the effects of cellular stresses and an increased stress response. The aging in the brain includes structural and functional changes, which together cause brain pathologies in the elderly. These changes are also thought to be critical risk factors in the development of cognitive disorders [1, 2]. It is well known that the cerebrovascular system supports brain function [3]. Vascular phenotypic and functional changes caused by aging make the brain more susceptible to neurodegenerative diseases, particularly to cognitive decline [4]. Dysregulation of cerebral blood flow (CBF) is one factor in the pathogenesis of vascular cognitive impairment (VCI) [5]. However, definition, diagnostic criteria, and treatments for VCI have not been firmly established. Thus, strategies in translational medicine and the clinical approach to VCI patients and the current aged society need to be established. This is because according to the World Alzheimer Report 2015, it was estimated that 46.8 million people worldwide suffer from dementia, and this number is expected to increase to 74.7 million by 2030 and 131.5 million by 2050 [6]. The report also stated that the incidence of dementia, including Alzheimer's disease (AD) and vascular dementia (VaD), will increase by 45%. As a result of the increase in the size of the aging population, the incidence of dementia and the onset or prevalence of neurodegenerative diseases are increasing. These diseases have become important social concerns and represent both a current and a future social and economic burden.

In the aging process, age-related cerebrovascular dysfunction results from multiple pathophysiological changes. The first of them is oxidative stress and inflammation. Excessive oxidative stress is well known to contribute to vascular aging in both animals [4, 7–10] and humans [11, 12]. It is an overproduction of reactive oxygen species (ROS) rather than accumulation of ROS. In cellular senescence, inflammatory mediators such as chemokines and cytokines are secreted in an autocrine or paracrine manner. This is often referred to as the senescence-associated secretory phenotype (SASP) [13–15]. The second is the narrowing of the vascular lumen caused by atherosclerotic plaques, which is referred to as atherosclerosis in large vessels or arteriosclerosis in small vessels [16–18]. Technically a further factor is endothelial cell senescence induced by the SASP in the aging process. This arises as a result of the action of pro-inflammatory cytokines such as interleukin (IL)-1 and IL-6 [19]. Under aging, atherosclerotic plaques are prone to arise in the human aorta and coronary arteries, which contain senescent endothelial cells [20]. The senescent phenotypes of endothelial cells can be physiologically classified as having either an anti-inflammatory phenotype or a pro-inflammatory senescent phenotype [21]. Recently, numerous studies have focused on the status of the immune system during aging [22–24]. This chapter introduces the current knowledge about cognitive decline according to cerebrovascular aging relevant to cellular senescence and the changes in the SASPs. It also provides approaches on how senescent vessels exposed to the SASP enhance age-related cerebrovascular degeneration and vascular damage-derived cognitive impairment.

## 2. Aging and vessels

Cellular senescence is the state in which normal cells cease to divide. It can be thought of as a type of programmed cell cycle arrest. The senescent cells go through changes in gene expression and secretion of soluble factors in response to excessive stresses [25]. The secreted soluble factors from senescent cells are referred to as the SASP [26–28]. The SASP includes interleukins (IL) and chemokines such as IL-1, IL-6, IL-8, monocyte chemoattractant protein (MCP)-2, and macrophage inflammatory protein (MIP)-1 [29]. In addition, nitric oxide, growth factors, and several matrix metalloproteinases have also been identified in the SASP [14]. Several studies have reported that SASP factors have roles in inducing normal cells to acquire a senescent phenotype and can act in a paracrine manner to affect the activity of other nearby cells [30]. This might suggest that SASP factors do not merely arise as a result of cell senescence but could rather act to promote the senescence phenotype in normal cells.

Although it still remains equivocal whether neurodegenerative diseases arise as a result of, or from, aging-related changes, it is clear, however, that the prevalence of neurodegenerative diseases that show a cognitive decline is positively associated with aging. Increases in oxidative stress and inflammation in response to aging trigger cellular senescence and the appropriate downstream responses. A series of these insults can aggravate age-related or neurodegenerative pathogenesis with several vascular diseases [31].

### 2.1 Endothelium

The endothelium is one of the vessel constituents and is important in vascular structure because of its high versatility. The endothelium has multifunctional roles in maintaining blood fluidity and metabolic homeostasis. The features are important in regulating the delivery of water and nutrients through the whole body [32]. The endothelium also plays an important role in the resolution of inflammatory responses. Morphological and functional changes in the endothelium are also involved in the development of numerous pathological disorders [33, 34]. Endothelial cells are located in the inner layer of the vasculature and can come into contact with blood-containing macrophages. Therefore, endothelial cells are the first target of cytokines circulating in the blood. Simultaneously, endothelial cells also secrete pro-inflammatory cytokines, such as IL-1, IL-6, IL-8, IL-15, MCP-1, and tumor necrosis factor (TNF)-α [29]. In fact, endothelial cell-derived pro-inflammatory cytokines and chemokines are important in recruiting immune cells to the site and play a role in wound healing, angiogenesis, and inflammatory diseases. In addition to their inflammatory function, endothelial cells also produce pro-thrombotic mediators and cellular adhesion molecules (ICAM-1, intercellular adhesion molecule-1; PAI-1, plasminogen activator inhibitor-1) and enhance the adhesion and transmigration of immune cells into underlying tissues. It has also been reported that senescent endothelial cells have reduced expression levels of nitric oxide (NO) as well as reduced expression levels and phosphorylation of endothelial NO synthase (eNOS) [35, 36].

It is well accepted that senescence in vascular endothelial cells is a common factor in various age-related diseases. Associated with aging, endothelial cells dynamically change the inflammatory phenotype to SASP [21]. A recent study has demonstrated that alterations in toll-like receptor (TLR) and TLR ligands during aging might determine the state of the inflammatory process [29]. Since endothelial cells are not immune cells, they cannot recognize foreign antigens via TLRs or present antigens through MHC II molecules to T and B cells [37]. On the other hand, endothelial cells have been shown to upregulate the mRNA levels of TLR-2, TLR-4, TLR-7, TLR-8, TLR-9, and TLR-10 during aging [38]. Since aging is a chronic inflammatory condition in the lower level, nonimmune endothelial cells could play a role in controlling and maintaining immune homeostasis. Taken these reasons, endothelial cells could be a therapeutic target to allow for recovery of a disruption in immune homeostasis.

Endothelial cells derived from patients with severe coronary artery disease have also been shown to be mostly senescent endothelial cells with reduced levels of telomeric DNA-binding factor 1 (TRF1) and increased telomere oxidation [20]. When TRF1 was overexpressed in a cellular aging model, namely, human umbilical vein endothelial cells' (HUVECs) passage for a long period of time, the telomere-associated DNA damage foci and the SASP were decreased [39, 40]. These results suggest that telomere dysfunction and the SASP occur prior to cellular senescence and induce vascular dysfunction following cardiovascular disease (CVD) development.

### 2.2 Atherosclerosis

Atherosclerosis and its associated clinical outcomes such as vascular stiffness are initiated and progressed through dysfunction in senescent endothelial cells [29]. During oxidation in the vessel, there are changes in its physicochemical properties including lipid charge, size, and content. Oxidized low-density lipid (oxLDL) becomes different from natural LDL. The oxLDL stimulates endothelial cells to induce the expression of adhesion molecules such as E-selectin and vascular cell adhesion molecule-1 (VCAM-1) on the surface of the artery [41]. Numerous senescent endothelial cells are detected in the aorta of the human with atherosclerotic plaques [42, 43]. The formation of atherosclerotic plaques is initiated by macrophages that infiltrate into the arterial intima in response to oxLDL present in the vessel [69]. Lipid-laden foam cells become pro-inflammatory, and macrophages secrete pro-inflammatory cytokines. The recruited macrophages move into the artery, and consequently, the atherosclerotic plaque size and complexity are getting larger [44].

Atherosclerosis occurs following chronic exposure to cellular stressors. It has been reported that SASP can be restrained simply by inhibiting TNF-α without any transmission of senescence signals in an autocrine or paracrine manner [45]. Anti-TNF-α treatment has been demonstrated to physiologically reduce the non-cell autonomous effects of SASP. In patients treated with adalimumab (Humira, a human monoclonal antibody against TNF-α), epigenetic modifications were triggered. The molecular mechanisms are identified as TNF-α signaling in senescent endothelial cells, which raises the possibility of therapeutic approaches for age-associated diseases. In senescent human umbilical vein endothelial cells (HUVECs), the levels of miR-146a-5p and miR-126-3p show higher than younger HUVECs. Additionally, the levels of miR-146a-5p are increased in both senescent and young HUVECs following lipopolysaccharide (LPS) exposure, whereas the level of miR-126-3p is decreased only in senescent HUVECs and is unchanged in young HUVECs [45]. This study also showed that changes in the levels of several microRNAs (miRNAs) do not arise as a result of just treatment with LPS or an anti-TNF-α antibody. These data suggest that some miRNAs work in an age-dependent manner in vessels and endothelial cells.

### 2.3 Vascular aging

From a classical perspective, the aged vasculature is viewed as having worsened vasodilation, arterial stiffness, remodeling of the extracellular matrix, intimal thickening, and endothelial cell dysfunction [46]. The effects of vascular aging have been explored extensively and have been attributed to the number of different causes with genome instability and mTOR being two of the major causes. Studies with mTOR-inhibiting drugs in vessels have shown that such drugs have a deleterious effect on endothelial function in patients who have advanced arterial aging and inserted coronary stents [47–49]. Compared to human studies, cultured endothelial cells have augmented anti-inflammatory effects to mTOR inhibitors with a dose-dependent manner and have increased cytostatic effect [50]. It also showed that rapamycin, an mTOR inhibitor, induces the expression of PAI-1 in mice as well as in cultured endothelial cells [51]. When the Atg7 gene, one of the mediators of the autophagic process, is deleted in mice, vascular aging is accelerated [52]. In a mouse model of Hutchinson-Gilford progeria, autophagy is activated by AMPK activation and inhibition of mTOR [53]. These results showed that the mTOR–AMPK signaling pathway might be a link to the regulation of autophagy in age-related diseases. Based on the results described above, it is hard to firmly establish that rapamycin plays a preventive role on cellular senescence.

Telomere shortening is known to be a hallmark of cellular senescence. Telomeres are significantly shorter in several endothelial cells and vascular smooth muscle cells (VSMCs), which is a clear marker of SASP in aged vasculature. The shortened telomeres in mouse vascular tissue have been shown to be sufficient to induce endothelial dysfunction [54], whereas human VSMCs still have a normal phenotype sustaining plaque stability regardless of telomere length [55]. Although telomere shortening is common in vascular aging and CVD, it remains unclear whether telomere shortening is sufficient to lead to cellular senescence and vascular degeneration in aged vessels [56].

In the patients with severe coronary artery disease, most of endothelial cells demonstrated the features of senescent endothelial cells that reduced levels of telomeric DNA-binding factor 1 (TRF1) and increased telomere oxidation as mentioned above [20, 39, 40]. These results suggest that telomere dysfunction and the SASP occur prior to cellular senescence and induce vascular dysfunction following CVD development.

The causes of vascular aging and vascular aging-related phenotypes can be summarized as follows:

i. Oxidative DNA damage: during aging, the onset of CVD led by changes in vascular endothelial cells results in an impairment of endothelium-dependent vasodilation, an overproduction of pro-inflammatory and pro-thrombotic factors, and an increase in oxidative stress [57]. In the human population, age is an important and independent risk factor for CVD [58].

ii. Telomere shortening: an association between telomere shortening and CVD risk factors has been found in atherosclerosis, arterial stiffness, type 1 and type 2 diabetes, and obesity [59–62].

iii. Genome instability: a failure in DNA damage repair occurs in cells and tissues during the aging process [63].

## 3. Aging and cerebrovascular function

As aging progresses, cerebrovascular function declines which can increase the possibility for ischemic stroke, intracerebral hemorrhages (ICHs), microbleeds, and cognitive decline [64]. Healthy functional cerebral vessels can coordinate with CBF and appropriately supply blood to the brain [65]. However, cerebrovascular aging has the following features, which can lead to age-related cerebrovascular diseases: (i) endothelial senescence, (ii) oxidative stress and inflammation, (iii) microvascular rarefaction, (iv) arterial stiffness, (v) vascular lumen narrowness, and (vi) CBF reduction. Each feature according to cerebrovascular aging is described in detail in the following subsections.

### 3.1 Cerebral vasculature

Cerebral vessels play a critical role in mediating between the whole body and the brain by transporting molecules between the blood and brain [5]. The brain vasculature that supplies blood to the brain tissue consists of two blood supply systems. One is the internal carotid artery system. This system is responsible for approximately 70% of the total CBF. The other system is the vertebral artery system, which is responsible for approximately 30% of the total CBF. These two major blood systems converge at Willis' circle, which allows communication between the left and right brain hemispheres, and branch out into the whole brain through cerebral arteries [66]. The most common structural feature of cerebral vessels is the blood–brain barrier (BBB), which comprises tight junctions and adherens junctions [5]. These tight junctions exist between endothelial cells, the basal membrane, pericytes, and the astrocyte end feet [67].

The BBB is important because it prevents harmful molecules from entering the brain tissue from the systemic circulation. Accordingly, a malfunction in BBB permeability has been reported in neurodegenerative disorders and cognitive decline that leads to dementia [68–70]. CBF is regulated in response to blood pressure through cerebral autoregulation. It was demonstrated that there were minor differences between CBF and blood pressure (within 10 mmHg of blood pressure) among healthy humans in the plateau region [71]. The report also suggested that hypertension and a higher pulsatile rate might disrupt cerebral autoregulation, which make subjects prone to neurodegenerative diseases because the aging brain is subject to hypoperfusion [71].

### 3.2 Cerebral vascular aging

Healthy functional cerebral vessels can coordinate with CBF and appropriately supply blood to the brain [65]. As aging progresses, however, cerebrovascular function declines, which can increase the possibility of ischemic stroke, intracerebral hemorrhages (ICHs), microbleeds, and cognitive decline [64]. Cerebrovascular aging has the following features, which can lead to age-related cerebrovascular diseases:

i. Endothelial senescence: many studies have shown the presence of senescent endothelial cells in aged cerebrovascular lesions, which is triggered by the accumulation of ROS [31] and modulated by inflammatory factors, as described above.

ii. Oxidative stress and inflammation: in vessels' walls, ROS increase nicotinamide adenine dinucleotide phosphate (NADPH) oxidase activity associated with aging [7, 72, 73]. These findings have been reported in both nonclinical and clinical studies. It is also well known that the vasculature can be easily damaged by vasculopathy, including atherosclerosis [74–76].

iii. Microvascular rarefaction: this is a condition where the microvascular network and its density are reduced. Rarefaction has been detected in some brain subregions, particularly in the hippocampus. Since the hippocampus is involved in memory, it could lead to memory loss [77, 78]. Circulating endothelial progenitor cells have been shown to be diminished by aging, which is linked to white matter changes and a decline in cognitive function [79, 80].

iv. Arterial stiffness: this is a major characteristic of vascular aging. Vascular stiffness increases blood flow velocity and blood pressure. Arterial stiffness results in an increase in systolic pressure and a decrease in diastolic pressure.

v. Vascular lumen narrowness: the accumulation of toxic molecules in the vessel walls makes the vascular lumen narrow. There have been clinical studies such as cerebral autosomal dominant arteriopathy with subcortical infarcts and leukoencephalopathy (CADASIL) that have examined Notch3 molecules in cerebral autosomal dominant arteriopathy with subcortical infarcts and leukoencephalopathy. The high-temperature requirement A serine peptidase 1 (HTRA1) is also explored in cerebral autosomal recessive arteriopathy and leukoencephalopathy [81–83].

vi. CBF reduction: generally, hypoperfusion in the cerebral circulation is suggested to lead to cognitive impairment [84]. In cases of mild hypoperfusion, synaptic plasticity is impaired by a reduction in protein synthesis during learning and memory consolidation [2]. Under severe hypoperfusion, there is failure in the formation of the action potential, disruption in the acid–base balance, occurrence of neuronal edema, and accumulation of neurotic molecules [85].

With respect to neural activity, cerebrovascular reactivity (CVR) can be used to measure the response levels of brain blood vessels to various stimuli. Very recent evidence has shown that cerebral vessel contractility and dilation decrease as aging progresses and have effects on the neurovascular damage mediated by NO [86]. In addition, there is an induction of vasoconstrictive factors in the cerebral endothelium [87]. Since the vessel wall undergoes structural changes through the normal aging process, it is a natural and frequently found phenomenon that the basement membrane becomes thicker but smooth muscle cells and elastin layer are thinner [88]. These different responses between young and old adults have been demonstrated using blood-oxygen-level-dependent functional MRI (BOLD fMRI) data [89]. As a result of these collective findings, it is now considered that the vasculature plays a critical secondary cause in many neurodegenerative diseases, particularly in neurovascular dysfunction. Therefore, there needs to be an increase in recognition and a focus on cognitive decline after vascular damage to develop newer therapeutic approaches.

## 4. Aging and vessel-related cognitive decline

Dementia is an irreversible cognitive condition. According to a statistical report, 7.7 million people are newly diagnosed with dementia every year [90]. Among these, patients with vascular cognitive impairment and dementia (VCID) compose over 20% of the total dementia patient population [91]. By 2030, the number of older people (>60 years of age) is predicted to increase by 56% compared to the number in 2015, and it will continue to grow year by year. Finally, by 2050, our society will become a superaged society, and it is evident that the prevalence of neurodegenerative diseases will increase. Cognitive-related diseases, such as AD or VaD, will increase by 45% in 2050 compared to 2015 [92].

Mild cognitive impairment (MCI) is included as a cognitive-related disease in the older population. Although MCI is also considered as a pre-step proceeding to dementia, patients with MCI still fortunately have a chance of recovery or at least have a chance to delay the progression of the disease. Therefore, new strategies are urgently needed to diagnose and treat patients with MCI. Some blood factors such as MCP-1 or IL-6 have been suggested to be biomarkers for estimating the progression in cognitive decline because the vascular blood factors are modified in patients with MCI [93]. Some clinical studies have shown that VCID occurs in 25–30% of aged people who have had a previous stroke [94, 95]. Stroke is known to be the second leading cause of cognitive dysfunction. Furthermore, a clinical history of stroke increases the risk of cognitive dysfunction up to fivefold [96, 97]. Therefore, the symptoms of poststroke dementia could be related to the occlusion site, occlusion type, occlusion numbers, and lesion volume in the brain. There are studies that have shown that poststroke cognitive decline is related to the pathology of cerebrovascular disease and dementia, although the mechanisms involved in poststroke dementia are complex [90, 98].

Aging is complex and vulnerable to cognitive decline as well as brain disorders [99]. A recent study concluded that cognitive impairment in aged adults with depression is correlated with the SASP profile [100]. This study showed that the levels of the SASP were highest in participants with both late-life depression (LLD) and MCI (**Figure 1**). This study suggests that cognitive impairment in LLD is linked to an aging-specific molecular profile, which might be an indicator for aging people with LLD who develop dementia [100]. Recent clinical studies have reported that depression and cognitive impairment in aging are associated with the regulation of the SASP: immune-inflammatory response [101], proteostasis [102], signal transduction, and oxidative stress [103].

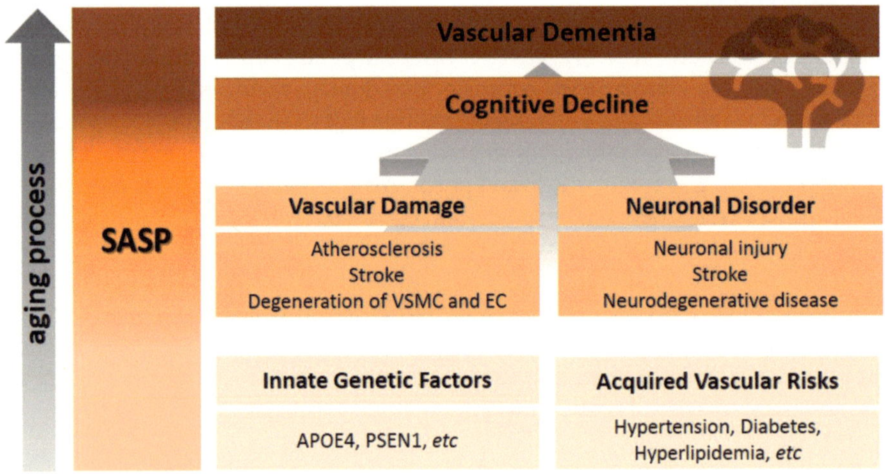


**Figure 1.**
*Aging, cerebrovascular burden, and developing cognitive decline to vascular dementia. With aging, the number of resident senescent cells displaying SASP increases. The familial genetic backgrounds and vascular risk factors acquired through individual lifestyle or harmful habits, such as smoking, increase vulnerability to vascular damage and neuronal dysfunction. Combined with aging factors, such as SASP, during the aging process, vascular damage and neuronal diseases could lead to susceptibility to cognitive decline, which consequently contributes to the progression of vascular dementia. Abbreviations: SASP, senescence-associated secretory phenotype; APOE4, apolipoprotein E4; PSEN1, presenilin 1; VSMC, vascular smooth muscle cell; EC, endothelial cell.*

## 5. Conclusions

Clinically and pathologically, vessel diseases including atherosclerosis are important diseases in a rapidly aging world. Age-related cerebrovascular dysfunctions result from multiple pathophysiological alterations. The clear one thing is that vascular aging and the aged brain vessels are vulnerable to damages and harmful factors such as the SASPs. Once the cerebral vessels have experienced insults, cognitive decline is eventually followed. The source of insults can be SASP particularly in the aging process. Despite efforts to develop therapeutic targets, it is not possible to identify the processes contributing to the onset of vascular disease and its progression of cognitive decline. Our aging society needed more fundamental approaches for treating aging-related neurodegenerative diseases containing dementia. Preferential treatment might be a preventive chance to neurodegenerative diseases. In the present time when dementia becomes an important issue in public heath, economics, social aspects, as well as the political fields, it should be possible to develop preventing and also therapeutic strategies against progressive dementia with a careful focus on treating vascular health by modulating the SASP.

## Acknowledgements

This study was supported by the Basic Science Research Program through the National Research Foundation of Korea (NRF) funded by the Ministry of Education (NRF-2018R1D1A1B07048587).

## Conflict of interest

The authors declare no conflict of interest.

## Author details

Kyoungjoo Cho
Department of Life Science, Kyonggi University, Suwon, South Korea

*Address all correspondence to: kcho0611@kgu.ac.kr

## References

[1] Kalaria RN. Linking cerebrovascular defense mechanisms in brain ageing and Alzheimer's disease. Neurobiology of Aging. 2009;**30**(9):1512-1514

[2] Iadecola C, Park L, Capone C. Threats to the mind: Aging, amyloid, and hypertension. Stroke. 2009;**40** (3 Suppl):S40-S44

[3] Catchlove SJ, Parrish TB, Chen Y, Macpherson H, Hughes ME, Pipingas A. Regional cerebrovascular reactivity and cognitive performance in healthy aging. Journal of Experimental Neuroscience. 2018;**12**:1179069518785151

[4] Ungvari Z, Kaley G, de Cabo R, Sonntag WE, Csiszar A. Mechanisms of vascular aging: New perspectives. The Journals of Gerontology Series A, Biological Sciences and Medical Sciences. 2010;**65**(10):1028-1041

[5] Yang T, Sun Y, Lu Z, Leak RK, Zhang F. The impact of cerebrovascular aging on vascular cognitive impairment and dementia. Ageing Research Reviews. 2017;**34**:15-29

[6] Mijaljica D, Prescott M, Devenish RJ. Microautophagy in mammalian cells: Revisiting a 40-year-old conundrum. Autophagy. 2011;**7**(7):673-682

[7] Csiszar A, Labinskyy N, Orosz Z, Xiangmin Z, Buffenstein R, Ungvari Z. Vascular aging in the longest-living rodent, the naked mole rat. American Journal of Physiology Heart and Circulatory Physiology. 2007;**293**(2):H919-H927

[8] Hamilton CA, Brosnan MJ, McIntyre M, Graham D, Dominiczak AF. Superoxide excess in hypertension and aging: A common cause of endothelial dysfunction. Hypertension. 2001;**37**(2 Pt 2):529-534

[9] Sun D, Huang A, Yan EH, Wu Z, Yan C, Kaminski PM, et al. Reduced release of nitric oxide to shear stress in mesenteric arteries of aged rats. American Journal of Physiology Heart and Circulatory Physiology. 2004;**286**(6):H2249-H2256

[10] van der Loo B, Labugger R, Skepper JN, Bachschmid M, Kilo J, Powell JM, et al. Enhanced peroxynitrite formation is associated with vascular aging. The Journal of Experimental Medicine. 2000;**192**(12):1731-1744

[11] Donato AJ, Eskurza I, Silver AE, Levy AS, Pierce GL, Gates PE, et al. Direct evidence of endothelial oxidative stress with aging in humans: Relation to impaired endothelium-dependent dilation and upregulation of nuclear factor-kappaB. Circulation Research. 2007;**100**(11):1659-1666

[12] Jablonski KL, Seals DR, Eskurza I, Monahan KD, Donato AJ. High-dose ascorbic acid infusion abolishes chronic vasoconstriction and restores resting leg blood flow in healthy older men. Journal of Applied Physiology. 2007;**103**(5):1715-1721

[13] Campisi J. Senescent cells, tumor suppression, and organismal aging: Good citizens, bad neighbors. Cell. 2005;**120**(4):513-522

[14] Coppe JP, Desprez PY, Krtolica A, Campisi J. The senescence-associated secretory phenotype: The dark side of tumor suppression. Annual Review of Pathology. 2010;**5**:99-118

[15] Freund A, Orjalo AV, Desprez PY, Campisi J. Inflammatory networks during cellular senescence: Causes and consequences. Trends in Molecular Medicine. 2010;**16**(5):238-246

[16] Jellinger KA. Morphologic diagnosis of "vascular dementia" - a critical

update. Journal of the Neurological Sciences. 2008;**270**(1-2):1-12

[17] Jellinger KA. Pathology and pathogenesis of vascular cognitive impairment-a critical update. Frontiers in Aging Neuroscience. 2013;**5**:17

[18] Yurdagul A Jr, Finney AC, Woolard MD, Orr AW. The arterial microenvironment: The where and why of atherosclerosis. The Biochemical Journal. 2016;**473**(10):1281-1295

[19] Bachstetter AD, Xing B, de Almeida L, Dimayuga ER, Watterson DM, Van Eldik LJ. Microglial p38alpha MAPK is a key regulator of proinflammatory cytokine up-regulation induced by toll-like receptor (TLR) ligands or beta-amyloid (Abeta). Journal of Neuroinflammation. 2011;**8**:79

[20] Voghel G, Thorin-Trescases N, Farhat N, Nguyen A, Villeneuve L, Mamarbachi AM, et al. Cellular senescence in endothelial cells from atherosclerotic patients is accelerated by oxidative stress associated with cardiovascular risk factors. Mechanisms of Ageing and Development. 2007;**128**(11-12):662-671

[21] Coleman PR, Chang G, Hutas G, Grimshaw M, Vadas MA, Gamble JR. Age-associated stresses induce an anti-inflammatory senescent phenotype in endothelial cells. Aging. 2013;**5**(12):913-924

[22] Barnes PJ. Mechanisms of development of multimorbidity in the elderly. The European Respiratory Journal. 2015;**45**(3):790-806

[23] Macaulay R, Akbar AN, Henson SM. The role of the T cell in age-related inflammation. Age. 2013;**35**(3):563-572

[24] Ostan R, Bucci L, Capri M, Salvioli S, Scurti M, Pini E, et al. Immunosenescence and immunogenetics of human longevity. Neuroimmunomodulation. 2008;**15**(4-6):224-240

[25] Bianchi ME. DAMPs, PAMPs and alarmins: All we need to know about danger. Journal of Leukocyte Biology. 2007;**81**(1):1-5

[26] Campisi J, d'Adda di Fagagna F. Cellular senescence: When bad things happen to good cells. Nature Reviews Molecular Cell Biology. 2007;**8**(9):729-740

[27] Purcell M, Kruger A, Tainsky MA. Gene expression profiling of replicative and induced senescence. Cell Cycle. 2014;**13**(24):3927-3937

[28] Zhu Y, Armstrong JL, Tchkonia T, Kirkland JL. Cellular senescence and the senescent secretory phenotype in age-related chronic diseases. Current Opinion in Clinical Nutrition and Metabolic Care. 2014;**17**(4):324-328

[29] Pantsulaia I, Ciszewski WM, Niewiarowska J. Senescent endothelial cells: Potential modulators of immunosenescence and ageing. Ageing Research Reviews. 2016;**29**:13-25

[30] Hubackova S, Krejcikova K, Bartek J, Hodny Z. IL1- and TGFbeta-Nox4 signaling, oxidative stress and DNA damage response are shared features of replicative, oncogene-induced, and drug-induced paracrine 'bystander senescence. Aging. 2012;**4**(12):932-951

[31] Erusalimsky JD. Vascular endothelial senescence: From mechanisms to pathophysiology. Journal of Applied Physiology. 2009;**106**(1):326-332

[32] Aird WC. Endothelial cell heterogeneity. Cold Spring Harbor Perspectives in Medicine. 2012;**2**(1):a006429

[33] Mordi I, Tzemos N. Is reversal of endothelial dysfunction still an attractive target in modern cardiology? World Journal of Cardiology. 2014;**6**(8):824-835

[34] Niwano S. Role of endothelial dysfunction in thrombus formation in the left atrium-protective role of nitric oxide synthesis in the surface of atrium. Circulation Journal: Official Journal of the Japanese Circulation Society. 2014;**78**(8):1841-1842

[35] Hayashi T, Yano K, Matsui-Hirai H, Yokoo H, Hattori Y, Iguchi A. Nitric oxide and endothelial cellular senescence. Pharmacology & Therapeutics. 2008;**120**(3):333-339

[36] Toda N. Age-related changes in endothelial function and blood flow regulation. Pharmacology & Therapeutics. 2012;**133**(2):159-176

[37] Boehmer ED, Goral J, Faunce DE, Kovacs EJ. Age-dependent decrease in toll-like receptor 4-mediated proinflammatory cytokine production and mitogen-activated protein kinase expression. Journal of Leukocyte Biology. 2004;**75**(2):342-349

[38] Fitzner N, Clauberg S, Essmann F, Liebmann J, Kolb-Bachofen V. Human skin endothelial cells can express all 10 TLR genes and respond to respective ligands. Clinical and Vaccine Immunology. 2008;**15**(1):138-146

[39] Rothkamm K, Barnard S, Moquet J, Ellender M, Rana Z, Burdak-Rothkamm S. DNA damage foci: Meaning and significance. Environmental and Molecular Mutagenesis. 2015;**56**(6):491-504

[40] Hohensinner PJ, Kaun C, Buchberger E, Ebenbauer B, Demyanets S, Huk I, et al. Age intrinsic loss of telomere protection via TRF1 reduction in endothelial cells. Biochimica et Biophysica Acta. 2016;**1863**(2):360-367

[41] Hansson GK, Hermansson A. The immune system in atherosclerosis. Nature Immunology. 2011;**12**(3):204-212

[42] Farhat N, Thorin-Trescases N, Voghel G, Villeneuve L, Mamarbachi M, Perrault LP, et al. Stress-induced senescence predominates in endothelial cells isolated from atherosclerotic chronic smokers. Canadian Journal of Physiology and Pharmacology. 2008;**86**(11):761-769

[43] Tian XL, Li Y. Endothelial cell senescence and age-related vascular diseases. Journal of Genetics and Genomics = Yi chuan xue bao. 2014;**41**(9):485-495

[44] Sergin I, Razani B. Self-eating in the plaque: What macrophage autophagy reveals about atherosclerosis. Trends in Endocrinology and Metabolism: TEM. 2014;**25**(5):225-234

[45] Prattichizzo F, Giuliani A, Recchioni R, Bonafe M, Marcheselli F, De Carolis S, et al. Anti-TNF-alpha treatment modulates SASP and SASP-related microRNAs in endothelial cells and in circulating angiogenic cells. Oncotarget. 2016;**7**(11):11945-11958

[46] North BJ, Sinclair DA. The intersection between aging and cardiovascular disease. Circulation Research. 2012;**110**(8):1097-1108

[47] Trapp A, Weis M. The impact of immunosuppression on endothelial function. Journal of Cardiovascular Pharmacology. 2005;**45**(1):81-87

[48] Habib A, Karmali V, Polavarapu R, Akahori H, Cheng Q, Pachura K, et al. Sirolimus-FKBP12.6 impairs endothelial barrier function through protein kinase C-alpha activation and disruption of the p120-vascular endothelial cadherin interaction. Arteriosclerosis, Thrombosis, and Vascular Biology. 2013;**33**(10):2425-2431

[49] Clever YP, Cremers B, Speck U, Dietz U, Bohm M, Scheller B. Influence of a paclitaxel coated balloon in combination with a bare metal stent on restenosis and endothelial function: Comparison with a drug eluting stent and a bare metal stent. Catheterization and Cardiovascular Interventions: Official Journal of the Society for Cardiac Angiography & Interventions. 2014;**84**(2):323-331

[50] Lehle K, Birnbaum DE, Preuner JG. Predominant inhibition of interleukin-6 synthesis in patient-specific endothelial cells by mTOR inhibitors below a concentration range where cell proliferation is affected and mitotic arrest takes place. Transplantation Proceedings. 2005;**37**(1):159-161

[51] Muldowney JA 3rd, Stringham JR, Levy SE, Gleaves LA, Eren M, Piana RN, et al. Antiproliferative agents alter vascular plasminogen activator inhibitor-1 expression: A potential prothrombotic mechanism of drug-eluting stents. Arteriosclerosis, Thrombosis, and Vascular Biology. 2007;**27**(2):400-406

[52] Grootaert MO, da Costa Martins PA, Bitsch N, Pintelon I, De Meyer GR, Martinet W, et al. Defective autophagy in vascular smooth muscle cells accelerates senescence and promotes neointima formation and atherogenesis. Autophagy. 2015;**11**(11):2014-2032

[53] Marino G, Ugalde AP, Salvador-Montoliu N, Varela I, Quiros PM, Cadinanos J, et al. Premature aging in mice activates a systemic metabolic response involving autophagy induction. Human Molecular Genetics. 2008;**17**(14):2196-2211

[54] Bhayadia R, Schmidt BM, Melk A, Homme M. Senescence-induced oxidative stress causes endothelial dysfunction. The Journals of Gerontology Series A, Biological sciences and Medical Sciences. 2016;**71**(2):161-169

[55] Matthews C, Gorenne I, Scott S, Figg N, Kirkpatrick P, Ritchie A, et al. Vascular smooth muscle cells undergo telomere-based senescence in human atherosclerosis: Effects of telomerase and oxidative stress. Circulation Research. 2006;**99**(2):156-164

[56] Liu Y, Bloom SI, Donato AJ. The role of senescence, telomere dysfunction and shelterin in vascular aging. Microcirculation. 2018;**26**(2):e12487

[57] Hadi HA, Carr CS, Al Suwaidi J. Endothelial dysfunction: Cardiovascular risk factors, therapy, and outcome. Vascular Health and Risk Management. 2005;**1**(3):183-198

[58] Cooney MT, Dudina AL, Graham IM. Value and limitations of existing scores for the assessment of cardiovascular risk: A review for clinicians. Journal of the American College of Cardiology. 2009;**54**(14):1209-1227

[59] Ogami M, Ikura Y, Ohsawa M, Matsuo T, Kayo S, Yoshimi N, et al. Telomere shortening in human coronary artery diseases. Arteriosclerosis, Thrombosis, and Vascular Biology. 2004;**24**(3):546-550

[60] Valdes AM, Andrew T, Gardner JP, Kimura M, Oelsner E, Cherkas LF, et al. Obesity, cigarette smoking, and telomere length in women. Lancet. 2005;**366**(9486):662-664

[61] Vasan RS, Demissie S, Kimura M, Cupples LA, Rifai N, White C, et al. Association of leukocyte telomere length with circulating biomarkers of the renin-angiotensin-aldosterone system: The Framingham heart study. Circulation. 2008;**117**(9):1138-1144

[62] Jeanclos E, Krolewski A, Skurnick J, Kimura M, Aviv H, Warram JH, et al. Shortened telomere length in white blood cells of patients with IDDM. Diabetes. 1998;**47**(3):482-486

[63] Gelino S, Hansen M. Autophagy - An Emerging Anti-Aging Mechanism. Journal of Clinical & Experimental Pathology. 2012;(Suppl 4):1-24

[64] Vasilevko V, Passos GF, Quiring D, Head E, Kim RC, Fisher M, et al. Aging and cerebrovascular dysfunction: Contribution of hypertension, cerebral amyloid angiopathy, and immunotherapy. Annals of the New York Academy of Sciences. 2010;**1207**:58-70

[65] Bolduc V, Thorin-Trescases N, Thorin E. Endothelium-dependent control of cerebrovascular functions through age: Exercise for healthy cerebrovascular aging. American Journal of Physiology. Heart and Circulatory Physiology. 2013;**305**(5):H620-H633

[66] Willie CK, Tzeng YC, Fisher JA, Ainslie PN. Integrative regulation of human brain blood flow. The Journal of Physiology. 2014;**592**(5):841-859

[67] Abbott NJ, Patabendige AA, Dolman DE, Yusof SR, Begley DJ. Structure and function of the blood-brain barrier. Neurobiology of Disease. 2010;**37**(1):13-25

[68] Farrall AJ, Wardlaw JM. Blood-brain barrier: Ageing and microvascular disease--systematic review and meta-analysis. Neurobiology of Aging. 2009;**30**(3):337-352

[69] Skoog I, Wallin A, Fredman P, Hesse C, Aevarsson O, Karlsson I, et al. A population study on blood-brain barrier function in 85-year-olds: Relation to Alzheimer's disease and vascular dementia. Neurology. 1998;**50**(4):966-971

[70] Zlokovic BV. The blood-brain barrier in health and chronic neurodegenerative disorders. Neuron. 2008;**57**(2):178-201

[71] Tan CO. Defining the characteristic relationship between arterial pressure and cerebral flow. Journal of Applied Physiology. 2012;**113**(8):1194-1200

[72] Adler A, Messina E, Sherman B, Wang Z, Huang H, Linke A, et al. NAD(P)H oxidase-generated superoxide anion accounts for reduced control of myocardial O2 consumption by NO in old Fischer 344 rats. American Journal of Physiology. Heart and Circulatory Physiology. 2003;**285**(3):H1015-H1022

[73] Jacobson A, Yan C, Gao Q, Rincon-Skinner T, Rivera A, Edwards J, et al. Aging enhances pressure-induced arterial superoxide formation. American Journal of Physiology. Heart and Circulatory Physiology. 2007;**293**(3):H1344-H1350

[74] Csiszar A, Wang M, Lakatta EG, Ungvari Z. Inflammation and endothelial dysfunction during aging: Role of NF-kappaB. Journal of Applied Physiology. 2008;**105**(4):1333-1341

[75] Franceschi C, Bonafe M, Valensin S, Olivieri F, De Luca M, Ottaviani E, et al. Inflamm-aging. An evolutionary perspective on immunosenescence. Annals of the New York Academy of Sciences. 2000;**908**:244-254

[76] O'Brien JT, Thomas A. Vascular dementia. Lancet. 2015;**386**(10004):1698-1706

[77] Riddle DR, Sonntag WE, Lichtenwalner RJ. Microvascular plasticity in aging. Ageing Research Reviews. 2003;**2**(2):149-168

[78] Sonntag WE, Lynch CD, Cooney PT, Hutchins PM. Decreases in cerebral microvasculature with age are associated with the decline in growth hormone and insulin-like growth factor 1. Endocrinology. 1997;**138**(8):3515-3520

[79] Hajjar I, Goldstein FC, Waller EK, Moss LD, Quyyumi A. Circulating progenitor cells is linked to cognitive

decline in healthy adults. The American Journal of the Medical Sciences. 2016;**351**(2):147-152

[80] Hayakawa K, Miyamoto N, Seo JH, Pham LD, Kim KW, Lo EH, et al. High-mobility group box 1 from reactive astrocytes enhances the accumulation of endothelial progenitor cells in damaged white matter. Journal of Neurochemistry. 2013;**125**(2):273-280

[81] Joutel A, Corpechot C, Ducros A, Vahedi K, Chabriat H, Mouton P, et al. Notch3 mutations in CADASIL, a hereditary adult-onset condition causing stroke and dementia. Nature. 1996;**383**(6602):707-710

[82] Henshall TL, Keller A, He L, Johansson BR, Wallgard E, Raschperger E, et al. Notch3 is necessary for blood vessel integrity in the central nervous system. Arteriosclerosis, Thrombosis, and Vascular Biology. 2015;**35**(2):409-420

[83] Fukutake T. Cerebral autosomal recessive arteriopathy with subcortical infarcts and leukoencephalopathy (CARASIL): From discovery to gene identification. Journal of Stroke and Cerebrovascular Diseases : The Official Journal of National Stroke Association. 2011;**20**(2):85-93

[84] O'Sullivan M, Lythgoe DJ, Pereira AC, Summers PE, Jarosz JM, Williams SC, et al. Patterns of cerebral blood flow reduction in patients with ischemic leukoaraiosis. Neurology. 2002;**59**(3):321-326

[85] Kalaria RN. Vascular basis for brain degeneration: Faltering controls and risk factors for dementia. Nutrition Reviews. 2010;**68**(Suppl 2):S74-S87

[86] Tarantini S, Hertelendy P, Tucsek Z, Valcarcel-Ares MN, Smith N, Menyhart A, et al. Pharmacologically-induced neurovascular uncoupling is associated with cognitive impairment in mice. Journal of Cerebral Blood Flow and Metabolism: Official Journal of the International Society of Cerebral Blood Flow and Metabolism. 2015;**35**(11):1871-1881

[87] Farkas E, Luiten PG. Cerebral microvascular pathology in aging and Alzheimer's disease. Progress in Neurobiology. 2001;**64**(6):575-611

[88] Kalaria RN. Cerebral vessels in ageing and Alzheimer's disease. Pharmacology & Therapeutics. 1996;**72**(3):193-214

[89] D'Esposito M, Deouell LY, Gazzaley A. Alterations in the BOLD fMRI signal with ageing and disease: A challenge for neuroimaging. Nature Reviews. Neuroscience. 2003;**4**(11):863-872

[90] Iadecola C. The pathobiology of vascular dementia. Neuron. 2013;**80**(4):844-866

[91] Gorelick PB, Scuteri A, Black SE, Decarli C, Greenberg SM, Iadecola C, et al. Vascular contributions to cognitive impairment and dementia: A statement for healthcare professionals from the american heart association/ american stroke association. Stroke. 2011;**42**(9):2672-2713

[92] Serra L, Musicco M, Cercignani M, Torso M, Spano B, Mastropasqua C, et al. Cognitive reserve and the risk for Alzheimer's disease: A longitudinal study. Neurobiology of Aging. 2015;**36**(2):592-600

[93] Clarke MC, Figg N, Maguire JJ, Davenport AP, Goddard M, Littlewood TD, et al. Apoptosis of vascular smooth muscle cells induces features of plaque vulnerability in atherosclerosis. Nature Medicine. 2006;**12**(9):1075-1080

[94] Allan LM, Rowan EN, Firbank MJ, Thomas AJ, Parry SW, Polvikoski TM,

et al. Long term incidence of dementia, predictors of mortality and pathological diagnosis in older stroke survivors. Brain: A Journal of Neurology. 2011;**134**(Pt 12):3716-3727

[95] Savva GM, Stephan BC, Alzheimer's Society Vascular Dementia Systematic Review G. Epidemiological studies of the effect of stroke on incident dementia: A systematic review. Stroke. 2010;**41**(1):e41-e46

[96] Merino JG. Dementia after stroke: High incidence and intriguing associations. Stroke. 2002;**33**(9):2261-2262

[97] Qu Y, Zhuo L, Li N, Hu Y, Chen W, Zhou Y, et al. Prevalence of post-stroke cognitive impairment in China: A community-based, cross-sectional study. PLoS One. 2015;**10**(4):e0122864

[98] Deramecourt V, Pasquier F. Neuronal substrate of cognitive impairment in post-stroke dementia. Brain: A Journal of Neurology. 2014;**137**(Pt 9):2404-2405

[99] Lopez-Otin C, Blasco MA, Partridge L, Serrano M, Kroemer G. The hallmarks of aging. Cell. 2013;**153**(6):1194-1217

[100] Diniz BS, Reynolds CF 3rd, Sibille E, Lin CW, Tseng G, Lotrich F, et al. Enhanced molecular aging in late-life depression: The senescent-associated secretory phenotype. The American Journal of Geriatric Psychiatry: Official Journal of the American Association for Geriatric Psychiatry. 2017;**25**(1):64-72

[101] Diniz BS, Sibille E, Ding Y, Tseng G, Aizenstein HJ, Lotrich F, et al. Plasma biosignature and brain pathology related to persistent cognitive impairment in late-life depression. Molecular Psychiatry. 2015;**20**(5):594-601

[102] Stelzhammer V, Haenisch F, Chan MK, Cooper JD, Steiner J, Steeb H, et al. Proteomic changes in serum of first onset, antidepressant drug-naive major depression patients. The International Journal of Neuropsychopharmacology. 2014;**17**(10):1599-1608

[103] Bot M, Chan MK, Jansen R, Lamers F, Vogelzangs N, Steiner J, et al. Serum proteomic profiling of major depressive disorder. Translational Psychiatry. 2015;**5**:e599

## Section 2

# Pathophysiology

Chapter 2

# Hemodynamics in Ruptured Intracranial Aneurysms

*Hejčl Aleš, Stratilová Mária, Švihlová Helena, Alena Sejkorová, Radovnický Tomáš, Hron Jaroslav, Feletti Alberto, Koblížek Miroslav, Zámečník Josef, Beneš Vladimír, Dragomir-Daescu Dan and Sameš Martin*

## Abstract

Incidental detection of unruptured intracranial aneurysms (UIA) has increased in the recent years. There is a need in the clinical community to identify those that are prone to rupture and would require preventive treatment. Hemodynamics in cerebral blood vessels plays a key role in the lifetime cycle of intracranial aneurysms (IA). Understanding their initiation, growth, and rupture or stabilization may identify those hemodynamic features that lead to aneurysm instability and rupture. Modeling hemodynamics using computational fluid dynamics (CFD) could aid in understanding the processes in the development of IA. The neurosurgical approach during operation of IA allows direct visualization of the aneurysm sac and its sampling in many cases. Detailed analysis of the quality of the aneurysm wall under the microscope, together with histological assessment of the aneurysm wall and CFD modeling, can help in building complex knowledge on the relationship between the biology of the wall and hemodynamics. Detailed CFD analysis of the rupture point can further strengthen the association between hemodynamics and rupture. In this chapter we summarize current knowledge on CFD and intracranial aneurysms.

**Keywords:** intracranial aneurysm, hemodynamics, rupture, cerebral blood flow, computational fluid dynamics

## 1. Introduction

Intracranial aneurysm (IA), a pathological dilation of the vessel wall, is the result of hemodynamic forces on the wall of the intracranial artery. It is characterized by mild to moderate structural changes of the vessel wall, which may result in aneurysm rupture, leading to a severe form of hemorrhagic stroke [1].

In the last 15 years, there has been increasing incidental detection of unruptured intracranial aneurysms (UIA) due to an increasing use of noninvasive radiological examinations, such as computed tomography angiography (CTA) and magnetic resonance angiography (MRA) [2]. The increasing use of these noninvasive techniques for various non-specific complaints results in higher detection and increasing treatment of UIA. While 20% of individuals operated on for an IA in 1998 were carrying a UIA, in more recent years, the number has increased to more than 50% of all patients operated on for IA in the Department of Neurosurgery of the Jan Evangelista Purkyně, Masaryk Hospital in Ústí nad Labem, Czech Republic. Concurrently, there have been an increasing number of patients that we monitor for UIA who do not receive treatment. Should the aneurysm not rupture, which occurs in the majority of IA cases, very few become symptomatic in other ways. If it does rupture, it results in severe consequences including death, various levels of neurological disabilities, and cognitive or social difficulties.

The decision on whether to treat an individual with a UIA is based on the balance between the risk of treatment and the risk of the natural history of the aneurysm. If the aneurysm does not rupture, the risk of other clinical symptoms is quite low. These symptoms may appear as compression of the nervous structures (the optic nerve may be compressed by an ophthalmic aneurysm, the oculomotor nerve by a posterior communicating artery aneurysm, or the brain stem may be compressed by a large basilar aneurysm). Other symptoms may result from embolization of thrombi from the sac of an aneurysm; this is, however, very rare [3]. The worst outcome is that patients may experience aneurysm rupture. Overall, this risk is low in most patients and therefore does not occur in the vast majority of them in their lifetime [4]. The risk of rupture is associated with many factors; some of them are inherent (higher risk of rupture in females, some nations, such as Japanese); other factors are modifiable (higher risks are associated with hypertension or smoking). The rupture leads to a severe form of hemorrhagic stroke or even death. The risk of death after rupture is somewhere between 26 and 36% of patients [5]. The improved care of patients with SAH in specialized neurovascular centers improves survival rates [6]. Alternatively, about 15% of patients die immediately after rupture or before they are transported to hospital. Approximately 20% of those that survive develop a global cognitive deficit [7].

Contrarily the treatment, even in selected UIA, may carry the risk of severe complications may be as high as 16% of patients; the risk of mortality being 0–3.2% and the chance of not being discharged home almost 20% [8]. All the scoring systems used for analyzing the risk of rupture are based on data from large population studies. These factors include the size of the aneurysm, its location within the circle of Willis, its shape, etc. However, the size or the shape of the aneurysm is a result of forces that themselves lead to aneurysm initiation, its growth, and eventual rupture (or stability with no rupture). This is the result of the balance between hemodynamic forces and the quality of the blood vessel wall at the site of the aneurysm. Immediately when the hemodynamic forces overcome the strength of the aneurysm wall, it will rupture. Consequently an understanding of the hemodynamics within the cerebral blood vessels and the aneurysm itself may help with understanding its initiation, growth, and eventual rupture. The ability to model the hemodynamics within the aneurysm could also possibly assist with predicting their risk element and the direction to preventive treatment. It may also be possible to securely monitor aneurysms with a non-risky hemodynamic profile.

In this chapter we aim to provide current information on aneurysm hemodynamic modeling, using CFD. We will focus on ruptured and unruptured aneurysms, the hemodynamic characteristics at the point of rupture and the difference between ruptured and unruptured IA. We will discuss the issue from the perspective of neurosurgery and its possible contribution to clinical practice. We will summarize our 8 years of experience with CFD modeling in intracranial aneurysms, as well as the current literature.

## 2. The pathophysiology of the life cycle of intracranial aneurysms

During physiological conditions, the cerebral blood vessels consist of three layers: (1) tunica intima with a basal membrane, endothelial cells, and the internal elastic lamina; (2) tunica media, which consists of circumferentially oriented smooth muscle cells inside a dense network of collagen and elastin fibers; and (3) tunica adventitia, which consists mostly of collagen providing strength for the vessel wall. Tunica intima and tunica media are separated by a layer of lamina elastica interna, which is the key structure and has to degrade for the intracranial aneurysm to develop [9]. Cerebral blood vessels differ from extracranial blood vessels in that they have a thicker internal elastic lamina, less elastin, and smooth muscle cells in the media; in addition, they have no lamina elastica externa and a thinner layer of adventitia. There is minimum perivascular tissue in the subarachnoid space. The bifurcations of cerebral blood vessels contain irregularities in the vessel wall. The bifurcations are the typical areas of aneurysm development [10, 11]. Due to the small diameter of intracranial blood vessels, the wall shear stress plays a significant role in the degeneration of blood vessels and development of IA. The small diameter of cerebral blood vessels is also influenced by pathological forces induced, for example, by hypertension, and these lead to the development of IA. On the other hand, it is not quite clear what is the character of hemodynamic forces that lead to the development and rupture of IA. Some hypotheses describe the pathological influence of low wall shear stress leading to blood flow stagnation and the accumulation of blood elements (erythrocytes, leukocytes, thrombocytes), causing degeneration of the vessel wall together with inflammatory changes [12]. Another theory is based on high wall shear stress (WSS) causing damage of the endothelium, remodeling of the blood vessel wall, and its eventual degradation. It seems that possibly both scenarios could play a role [13].

## 3. Computational fluid dynamics (CFD) of intracranial aneurysms

The actual process of modeling hemodynamic parameters consists of several steps. Creating a 3D model is done by manual or semiautomatic segmentation (**Figure 1**). Angiographic examinations (3D angiography, CT angiography, or MR angiography) are used as the source data. Each radiological method has its own limitations (calcifications, flow artifacts, etc.). Several studies have tried to assess the relationship between different imaging examinations [14, 15]. In one such study, the authors compared the results of CFD obtained from CTA or DSA [14]. In conclusion, the authors state that, despite the quantitative differences in the individual hemodynamic parameters between the CTA and the DSA segmented group, the basic flow characteristics of both groups were identical.

In the next step, a calculation is performed using the Navier-Stokes equations, which describe the flow of incompressible fluid with constant viscosity. The use of the numerical solution of the Navier-Stokes equations calculates with assumption of blood having laminar flow. Possible influences of phenomena not captured by this model are further investigated, such as the influence of turbulent flow or viscosity change depending on the shear stress [16–19].

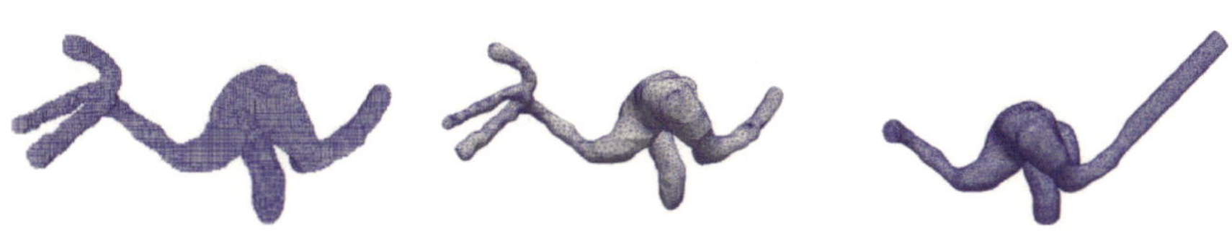

**Figure 1.**
*The process of obtaining patient-specific geometry from the CT or MR scan with high resolution includes accurate voxel segmentation of the vessel, generating surface mesh, and finally smoothing, generating volumetric mesh, and prescribing inlets and outlets with possible shortening and elongating of the outputs.*

These calculations characterize the flow, i.e., they provide information about fluid velocity and pressure on the vessel wall and the quantities derived there from such a stress tensor. Due to the uncertainty in the description of the area, as well as the specified boundary conditions, the inconsistency of these variables may be significant, but certain global-derived quantities—wall shear stress and oscillatory shear index (OSI)—are identical for a certain variation in the accuracy of numerical solutions [20]. WSS is defined as the pressure that acts in parallel with the blood vessel lumen. The OSI then describes the difference between the WSS vector and the blood flow during the cardiac cycle. When interpreting the data, we always need to bear in mind the approximations and assumptions during the process of CFD modeling.

The development of intracranial aneurysm can be divided into three phases: initiation, growth, and stabilization. Only a small percentage of aneurysms are unstable, progressing, and eventually resulting in rupture. The growth, shape change, and rupture of the aneurysm are the situations that we try to understand by mathematical modeling and to estimate the risk of these critical phases of development.

### 3.1 CFD in ruptured vs. unruptured intracranial aneurysms

One way to determine the risk of intracranial aneurysms is to compare the hemodynamic characteristics between ruptured and unruptured aneurysms. We can either compare non-specific aneurysms based on the status of rupture or only compare ruptured and unruptured aneurysms either at specific locations (MCA, PCom, etc.) or the so-called "mirror" aneurysms (right and left PCom or MCA aneurysms) [21, 22].

To date, several studies have been conducted to compare ruptured and unruptured aneurysms [22, 23]. Some of them were performed on a large number of aneurysms; others were focused on a small number of aneurysms at a specific location [22, 24–26]. The aim of these studies was to find differences between morphological and hemodynamic parameters, which would distinguish both groups. The characteristics of ruptured aneurysms could then help to identify the risky ones.

In one of the largest studies on 119 aneurysms, the authors found differences in 4 morphological and 6 hemodynamic parameters between ruptured and unruptured intracranial aneurysms [27]. The multivariate logistic regression analysis revealed that the morphological factor of size ratio and two hemodynamic factors, WSS and OSI, were independent factors of rupture risk. In 2017, a meta-analysis was published which, based on 1257 aneurysms from 22 studies, evaluated differences in hemodynamic parameters between ruptured and unruptured aneurysms. It showed that in ruptured aneurysms, WSS is significantly lower than in unruptured ones [28]. The same result was shown on 106 ACM aneurysms [22]. Alternatively, the largest ever study comparing ruptured and unruptured aneurysms has shown that wall shear stress is higher than those in unruptured aneurysms [29].

Previous results must therefore be given careful consideration as many factors have a significant influence on WSS. The meta-analysis itself shows, for example, the difference in WSS in aneurysms at different locations (the lowest is in the aneurysms of the apex of the basilar artery). One way to eliminate the influence of different localizations is to compare either the so-called mirror aneurysms (right and left IA MCA or PCom) or aneurysms of one localization in general (ACom, ICA, MCA, PCom, etc.).

Another important factor affecting IA hemodynamics is their size [13, 30]. We compared hemodynamic factors in small and large aneurysms based on the largest diameter of 10 mm (small <10 mm, large >10 mm) as this is commonly used to differentiate between small and large aneurysms in clinical practice (publication in preparation). We have found that size significantly influences the WSS within the aneurysm, independent of its rupture status. WSS in small aneurysms was significantly smaller. The only similar study used a volume of the sac to differentiate small and large aneurysms [30]. However, in clinical practice, the volume of the sac is not assessed on a regular basis, and its use is less practical in clinics. Nonetheless the results of both studies emphasize the importance of aneurysm size assessment with respect to evaluation of hemodynamic factors; generally it is necessary to compare hemodynamic parameters in equally sized aneurysms. One possible way to circumvent this effect is to use the so-called WSS statistical maps to convert the results to the surface of the aneurysm sac [31].

Specific limitations of studies comparing ruptured and unruptured aneurysms result from the fact that we already assess the condition given by rupture, not the aneurysm at risk, before rupture. Therefore, altered morphology of the aneurysm after rupture can lead to erroneous results or misinterpretations [32]. Another limitation in these studies is that we usually do not possess the individual boundary conditions for each aneurysm and need to use literature-based information.

### 3.2 CFD in ruptured intracranial aneurysms

The study of hemodynamics in ruptured aneurysms provides a chance to link the hemodynamic parameters with rupture (**Figure 2A–D**). Most studies have focused on the aneurysm sac as a whole. However, the aneurysm sac in ruptured aneurysms may be divided into the site of the rupture and the surrounding part of the sac. In these rare cases when we are able to differentiate those two parts of the aneurysm sac, we can combine our knowledge with local hemodynamic parameters. There are two types of studies in which the authors were able to identify the point of rupture. Firstly, there are surgical series when the neurosurgeon perioperatively identifies the site of rupture (perioperative rupture, apparent wall rupture during inspection of the sac usually before clip deployment, etc.) [33, 34]. Secondly, there are mostly case reports when the rupture in the angiographic room occurs, and the leakage of blood from the sac is thus identifiable during the interventional procedure [35, 36].

The site of rupture may show specific hemodynamic features (**Figure 2D**). So far there have been few studies with altogether a low number of patients (around 40 in total). The results are rather contradictory as it is apparent from the table; thus, it is difficult to make any straightforward general conclusions (**Table 1**).

It seems that the site of rupture is associated either with concentrated jet flow and high WSS (**Figure 2D**) or, on the other hand, a slow flow and low WSS. Both types of flow can lead to degeneration of the blood vessel wall but via a different mechanism [13]. Whereas low WSS and high OSI may lead to the activation of inflammatory cells and impairment of vessel wall structure, high WSS leads to the activation of cells in the vessel wall, leading to the growth of aneurysm sacs and rupture in small sacs or blebs. Reaching a certain size of the aneurysm sac during its growth leads to slowing the flow and recirculations, resulting in WSS decrease. In the IA itself, the highest WSS is usually around the neck and it decreases toward the apex. The low WSS can lead to degradation of the internal structure of the vessel wall and a further increase in the size of the sac. Most ruptures take place just in the apex of the aneurysm sac.

The disadvantage of all studies evaluating local hemodynamic parameters relative to the rupture site is the same as in all studies evaluating ruptured aneurysms. As mentioned above ruptured aneurysms may have a different shape after rupture, which can influence the results of hemodynamic modeling parameters as compared to the pre-rupture situation [32, 37]. Studies in which a hemodynamic analysis was

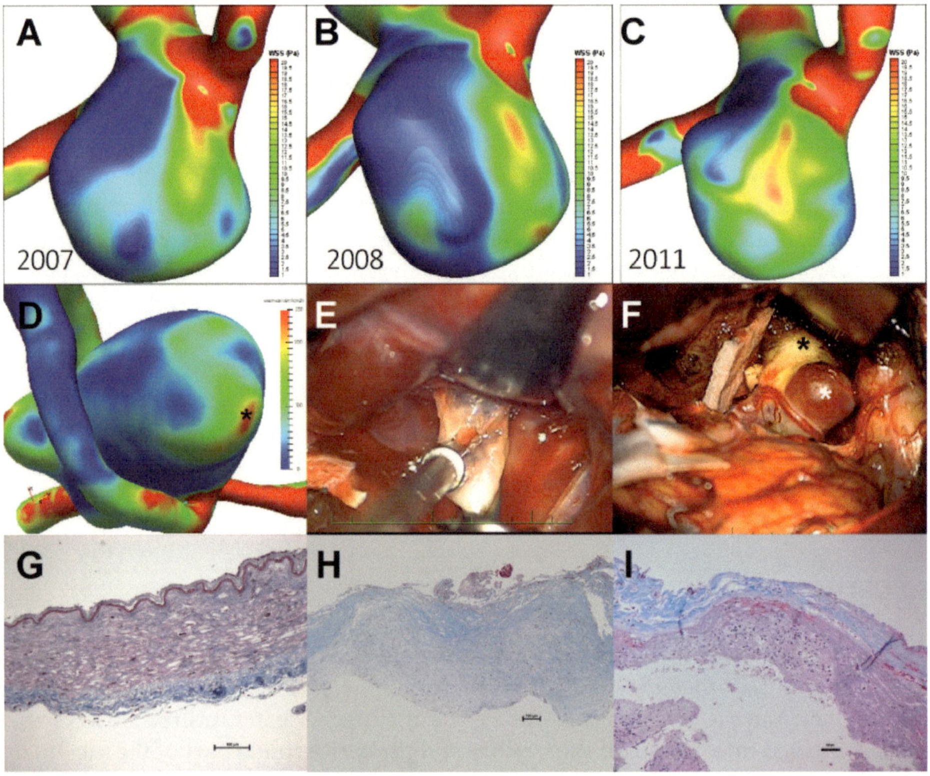


**Figure 2.**

*(A–C) Development of WSS over time in an IA that eventually ruptured. The WSS gradually decreased between the years 2007 and 2011. (D) A ruptured ACom aneurysm. The point of rupture (*) was confirmed during surgery. It was associated with increased WSS. (E) A perioperative image showing a ruptured MCA aneurysm. The point of rupture is in the weak part of the aneurysm wall. (F) A perioperative image showing an unruptured MCA aneurysm with heterogenous wall, an atherosclerotic part with a thrombus inside (black asterisk) and a red thin wall (white asterisk). (G) A histological image showing in detail the vessel wall of the Willis's circle without an aneurysm: the structure consists of the tunica intima with endothelial cells, which is separated from the tunica media by the internal elastic lamina (IEL), the tunica media with linear layer of smooth muscle cells, and the tunica adventitia, the outermost layer, which comprise mainly of collagen. (H) An UIA: moderate structural changes of the vessel wall, mainly fibrosis across the vessel wall without layers and the internal elastic lamina. (I) A ruptured IA: severe structural changes of the vessel wall. The wall is thinner, without tunica intima, and linear layer of smooth muscle cells, with the presence of organized thrombus (Masson trichrome staining in all three histological images).*

performed shortly before rupture avoid this limitation and may be helpful [35, 38]. These studies are rare, but their results are important, as they provide a hemodynamic characteristic within an extremely vulnerable aneurysm (which will soon rupture). Zhang et al. described three cases of large carotid aneurysms just before their rupture (2–5 days before SAK from aneurysm) and compared them with the same large eight unruptured ones [35]. They found that all ruptured aneurysms had an irregular shape and a higher aspect ratio (AR), and the WSS was lower than in the parent artery, as opposed to ruptured aneurysms. Additionally, in another study where the hemodynamic study of the basilar artery apex was performed 2 hours before the aneurysm rupture, the authors also found that in this aneurysm, WSS was lower than the parent artery [38]. However, the actual rupture site was associated with high WSS at the point of the blood jet into the sac. We found a similar flow characteristic in our case report where the site of rupture correlated with concentrated jet flow accompanied with high WSS and high normal pressure [39].

Understanding the changes in hemodynamics in ruptured aneurysms over time before the moment of rupture is of great importance; such studies are obviously quite

| Author, year | No. of cases | Identification of rupture | Hemodynamics at the site of rupture |
|---|---|---|---|
| Kono et al., 2012 [33] | 1 | 3DRA | Low WSS at diastole and high pressure at systole |
| Omodaka et al., 2012 [56] | 6 | Periop finding | Low WSS and high OSI |
| Hodis et al., 2013 [36] | 1 | 2DA | Jet flow, elevated WSS, and pressure at systole |
| Fukazawa et al., 2015 [34] | 12 | Periop finding | Low WSS and slow flow |
| Cebral et al., 2015 [57] | 9 | 3DRA and CT | High WSS |
| Hejčl et al., 2017 [39] | 1 | Periop finding | Jet flow and high WSS |
| Wang et al., 2018 [58] | 1 | Periop finding | Low WSS and high OSI |
| Suzuki et al. 2019 [59] | 7 | Periop finding | Max pressure areas, then decreased WSS |

**Table 1.**
*CFD studies evaluating hemodynamic parameters at the known site of rupture.*

rare [32, 40]. Our own study showed that a secondary aneurysm, a frequent rupture site, was observed in the aneurysm that subsequently ruptured (**Figure 2A-C**) [40]. WSS was reduced and the flow was slow at the rupture point. Over time, the area of low WSS increases in aneurysms that rupture (Sejkorová et al., in preparation). Such studies are vital for identifying the hemodynamic factors associated with the increased risk of rupture and may possibly be used in the future as an indicator for the active treatment of monitored UIA.

### 3.3 Correlating hemodynamics with the histology of the wall of intracranial aneurysms

One of the shortcomings of mathematical modeling is that we still know little about the relationship between hemodynamics and its influence of the biology of the vessel wall [41]. Understanding the balance between the flow and the biology of the aneurysm wall is the key factor in the life cycle intracranial aneurysms. The aneurysm wall ruptures when there is an imbalance between the aneurysm wall thickness and hemodynamic forces; both reciprocities are influenced. Modeling the relationship between histological changes and hemodynamic parameters is a logical way of research development (**Figure 2E–I**). The correlation of histological changes with mathematical models can help to verify the accuracy of mathematical models of hemodynamics, to improve understanding of the acquired data, and to transfer this methodology closer to practice in clinical neurosurgery. The correlation of histological changes and hemodynamics avoids errors related to CFD parameter evaluation in relation to, for example, aneurysm rupture; while the ruptured one was not ruptured prior to the event, the unruptured one could be ruptured in a few hours.

Frösen et al. classified four types of histological wall structures of aneurysms, based on disorganization of the vessel wall structure, myointimal hyperplasia or hypocellularity of the vessel wall, smooth muscle cell (SMC) proliferation, and the presence of organized thrombus [42]. The ruptured aneurysm wall is more often characterized by being disorganized, thinner, hypocellular, with an organized thrombus present (**Figure 2I**). Different types of wall structures can be found within one aneurysm sac. One of the first studies to correlate hemodynamic parameters with the pattern of the vessel wall has recently been published [43]. Quite

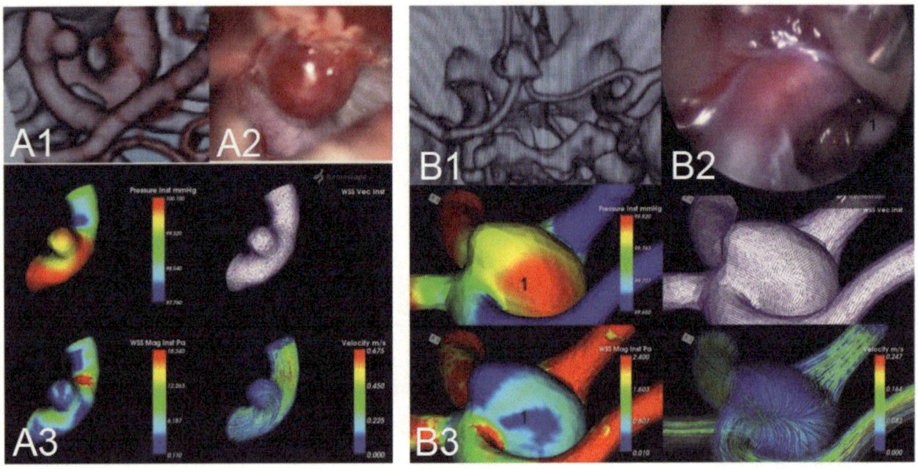


**Figure 3.**
*(Left panel) Red, thin areas on aneurysm wall are more often associated with low WSS. (A1) Right ICA aneurysm. (A2) Intraoperative microscopical view. (A3) CFD analysis. (Right panel) Yellow, atherosclerotic areas on aneurysm wall are more often associated with low WSS, high pressure, diverging WSS vectors, direct impact of streamlines with high-velocity flow (labeled with "1" in the figure). (B1) Anterior communicating artery aneurysm. (B2) Intraoperative endoscopic view. (B3) CFD analysis.*

surprisingly, the authors found that the high WSS and high-velocity flow were associated with the appearance of inflammatory changes in the aneurysm wall, while low flow areas were associated with degenerative changes in the aneurysm wall and loss of smooth muscle and pericytes. This finding is quite different from the previous studies, which did not correlate hemodynamics and histological characteristics. The correlation of histological changes and hemodynamics avoids the risk of error in comparing ruptured and unruptured aneurysms. There will most likely be a difference between an aneurysm that never ruptures and an aneurysm whose rupture is imminent. However it is not known which aneurysms we are analyzing.

In a less elaborative way, CFD modeling can be correlated simply with the perioperative findings during surgery (**Figures 2E, F and 3**). The wall of many aneurysms can be heterogenous including thin red areas, calcifications, and the thick yellow atherosclerotic wall part. In one such study, red, thin aneurysm wall areas were more often associated with low WSS (**Figure 3A1–3**) [44]. A total of 39 areas were identified and directly visually inspected on the aneurysms walls. The study showed that red, thin aneurysm wall areas were more often associated with low WSS, high pressure, parallel WSS vectors, and curved streamlines (75%) [40]. On the other hand, the association of low WSS with high pressure, diverging WSS vectors, direct impact of streamlines, and high-velocity flow more frequently matched with yellow, atherosclerotic aneurysm walls (79%) (**Figure 3B1–3**). Although routinely used imaging techniques can provide information about morphology and anatomical relationships of the aneurysm with the surrounding structures, there is currently no way to predict the thickness of the aneurysm wall. CFD can potentially provide this kind of information, which would be valuable not only to assess rupture risk but also to improve the surgical strategy during clipping or coiling. The authors of this study hypothesize that direct, high-velocity impact of blood flow on a specific area of the aneurysm could trigger a remodeling of the wall, ultimately leading to a reactive thickening.

In our recent project, we evaluated histological changes in ruptured and unruptured intracranial aneurysms. According to our preliminary data on the first 30 samples of individuals with ruptured and unruptured IA together with some control samples from similar locations of the cadaver's Willis's circle, the wall was damaged by scarring, with the disappearance of the tunica intima and the internal elastic membrane, in patients with both ruptured and unruptured aneurysms (**Figure 2G–I**). In the classification according to Frösen et al., categories A to C were demonstrated for unruptured IA, i.e., minor to moderate structural changes, such as fibrosis and disorganization of SMC (**Figure 2H**). However, the wall of ruptured aneurysms was thin, hypocellular, and fibrotized, often with the presence of an organized thrombus (**Figure 2I**). In the classification according to Frösen, it corresponded to categories C and D, i.e., a significantly damaged wall.

The correlation of vessel wall biology in intracranial aneurysms also has limitations:

1. Resection of only a part of the aneurysm sac. The entire aneurysm cannot be taken for histological evaluation. Due to the need to close at least the neck, but often also significant parts of the dome with an aneurysm clip, it is often possible to remove only the apex bag, even for larger aneurysms. Often small aneurysms are all hidden within a clip. On the other hand, large aneurysms often have a wall that is altered by atherosclerosis, weakened or calcified, and thus requires the application of, for example, several parallel clips and often a minimal residue of free sac to allow for sampling. A possible, at least partial, solution is the correlation of hemodynamics with the perioperative description of the aneurysm wall character (thinned wall, calcification, thickened atherosclerotic wall, etc.) by a neurosurgeon.

2. 3D orientation of the histological sample against angiographic imaging. The problem is the orientation of the cut bag in 3D space or 3D neuroradiological mapping. The hemodynamic parameters are processed in a 3D image based on CTA or 3D DSA. However, after cutting off the tip of the bag, it is necessary to orient the specimen and mark it properly so that the histology of the vessel wall with hemodynamic results can be ideally correlated. So far, a methodological study has been published to address this topic. However, it is currently quite complicated to be applied in clinical practice.

Another disease that is also used to investigate the relationship between atherosclerosis and hemodynamics is the carotid plaque in the bifurcation of the common carotid artery (**Figure 4**) [45]. This model is more advantageous for several reasons. It can be removed completely without disturbing its structure and then prepared for histological examination in one piece. Due to the size of the plaque and a simple orientation in the 3D geometry of the carotid arteries, the spatial correlation of the plaque model relative to the 3D image of hemodynamic calculations is simple. Also mathematical calculations on the carotid arteries are significantly simpler due to the relatively flat shape of the vessels and the larger cross-sectional size of the arteries, which are thus less affected by minor inequalities and errors given by the neuroradiological images. Therefore, the histological studies of carotid plaques in correlation with hemodynamic characteristics in the common carotid bifurcation can be performed with fewer approximations and thus can contribute to the understanding of atherosclerosis and degenerative changes in the vascular wall.

### 3.4 Hemodynamics and the risk of intracranial aneurysm rupture

The degeneration of the aneurysm wall progresses from the neck toward the dome. Aneurysm rupture usually occurs at the apex, which is also often a low shear stress region. According to a large meta-analysis by Zhou et al., the low shear stress (0–1.5 Pa) in the aneurysm sac is a characteristic of ruptured aneurysms [28]. It

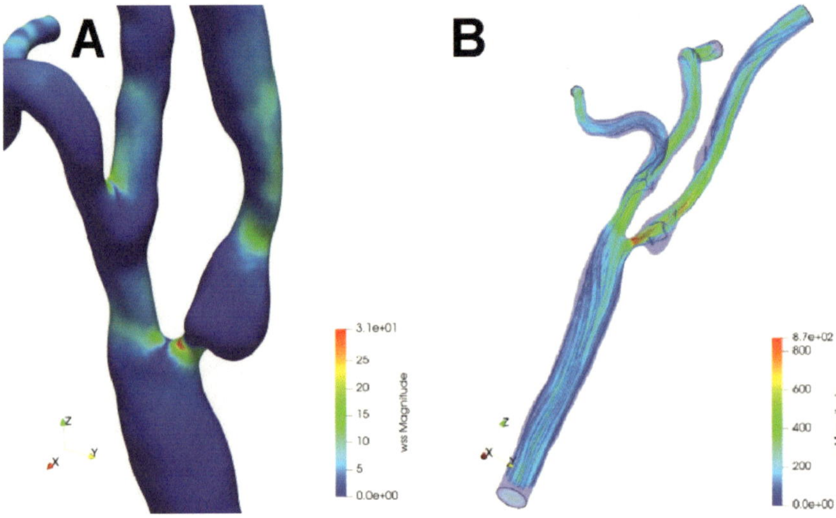


**Figure 4.**
*CFD in a model of carotid stenosis. WSS (A) and streamlines (B).*

is assumed that wall shear stress of approximately 2.0 N/m$^2$ (Pa) is most suitable for maintaining the integrity of the vessel wall. A shear stress of less than 1.5 N/m$^2$ results in endothelial cell apoptosis [46]. Takao et al. found that the minimum WSS value for ruptured aneurysms was half that of ruptured aneurysms [26]. Thus, low WSS may be an indicator of an increased risk of intracranial aneurysm rupture. Furthermore, several authors have demonstrated that in ruptured aneurysms, the low WSS region is greater than in unruptured aneurysms [21, 25, 47]. Similar results were found in our study (Sejkorová et al., in preparation), in which we have shown that the area of low wall shear stress (LSA) grows over time in those aneurysms that eventually ruptured. The nature of the flow and its properties are influenced by the shape of the sac. Inside the narrow neck aneurysms, there may be a slow flow with recirculations, resulting in low shear stress leading to increased vascular degeneration. Hemodynamic changes within the aneurysm lead to the production of biological signals in endothelial cells and may result in microscopic changes in the vessel wall [48]. Nitric oxide is a key mediator of low WSS and shear stress oscillation. The low shear stress further promotes the expression of adhesion molecules such as VCAM-1 and ICAM-1. These promote adhesion of leukocytes leading to inflammation and vascular changes. Therefore low WSS seems to be associated with degeneration of cerebral aneurysm vessel wall resulting in rupture. But the situation is probably more complex as in another study in a large number of aneurysms, the authors found that ruptured aneurysms were characterized by concentrated blood stream and a higher shear stress compared to unruptured ones [29].

### 3.5 Limitations of mathematical modeling of IA

Mathematical modeling performed in IA extends our knowledge on the pathophysiology of their initiation, growth, development, and rupture [13, 49]. At the same time, it is necessary to note that CFD modeling is usually based on many approximations and carries several limitations. In most studies, individual patient data are not available. This is particularly difficult to obtain in patients with ruptured aneurysms that require acute treatment, and there is usually no time for additional diagnostic examinations (TCD or PC-MR). The method that can partially reduce the disadvantage of missing individual data is to relate values in the aneurysm to the parent artery. Such value normalization reduces the impact of missing input data. Another limitation is that CFD represents mathematical models that are currently not able to describe all aspects of the biology of the cerebral aneurysms and cerebral blood vessels, their histology, atherosclerotic changes, pulsations, etc. Also during modeling, blood vessels are simplified as rigid tubes. The rheological properties of blood are simplified as incompressible Newtonian fluid.

Another aspect associated with limitations in CFD modeling is the use of different mathematical modeling algorithms among various groups working on CFD. This has been clearly shown in the CFD rupture challenge—phase I and phase II [50, 51]. In the rupture challenge, two MCA aneurysms, one ruptured and one unruptured IA, were evaluated using CFD analysis, and the status of the aneurysm was supposed to be identified by the research groups. In the second phase, several research groups were supposed to describe the hemodynamic parameters in one IA. The vast differences among the research groups confirmed the fact that various algorithms may lead to significant differences in the hemodynamic analysis [52]. In future it will be necessary to somehow unify the methodology in order to get more universally applicable results.

Another disadvantage of CFD modeling is the relatively complicated protocol with the need to include sophisticated and laborious calculations requiring supercomputers. Nonetheless, technological advances in imaging may provide hemodynamic modeling during regular MRI examinations [53]. If MRI allows precise evaluation of hemodynamic parameters in the future, it can be used even during initial MRI evaluation and during follow-ups without radiation burden.

## 4. Final remarks and future directions

The rationale for studying hemodynamics of IA is the increasing detection of UIA with the need to decide whether to treat or watch the aneurysm. Studying and modeling hemodynamics within an aneurysm provides more information on the pathophysiology of IA. We can evaluate the hemodynamic parameter at one time point or follow the aneurysm with CFD assessments over time [40, 54]. The method has been mostly developed by endovascular surgeons with the goal to assess the effect of various treatment modalities, such as flow diverters, stents, scarification of the parent vessel, etc. The neurosurgeons would mostly need information on aneurysm hemodynamics with respect to the rupture risk in the assessment of UIA [40]. The neurosurgeons themselves may provide unique information on aneurysm wall quality: direction visualization of the aneurysm sac under the operating microscope (calcifications, wall weakening, atherosclerotic changes, thrombosis), identification of the site of rupture, aneurysm sac harvesting after clipping, etc. The aneurysm sac wall may then be assessed histologically. Some pilot studies have already been published [43]. Despite an increasing number of CFD studies, there are, to date, still no conclusions with respect to hemodynamics and growth or rupture that would be universally accepted.

From a clinical point of view, the CFD data need to be clinically useful and relevant, such as in a study that points out the relationship between the hemodynamic factors and the risk of endovascular treatment failure in patients treated for a basilar apex aneurysm [55]. The CFD parameters more often mentioned with respect to clinical use are WSS and character of flow. Many studies show that aneurysms with low WSS and complex flow tend to be associated with a higher risk of rupture [27, 28]. Further developments are still required in CFD research before it may be considered clinically relevant in providing useful information on UIA and its assessment, with respect to the risk of rupture.

## Acknowledgements

Supported by Ministry of Health of the Czech Republic, grants nr. NV17-32872A and NV19-04-00270. 

## Author details

Hejčl Aleš[1,2,3*], Stratilová Mária[4], Švihlová Helena[5], Alena Sejkorová[1], Radovnický Tomáš[1], Hron Jaroslav[5], Feletti Alberto[6], Koblížek Miroslav[7], Zámečník Josef[7], Beneš Vladimír[8], Dragomir-Daescu Dan[9] and Sameš Martin[1]

1 Department of Neurosurgery, J. E. Purkyně University, Masaryk Hospital, Ústí nad Labem, Czech Republic

2 International Clinical Research Center, St. Anne's Hospital, Brno, Czech Republic

3 Department of Neuroregeneration, Institute of Experimental Medicine, Academy of Sciences of the Czech Republic, Prague, Czech Republic

4 Second Faculty of Medicine, Charles University, Prague, Czech Republic

5 Faculty of Mathematics and Physics, Mathematical Institute, Charles University, Prague, Czech Republic

6 Department of Neurosurgery, Verona, Italy

7 Department of Pathology and Molecular Medicine, Second Faculty of Medicine, Charles University and University Hospital Motol, Prague, Czech Republic

8 Department of Neurosurgery and Neuro-oncology, First Faculty of Medicine, Charles University, Military University Hospital Prague, Czech Republic

9 Department of Physiology and Biomedical Engineering, Mayo Clinic, Rochester, Minnesota, USA

*Address all correspondence to: ales.hejcl@gmail.com

## References

[1] Brisman JL, Song JK, Newell DW. Cerebral aneurysms. The New England Journal of Medicine. 2006;**355**(9): 928-939

[2] Gabriel RA, Kim H, Sidney S, et al. Ten-year detection rate of brain arteriovenous malformations in a large, multiethnic, defined population. Stroke. 2010;**41**(1):21-26

[3] Calviere L, Viguier A, Da Silva NA Jr, Cognard C, Larrue V. Unruptured intracranial aneurysm as a cause of cerebral ischemia. Clinical Neurology and Neurosurgery. 2011;**113**(1):28-33

[4] Rinkel GJ, Djibuti M, Algra A, van Gijn J. Prevalence and risk of rupture of intracranial aneurysms: A systematic review. Stroke. 1998;**29**(1):251-256

[5] Connolly ES Jr, Rabinstein AA, Carhuapoma JR, et al. Guidelines for the management of aneurysmal subarachnoid hemorrhage: A guideline for healthcare professionals from the American Heart Association/American Stroke Association. Stroke. 2012;**43**(6):1711-1737

[6] Rinaldo L, McCutcheon BA, Murphy ME, et al. Quantitative analysis of the effect of institutional case volume on complications after surgical clipping of unruptured aneurysms. Journal of Neurosurgery. 2017;**127**(6):1297-1306

[7] Springer MV, Schmidt JM, Wartenberg KE, Frontera JA, Badjatia N, Mayer SA. Predictors of global cognitive impairment 1 year after subarachnoid hemorrhage. Neurosurgery. 2009;**65**(6):1043-1050; discussion 1050-1041

[8] Kerezoudis P, McCutcheon BA, Murphy M, et al. Predictors of 30-day perioperative morbidity and mortality of unruptured intracranial aneurysm surgery. Clinical Neurology and Neurosurgery. 2016;**149**:75-80

[9] Lasheras JC. The biomechanics of arterial aneurysms. Annual Review of Fluid Mechanics. 2007;**39**:293-319

[10] Stehbens WE. Pathology and pathogenesis of intracranial berry aneurysms. Neurological Research. 1990;**12**(1):29-34

[11] Finlay HM, Whittaker P, Canham PB. Collagen organization in the branching region of human brain arteries. Stroke. 1998;**29**(8):1595-1601

[12] Crompton MR. Mechanism of growth and rupture in cerebral berry aneurysms. British Medical Journal. 1966;**1**(5496):1138-1142

[13] Meng H, Tutino VM, Xiang J, Siddiqui A. High WSS or low WSS? Complex interactions of hemodynamics with intracranial aneurysm initiation, growth, and rupture: Toward a unifying hypothesis. American Journal of Neuroradiology. 2014;**35**(7):1254-1262

[14] Geers AJ, Larrabide I, Radaelli AG, et al. Patient-specific computational hemodynamics of intracranial aneurysms from 3D rotational angiography and CT angiography: An in vivo reproducibility study. American Journal of Neuroradiology. 2011;**32**(3):581-586

[15] Ren Y, Chen GZ, Liu Z, Cai Y, Lu GM, Li ZY. Reproducibility of image-based computational models of intracranial aneurysm: A comparison between 3D rotational angiography, CT angiography and MR angiography. Biomedical Engineering Online. 2016;**15**(1):50

[16] Øyvind E, Mardal K-A. On the assumption of laminar flow in physiological flows: Cerebral aneurysms as an illustrative example, modeling the heart and the circulatory system. Modeling the Heart and the Circulatory System. 2015;**14**:177-195

[17] Hippelheuser JE, Lauric A, Cohen AD, Malek AM. Realistic non-Newtonian viscosity modelling highlights hemodynamic differences between intracranial aneurysms with and without surface blebs. Journal of Biomechanics. 2014;**47**(15):3695-3703

[18] Liepsch DSS, Frolov S. An impact of non-Newtonian blood viscosity on hemodynamics in a patient-specific model of a cerebral aneurysm. Journal of Physics: Conference Series. 2018;**2018**(1084):12001

[19] Xiang J, Tremmel M, Kolega J, Levy EI, Natarajan SK, Meng H. Newtonian viscosity model could overestimate wall shear stress in intracranial aneurysm domes and underestimate rupture risk. Journal of NeuroInterventional Surgery. 2012;**4**(5):351-357

[20] Evju O, Pozo JM, Frangi AF, Mardal KA. Robustness of common hemodynamic indicators with respect to numerical resolution in 38 middle cerebral artery aneurysms. PLoS One. 2017;**12**(6):e0177566

[21] Lu G, Huang L, Zhang XL, et al. Influence of hemodynamic factors on rupture of intracranial aneurysms: Patient-specific 3D mirror aneurysms model computational fluid dynamics simulation. American Journal of Neuroradiology. 2011;**32**(7):1255-1261

[22] Miura Y, Ishida F, Umeda Y, et al. Low wall shear stress is independently associated with the rupture status of middle cerebral artery aneurysms. Stroke. 2013;**44**(2):519-521

[23] Cebral JR, Mut F, Weir J, Putman CM. Association of hemodynamic characteristics and cerebral aneurysm rupture. American Journal of Neuroradiology. 2011;**32**(2):264-270

[24] Liu J, Xiang J, Zhang Y, et al. Morphologic and hemodynamic analysis of paraclinoid aneurysms: Ruptured versus unruptured. Journal of NeuroInterventional Surgery. 2014;**6**(9):658-663

[25] Jou LD, Lee DH, Morsi H, Mawad ME. Wall shear stress on ruptured and unruptured intracranial aneurysms at the internal carotid artery. American Journal of Neuroradiology. 2008;**29**(9):1761-1767

[26] Takao H, Murayama Y, Otsuka S, et al. Hemodynamic differences between unruptured and ruptured intracranial aneurysms during observation. Stroke. 2012;**43**(5):1436-1439

[27] Xiang J, Natarajan SK, Tremmel M, et al. Hemodynamic-morphologic discriminants for intracranial aneurysm rupture. Stroke. 2011;**42**(1):144-152

[28] Zhou G, Zhu Y, Yin Y, Su M, Li M. Association of wall shear stress with intracranial aneurysm rupture: Systematic review and meta-analysis. Scientific Reports. 2017;**7**(1):5331

[29] Cebral JR, Mut F, Weir J, Putman C. Quantitative characterization of the hemodynamic environment in ruptured and unruptured brain aneurysms. American Journal of Neuroradiology. 2011;**32**(1):145-151

[30] Lauric A, Hippelheuser J, Cohen AD, Kadasi LM, Malek AM. Wall shear stress association with rupture status in volume matched sidewall aneurysms. Journal of NeuroInterventional Surgery. 2014;**6**(6):466-473

[31] Goubergrits L, Schaller J, Kertzscher U, et al. Statistical wall shear stress maps of ruptured and unruptured middle cerebral artery aneurysms. Journal of the Royal Society Interface. 2012;**9**(69):677-688

[32] Schneiders JJ, Marquering HA, van den Berg R, et al. Rupture-associated

changes of cerebral aneurysm geometry: High-resolution 3D imaging before and after rupture. American Journal of Neuroradiology. 2014;**35**(7):1358-1362

[33] Kono K, Fujimoto T, Shintani A, Terada T. Hemodynamic characteristics at the rupture site of cerebral aneurysms: A case study. Neurosurgery. 2012;**71**(6):E1202-E1208; discussion 1209

[34] Fukazawa K, Ishida F, Umeda Y, et al. Using computational fluid dynamics analysis to characterize local hemodynamic features of middle cerebral artery aneurysm rupture points. World Neurosurgery. 2015;**83**(1):80-86

[35] Zhang Y, Jing L, Zhang Y, Liu J, Yang X. Low wall shear stress is associated with the rupture of intracranial aneurysm with known rupture point: Case report and literature review. BMC Neurology. 2016;**16**(1):231

[36] Hodis S, Uthamaraj S, Lanzino G, Kallmes DF, Dragomir-Daescu D. Computational fluid dynamics simulation of an anterior communicating artery ruptured during angiography. BML Case Reports. 2013;**2013**:pii: bcr2012010596

[37] Kono K, Tomura N, Yoshimura R, Terada T. Changes in wall shear stress magnitude after aneurysm rupture. Acta Neurochirurgica. 2013;**155**(8):1559-1563

[38] Cebral JR, Hendrickson S, Putman CM. Hemodynamics in a lethal basilar artery aneurysm just before its rupture. American Journal of Neuroradiology. 2009;**30**(1):95-98

[39] Hejčl A, Svihlova H, Sejkorova A, et al. Computational fluid dynamics of a fatal ruptured anterior communicating artery aneurysm. Journal of Neurological Surgery Part A: Central European Neurosurgery. 2017;**78**(6):610-616

[40] Sejkorova A, Dennis KD, Svihlova H, et al. Hemodynamic changes in a middle cerebral artery aneurysm at follow-up times before and after its rupture: A case report and a review of the literature. Neurosurgical Review. 2017;**40**(2):329-338

[41] Cebral JR, Detmer F, Chung BJ, et al. Local hemodynamic conditions associated with focal changes in the intracranial aneurysm wall. American Journal of Neuroradiology. 2019;**40**(3):510-516

[42] Frösen J, Piippo A, Paetau A, et al. Remodeling of saccular cerebral artery aneurysm wall is associated with rupture: Histological analysis of 24 unruptured and 42 ruptured cases. Stroke. 2004;**35**(10):2287-2293

[43] Cebral J, Ollikainen E, Chung BJ, et al. Flow conditions in the intracranial aneurysm lumen are associated with inflammation and degenerative changes of the aneurysm wall. American Journal of Neuroradiology. 2017;**38**(1):119-126

[44] Feletti A, Wang X, Talari S, et al. Computational fluid dynamics analysis and correlation with intraoperative aneurysm features. Acta Neurochirurgica Supplement. 2018;**129**:3-9

[45] Li CH, Gao BL, Wang JW, Liu JF, Li H, Yang ST. Hemodynamic factors affecting carotid sinus atherosclerotic stenosis. World Neurosurgery. 2019;**121**:e262-e276

[46] Shojima M, Oshima M, Takagi K, et al. Magnitude and role of wall shear stress on cerebral aneurysm: Computational fluid dynamic study of 20 middle cerebral artery aneurysms. Stroke. 2004;**35**(11):2500-2505

[47] Zhang Y, Yang X, Wang Y, et al. Influence of morphology and hemodynamic factors on rupture of multiple intracranial aneurysms:

Matched-pairs of ruptured-unruptured aneurysms located unilaterally on the anterior circulation. BMC Neurology. 2014;**14**:253

[48] Penn DL, Komotar RJ, Sander Connolly E. Hemodynamic mechanisms underlying cerebral aneurysm pathogenesis. Journal of Clinical Neuroscience. 2011;**18**(11):1435-1438

[49] Nixon AM, Gunel M, Sumpio BE. The critical role of hemodynamics in the development of cerebral vascular disease. Journal of Neurosurgery. 2010;**112**(6):1240-1253

[50] Janiga G, Berg P, Sugiyama S, Kono K, Steinman DA. The computational fluid dynamics rupture challenge 2013-phase I: Prediction of rupture status in intracranial aneurysms. American Journal of Neuroradiology. 2015;**36**(3):530-536

[51] Berg P, Roloff C, Beuing O, et al. The computational fluid dynamics rupture challenge 2013-phase II: Variability of hemodynamic simulations in two intracranial aneurysms. Journal of Biomechanical Engineering. 2015;**137**(12):121008

[52] Berg P, Voss S, Saalfeld S, et al. Multiple aneurysms anatomy challenge 2018 (MATCH): Phase I: Segmentation. Cardiovascular Engineering and Technology. 2018;**9**(4):565-581

[53] van Ooij P, Guedon A, Poelma C, et al. Complex flow patterns in a real-size intracranial aneurysm phantom: Phase contrast MRI compared with particle image velocimetry and computational fluid dynamics. NMR in Biomedicine. 2012;**25**(1):14-26

[54] Cornelissen BM, Schneiders JJ, Potters WV, et al. Hemodynamic differences in intracranial aneurysms before and after rupture. American Journal of Neuroradiology. 2015;**36**(10):1927-1933

[55] Sugiyama S, Niizuma K, Sato K, et al. Blood flow into basilar tip aneurysms: A predictor for recanalization after coil embolization. Stroke. 2016;**47**(10):2541-2547

[56] Omodaka S, Sugiyama S, Inoue T, et al. Local hemodynamics at the rupture point of cerebral aneurysms determined by computational fluid dynamics analysis. Cerebrovascular Diseases. 2012;**34**(2):121-129

[57] Cebral JR, Vazquez M, Sforza DM, et al. Analysis of hemodynamics and wall mechanics at sites of cerebral aneurysm rupture. Journal of NeuroInterventional Surgery. 2015;7(7):530-536

[58] Wang Y, Leng X, Zhou X, Li W, Siddiqui AH, Xiang J. Hemodynamics in a middle cerebral artery aneurysm before its growth and fatal rupture: Case study and review of the literature. World Neurosurgery. 2018;**119**:e395-e402

[59] Suzuki T, Stapleton CJ, Koch MJ, et al. Decreased wall shear stress at high-pressure areas predicts the rupture point in ruptured intracranial aneurysms. Journal of Neurosurgery. 2019:1-7

Chapter 3

# Serum Homocysteine and Intracranial Aneurysms

*Mei-Ling Sharon Tai, Tsun Haw Toh, Hafez Hussain and Kuo Ghee Ong*

## Abstract

Subarachnoid haemorrhage (SAH) occurs as a result of rupture of intracranial aneurysms. SAH causes significant morbidity and mortality. In addition, SAH leads to significant financial burden. In this chapter, we will look into the association between raised serum homocysteine and intracranial aneurysms. In a study on the Han Chinese patients with intracranial aneurysm who were admitted to the hospital, the mean serum total homocysteine level in the patient group with intracranial aneurysm was significantly higher than those in the control group. In the same study, the patients with raised serum homocysteine had 2.196 higher risk of developing intracranial aneurysms. Ren et al. proposed that homocysteine should be seen as an indicator of the risk of intracranial aneurysm and not a direct cause of intracranial aneurysm. In another study, homocysteine increases the development of intracranial aneurysms in rats. Endothelial damage is an early change in the walls of intracranial aneurysms. Polymorphisms of the genes coding for the various components of the vessel walls may be associated with the formation of intracranial aneurysms. In a previous animal study, the size of intracranial aneurysms is significantly smaller in the mice with inducible nitric oxide synthase (iNOS) compared with the mice without iNOS.

**Keywords:** homocysteine, aneurysm, intracranial, serum, subarachnoid haemorrhage

## 1. Introduction

### 1.1 Subarachnoid haemorrhage

Subarachnoid haemorrhage (SAH) is caused by rupture of intracranial aneurysms [1, 2]. Approximately 5–15% of the stroke patients have ruptured intracranial aneurysms [3, 4].

Aneurysmal SAH leads to a prolonged hospital stay [1]. Therefore, aneurysmal subarachnoid haemorrhage results in a significant financial burden in the USA [1]. In addition, aneurysmal SAH causes approximately 45% mortality in 30 days [3, 5]. As many as 30% of the patients who survived the SAH had moderate to severe neurological deficit and disability [3, 5].

### 1.2 Intracranial aneurysms

Saccular intracranial aneurysms are abnormal focal outpouchings of cerebral arteries [3]. The prevalence of intracranial aneurysms in the adult population in the USA is 1–5% [3, 6]. Most of the intracranial aneurysms are small [3]. Approximately 50–80% of all the intracranial aneurysms do not rupture [3, 7].

Intracranial aneurysms are usually sporadically acquired lesions [3]. A rare familial form is present, and this is associated with conditions such as cerebral arteriovenous malformations (AVMs), autosomal dominant polycystic kidney disease (ADPKD), fibromuscular dysplasia, Marfan syndrome and Ehlers-Danlos syndrome [3, 5]. Multiple genetic susceptibilities may be acting synergistically in the development of SAH [5, 8]. The increase in the familial risk of developing SAH is nearly four times higher among first-degree relatives [5, 9, 10].

Unruptured aneurysms can potentially result in cranial nerve palsies such as third cranial nerve palsy and rarely brainstem compression [3, 7, 11]. These patients have a higher risk of rupture of intracranial aneurysm [3, 7]. They have an annual risk of aneurysmal rupture of about 6% [3, 12].

### 1.3 Homocysteine

Homocysteine is an endogenous, nonstructural protein which contains sulphur [13]. Homocysteine is involved in the metabolism pathway of methionine and cysteine [13, 14]. Homocysteine can be irreversibly degraded to cysteine via the trans-sulphuration pathway or remethylated back to methionine [15]. The biochemistry of methionine is regulated by the enzymes controlling homocysteine concentration [15]. An elevated level of serum homocysteine is the intermediate product of methionine metabolism [16].

In addition, the metabolism of homocysteine is dependent on nutritional factors comprising of vitamin $B_{12}$ and folic acid [16, 17]. A reduction in the levels of vitamin $B_{12}$ and folic acid causes an increase in serum homocysteine levels [16]. Homocysteine also plays an important role in the metabolism of folic acid and catabolism of choline which are both vital for the regulation of methionine [15]. Homocysteine is very important for the cellular homeostasis [15].

Normal level of total concentration of homocysteine in plasma of healthy people is between 5.0 and 15.0 mmol/l. [13] Raised serum homocysteine is an independent risk factor for cardiovascular diseases [13, 15, 18]. Elevated serum homocysteine is associated with a rise in morbidity and mortality [18, 19].

An increase in serum homocysteine results in oxidative stress and systemic inflammation which in turn leads to an accelerated telomere shortening [13, 19]. Furthermore, elevated serum homocysteine damages endothelial cells [13]. As a result, the blood vessels are less flexible and the process of haemostasis is disturbed [13]. **An increase in serum homocysteine can be treated by folic acid, vitamin B12 and vitamin B6 supplements** [13, 15].

## 2. Homocysteine and intracranial aneurysm

Ren et al. conducted a study on the Han Chinese patients with intracranial aneurysm who were admitted to the hospital [17]. In this study, the mean serum total homocysteine level in the patient group with intracranial aneurysm was significantly higher than those in the control group [17]. In addition, homocysteine had an adjusted odds ratio of 2.196 ($P$ = 0.012) for the development of intracranial aneurysm [17].

Furthermore, raised serum homocysteine was reported to be an independent risk factor for development of intracranial aneurysms [17]. Ren et al. proposed that homocysteine should be seen as an indicator of the risk of intracranial aneurysm and not a direct cause of intracranial aneurysm [17].

In the same study, an association between serum total homocysteine and folate and vitamin $B_{12}$ in the patients with intracranial aneurysm was present [17]. The serum total homocysteine level was negatively correlated with folate and vitamin $B_{12}$ levels in the study by Ren et al. [17] Folic acid and vitamin $B_{12}$ are therefore found to be protective against formation of intracranial aneurysms [17]. This is due to the roles of vitamin $B_{12}$ and folic acid in the regulation of the metabolism of homocysteine [17]. In a previous study, insufficient plasma level of one or more B vitamins may potentially result in high levels of serum homocysteine [16].

In the study conducted by Xu et al., homocysteine increases the development of intracranial aneurysms in rats, possibly by the different effects on the expression of molecules which are essential for vascular wall modeling [20]. The formation of intracranial aneurysms is associated with chronic inflammation [20].

Endothelial damage is one of the early changes in the walls of intracranial aneurysms resulting from inflammation [20]. An increase in serum homocysteine has been reported to damage the vascular endothelium [20]. This in turn leads to the development of atherosclerosis [20].

## 3. Polymorphism

Interestingly, polymorphism of the genes coding for the various components of the vessel walls has been proposed to be associated with the development of intracranial aneurysms [5, 8].

Polymorphisms involving homocysteine metabolism can also promote formation of abdominal aortic aneurysms, dissection of the cervical arteries and atherosclerosis [5, 21, 22].

Moreover, the expression of matrix metalloproteinase-2 (MMP-2), endothelial nitric oxide synthase (eNOS), vascular endothelial growth factor (VEGF) and MMP-2 in the walls of intracranial aneurysm was increased by methionine treatment in Xu et al.'s study [20].

Furthermore, autosomal recessive deficiency in cystathionine-synthase is involved in homocysteine metabolism [5, 23]. This deficiency in cystathionine-synthase presents together with the development of intracranial aneurysms [5, 23].

In the study by Semmler et al., polymorphisms of homocysteine metabolism are possible risk factors for the formation of intracranial aneurysms [5]. The G-allele of RFC1c.80G→A and the insertion allele of DHFRc.594 + 59del19bp polymorphisms may result in intracranial aneurysm formation [5]. The G-allele of the missense polymorphism Tc2c.777C→G may protect from the development of intracranial aneurysm [5]. This G-allele of the Tc2c.777C→G polymorphism has been reported to affect the vitamin $B_{12}$ binding affinity and the ability to transport vitamin $B_{12}$ into tissues [5, 24–26]. This causes a decrease in remethylation of homocysteine to methionine by vitamin $B_{12}$-dependent MTR [5, 24–26].

## 4. Role of nitric oxide in homocysteine metabolism

Impairment of homocysteine metabolism may lead to an accumulation of asymmetric dimethylarginine [27, 28]. Asymmetric dimethylarginine.is a major endogenous inhibitor of nitric oxide (NO) and is a good predictor of early cardiovascular diseases and mortality [27–30]. In addition, the availability of NO is a major requirement for the development of intracranial aneurysms [5, 31].

In an animal study conducted in rodents, the development of intracranial aneurysm was prevented by inhibition of nitric oxide synthase (NOS) [5, 31]. Inducible nitric oxide synthase (iNOS) is expressed in human and rat cerebral aneurysms [2]. In another animal study, the size of intracranial aneurysms is significantly smaller in the mice with iNOS compared to the mice without iNOS [2, 5].

Aminoguanidine is a relatively selective inhibitor of iNOS [2]. Aminoguanidine reduces the number of the aneurysms in rats [2]. In the study by Sadamasa et al., iNOS possibly has management potential in the prevention of the progression of cerebral aneurysms, though it is not necessary for the initiation of cerebral aneurysm [2].

However, in another study, there was no association between homocysteine and intracranial aneurysms. Notably, this study was conducted comparing a case group (patients with intracranial aneurysms) with a control group consisting of patients with arteriovenous malformation (AVM) as well as no aneurysms [14].

## 5. Management

Raised serum homocysteine can be properly managed with dietary changes [17]. An increase in serum homocysteine can be treated by folic acid, vitamin $B_{12}$ and vitamin $B_6$ supplements [13, 15]. Folic acid and vitamin $B_{12}$ supplements can prevent the development and progression of intracranial aneurysm [17].

## 6. Conclusion

In conclusion, we believe that there is association between raised serum homocysteine and development or progression of intracranial aneurysms. In the future, more case-control research studies can be conducted to compare the patients with intracranial aneurysms and patients without intracranial aneurysms and AVM.

## Acknowledgements

We would like thank Dr. Abdul Rashid Mat Mahidin, Dr. Esther Yeow Kar Mun, Dr. Lattish Rao Threemurthy and Dr. Parathythasan a/l Rajaandra for their help.

## Funding source

This chapter is supported by the University of Malaya UMCares grant RU013-2017C.

## Author details

Mei-Ling Sharon Tai[1]*, Tsun Haw Toh[1], Hafez Hussain[2] and Kuo Ghee Ong[2]

1 Division of Neurology, Department of Medicine, Faculty of Medicine, University Malaya, Kuala Lumpur, Malaysia

2 SOCSO Tun Razak Rehabilitation Centre, Melaka, Malaysia

*Address all correspondence to: sharont1990@gmail.com

## References


[1] Modi S, Shah K, Schultz L, Tahir R, Affan M, Varelas P. Cost of hospitalization for aneurysmal subarachnoid hemorrhage in the United States. Clinical Neurology and Neurosurgery. 2019;**182**:167-170

[2] Sadamasa N, Nozaki K, Hashimoto N. Disruption of gene for inducible nitric oxide synthase reduces progression of cerebral aneurysms. Stroke. 2003;**34**:2980-2984

[3] Brisman JL, Song JK, Newell DW. Cerebral aneurysms. The New England Journal of Medicine. 2006;**355**:928-939

[4] Bederson JB, Awad IA, Wiebers DO, et al. Recommendations for the management of patients with unruptured intracranial aneurysms: A statement for healthcare professionals from the Stroke Council of the American Heart Association. Stroke. 2000;**31**:2742-2750

[5] Semmler A, Linnebank M, Krex D, Götz A, Moskau S, Ziegler A, et al. Polymorphisms of homocysteine metabolism are associated with intracranial aneurysms. Cerebrovascular Diseases. 2008;**26**(4):425-429

[6] Wiebers DO, Whisnant JP, Huston J III, et al. Unruptured intracranial aneurysms: Natural history, clinical outcome, and risks of surgical and endovascular treatment. Lancet. 2003;**362**:103-110

[7] Connolly ES, Solomon RA. Management of unruptured aneurysms. In: Le Roux PD, Winn HR, Newell DW, editors. Management of Cerebral Aneurysms. Philadelphia: Saunders; 2004. pp. 271-285

[8] Ruigrok YM, Rinkel GJ, Wijmenga C. Genetics of intracranial aneurysms. Lancet Neurology. 2005;**4**:179-189

[9] Teasdale GM, Wardlaw JM, White PM, Murray G, Teasdale EM, Easton V. The familial risk of subarachnoid haemorrhage. Brain. 2005;**128**:1677-1685

[10] Schievink WI, Schaid DJ, Michels VV, Piepgras DG. Familial aneurysmal subarachnoid hemorrhage: A community-based study. Journal of Neurosurgery. 1995;**83**:426-429

[11] Schievink WI. Intracranial aneurysms. The New England Journal of Medicine. 1997;**336**:28-40

[12] Wiebers DO, Whisnant JP, Sundt TM Jr, O'Fallon WM. The significance of unruptured intracranial saccular aneurysms. Journal of Neurosurgery. 1987;**66**:23-29

[13] Baszczuk A, Kopczyński Z. Hyperhomocysteinemia in patients with cardiovascular disease. Postępy Higieny i Medycyny Doświadczalnej (Online). 2014;**68**:579-589

[14] Rosi J, Morais BA, Pecorino LS, Oliveira AR, Solla DJF, Teixeira MJ, et al. Hyperhomocysteinemia as a risk factor for intracranial aneurysms: A case-control study. World Neurosurgery. 2018;**119**:e272-e275

[15] Tinelli C, Di Pino A, Ficulle E, Marcelli S, Feligioni M. Hyperhomocysteinemia as a risk factor and potential nutraceutical target for certain pathologies. Frontiers in Nutrition. 2019;**6**:49

[16] Selhub J, Jacques PF, Wilson PW, et al. Vitamin status and intake as primary determinants of homocysteinemia in an elderly population. JAMA. 1993;**270**:2693-2698

[17] Ren JR, Ren SH, Ning B, Wu J, Cao Y, Ding XM, et al. Hyperhomocysteinemia as a risk factor for saccular intracranial

aneurysm: A cohort study in a Chinese Han population. Journal of Stroke and Cerebrovascular Diseases. 2017;**26**(12):2720-2726

[18] Azad MAK, Huang P, Liu G, Ren W, Teklebrh T, Yan W, et al. Hyperhomocysteinemia and cardiovascular disease in animal model. Amino Acids. 2018;**50**(1):3-9

[19] Pusceddu I, Herrmann W, Kleber ME, Scharnagl H, Hoffmann MM, Winklhofer-Roob BM, et al. Subclinical inflammation, telomere shortening, homocysteine, vitamin $B_6$, and mortality: The Ludwigshafen Risk and Cardiovascular Health Study. European Journal of Nutrition. 2019;**25**. [Epub ahead of print]

[20] Xu Y, Tian Y, Wei HJ. Methionine diet-induced hyperhomocysteinemia accelerates cerebral aneurysm formation in rats. Neuroscience Letters. 2011;**494**:139-144

[21] Casas JP, Bautista LE, Smeeth L, Sharma P, Hingorani AD. Homocysteine and stroke: Evidence on a causal link from Mendelian randomisation. Lancet. 2005;**365**:224-232

[22] Arauz A, Hoyos L, Cantu C, Jara A, Martinez L, Garcia I, et al. Mild hyperhomocysteinemia and low folate concentrations as risk factors for cervical arterial dissection. Cerebrovascular Diseases. 2007;**24**:210-214

[23] Yap S, Boers GH, Wilcken B, Wilcken DE, Brenton DP, Lee PJ, et al. Vascular outcome in patients with homocystinuria due to cystathionine beta-synthase deficiency treated chronically: A multicenter observational study. Arteriosclerosis, Thrombosis, and Vascular Biology. 2001;**21**:2080-2085

[24] Afman LA, Lievers KJ, van der Put NM, Trijbels FJ, Blom HJ. Single nucleotide polymorphisms in the transcobalamin gene: Relationship with transcobalamin concentrations and risk for neural tube defects. European Journal of Human Genetics. 2002;**10**:433-438

[25] Afman LA, van der Put NM, Thomas CM, Trijbels JM, Blom HJ. Reduced vitamin $B_{12}$ binding by transcobalamin II increases the risk of neural tube defects. QJM. 2001;**94**:159-166

[26] Miller JW, Ramos MI, Garrod MG, Flynn MA, Green R, Transcobalamin II. 775G 1 C polymorphism and indices of vitamin $B_{12}$ status in healthy older adults. Blood. 2002;**100**:718-720

[27] Ito A, Tsao PS, Adimoolam S, Kimoto M, Ogawa T, Cooke JP. Novel mechanism for endothelial dysfunction: Dysregulation of dimethylarginine dimethylaminohydrolase. Circulation. 1999;**99**:3092-3095

[28] Stuhlinger MC, Tsao PS, Her JH, Kimoto M, Balint RF, Cooke JP. Homocysteine impairs the nitric oxide synthase pathway: Role of asymmetric dimethylarginine. Circulation. 2001;**104**:2569-2575

[29] Schnabel R, Blankenberg S, Lubos E, Lackner KJ, Rupprecht HJ, Espinola-Klein C, et al. Asymmetric dimethylarginine and the risk of cardiovascular events and death in patients with coronary artery disease: Results from the AtheroGene study. Circulation Research. 2005;**97**:e53-e59

[30] Cooke JP. Asymmetrical dimethylarginine: The uber marker? Circulation. 2004;**109**:1813-1818

[31] Fukuda S, Hashimoto N, Naritomi H, Nagata I, Nozaki K, Kondo S, et al. Prevention of rat cerebral aneurysm formation by inhibition of nitric oxide synthase. Circulation. 2000;**101**:2532-2525

Chapter 4

# Vascular Calcifications

*Mehmet Erin Tüysüz and Mehmet Dedemoğlu*


## Abstract

Calcium-phosphate levels have an effect on the vascular wall. Calcium is a cation in human body. It is has a crucial effect on intracellular and extracellular mechanisms. Extracellular calcium levels are more than intracellular levels. In total serum, the calcium level is approximately 8.8–10.4. Parathormone and vitamin D regulate blood calcium levels. Phosphorus is more common than calcium in the human body. Most of the phosphorus is present in the skeletal system. Phosphorus level is approximately 2.5–4.5 mg/dl in blood. It is often observed calcification in cardiovascular system in some diseases such as chronic renal failure due to increased calcium-phosphate levels. While the calcification seems in tunica intima layer of the vessel in atherosclerotic disease, it seems in tunica media layer of vessel in chronic renal failure with high uremic level. Vascular calcification is due to arterial stiffness, stenosis, and occlusion. Vascular and valvular calcifications are irreversible. Increased arterial stiffness destroys vascular compliance, causes left ventricular hypertrophy, and disrupts coronary perfusion. As a result, increased vascular calcification is associated with cardiovascular mortality.


**Keywords:** cardiovascular calcification, arterial stiffness, vascular compliance, hyperparathyroidism, hyperphosphatemia

## 1. Introduction

Cardiovascular pathologies are still one of the most serious diseases in the world and are also known to be an important reason of mortality and morbidity. Furthermore, they cause a significant burden on the health costs. The understanding of pathophysiology of cardiovascular diseases has an important role for the treatment success. In this chapter, vascular calcification mechanism and its results will be discussed.

There are several reasons leading to vascular calcifications (**Table 1**). Vascular calcifications often occur in the advanced stage of the atherosclerosis [1]. In addition to this, these calcifications may also occur as a complication of metabolic disorders in the end stage of chronic renal failure. Calcium deposits accumulate in vascular tissues as a result of secondary hyperparathyroidism that occurs in chronic renal failure [2, 3]. Another cause of vascular calcifications is familial hypercholesterolemia. Particularly severe aortic calcifications are seen in these patients [4]. Vascular calcifications associated with diabetes mellitus also affect the media and intima layer of vessels [5]. Hypertension is associated with calcifications in the abdominal aorta [6]. The other causes of vascular calcification include smoking [7], male gender [6], and older age [7]. Recently, it has been observed thanks to intravascular invasive images that the use of statins increases vascular calcification. Despite the antilipidemic and anti-inflammatory effects of it, statins cause an

| **Causes of vascular calcification** |
|---|
| • Atherosclerosis |
| • Chronic renal failure |
| • Familial hypercholesterolemia |
| • Diabetes mellitus |
| • Hypertension |
| • Smoking |
| • Male gender |
| • Older age |

**Table 1.**
*The causes of vascular calcification.*

increased calcification in vascular tissue with an unknown mechanism. This effect is defined as the statin paradox [8].

## 2. Pathophysiology

Vascular smooth muscle cells (VSMCs) play an important role in the pathology of vascular calcifications. Vascular smooth muscle cells are of mesenchymal origin. These cells may turn into osteoblasts and chondrocytes under stress. Osteoblast-like cells that contain hydroxyapatite crystals appear in the extracellular matrix during vascular smooth muscle calcification. Subsequently, the number of osteochondrogenic cells increases, and calcification inhibitors are suppressed; an increased regulation of bone mineralization regulating genes and the release of calcified membrane-dependent carriers from smooth muscle cells in these calcifications are observed. In addition, intracellular phosphate concentration increases in osteoblast-like cells due to developing hyperphosphatemia in chronic renal failure. Apoptosis in smooth muscle cells, oxidative stress, remodeling in extracellular matrix, and high levels of metalloproteinases increase vascular calcification, resulting in endothelial dysfunction [9].

Vascular smooth muscle cells are the predominant cell type in the arterial wall. VSMCs are mainly composed of the medial layer of the blood vessels, which are subjected to mechanical stress and pressure of blood flow, and maintain vascular tone and resistance [10]. Calcium functions as a stimulator, and under physiological conditions, intracellular calcium is present in VSCMs to regulate many biophysical and biochemical processes [11]. Although the agents responsible for production of vasospasm have not yet been clearly identified, recently the molecular mechanisms involved in the development of vasospasm mainly based on experimental data in canine two-hemorrhage model are reviewed. The blood products after subarachnoid hemorrhage most likely stimulate many cell membrane receptors to activate the tyrosine kinase pathway of WSCMs. The activation of the tyrosine kinase pathway is associated with continuous elevation of intracellular Ca++ levels and activation of mu-calpain. The increased intracellular Ca++ concentration stimulates Ca++/calmodulin and depends on myosin light-chain kinase to phosphorylate myosin light-chain continuously during vasospasms [12]. Cerebral vasospasm is the most frequent and troublesome complication after aneurysmal subarachnoid hemorrhage. Cerebral vasospasm is considered a treatable clinicopathological entity; it is still responsible for many deaths and serious disabilities among patients suffering from intracranial aneurysm rupture [13].

## 3. Classification

Vascular calcifications are divided into two subtypes (**Figure 1**). These are called intima and media calcifications according to the localization of calcification.

Intimal calcifications or the so-called atherosclerotic calcifications begin to occur in the presence of chronic inflammations and/or lipid accumulations. Lipid-loaded calcifications in the intima cause intimal thickening and subsequent narrowing of the lumen diameter.

Medial calcifications are characterized by concentric calcium deposits in the tunica media layer. Here, elastin lamellae occur between the smooth muscle cells and the elastin fibers. Medial calcifications cause loss of elasticity in the arteries, resulting in arterial stiffness [9].

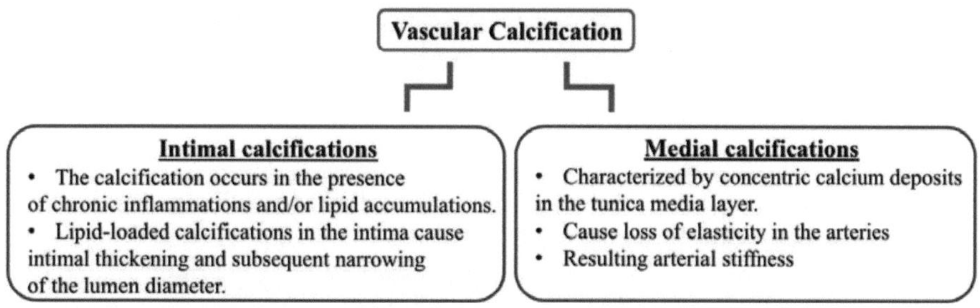


**Figure 1.**
*The classification of vascular calcification.*

## 4. Imaging methods

Various methods are used to visualize calcifications. Macrocalcifications can be seen in three ways:

1. Speckled: spotty calcification flecks, up to 50 μm diameters

2. Sheetlike fragments: linear or wide single focus of calcium, >2 mm in diameter

3. Diffuse: segments of continuous calcification, ≥5 mm in diameter

Imaging methods can be performed as noninvasive and invasive (**Table 2**).

### 4.1 Noninvasive methods

Computerized tomography (CT) is the gold standard for imaging calcifications. 400 μm of calcification can be shown as 2D and 3D with the help of CT. However, the calcifications sometimes can be seen as more exaggerated than usual because of the absorption of high X-rays by neighboring tissues in CT imaging. This exaggerated image (artifact) may mask parts of calcification in the proximal region of the lesions. In this case, the artifact can be distinguished from the surrounding soft tissue with the help of magnetic resonance imaging (MRI). MRI is also superior to CT in differentiating multiple components including the coexistence of lipid accumulation, fibrotic tissue, and calcifications.

Microcalcifications can be detected by the use of positron emission tomography (PET) which is one of the other noninvasive methods. Early microcalcifications are shown using indirect gamma rays with the aid of 18F-sodium fluoride. With the use

| The imaging methods for vascular calcification |
|---|
| *Noninvasive methods* |
| • Computerized tomography (CT) |
| • Magnetic resonance imaging (MRI) |
| • Positron emission tomography (PET) |
| *Invasive methods* |
| • Intravascular ultrasound (IVUS) |
| • Optical coherence tomography (OCT) |

**Table 2.**
*The imaging methods for vascular calcifications.*

of MRI or CT combined with PET, we can obtain more detailed information about the effects of calcifications, interactions with fibrotic tissue, and plaque geometry.

### 4.2 Invasive methods

In recent years, intravascular ultrasound (IVUS) has been widely used in the detection of vascular calcifications, and its success is 50% higher than CT imaging. However, in the vessels with severe calcifications, they may not be able to adequately measure volume and wall thickness due to acoustic shadowing and insufficient penetration into macrocalcific deposits.

Optical coherence tomography (OCT) is an alternative modality using infrared ray. The specificity and sensitivity of this method is higher than other methods. OCT also identifies superficial calcifications in the vessels. In addition, in the case of acute plaque rupture, OCT detects spot calcifications in the areas of plaque near the lumen and the thinning of the vessel wall [14].

## 5. Clinical properties

The calcifications may occur in all anatomic structures of the cardiovascular system. Pericardial calcifications occur secondary to inflammation. Calcification of this type is usually asymptomatic; however, the clinical findings are observed when it causes constrictive pericarditis [15].

Myocardial calcifications are metastatic or dystrophic calcifications. Metastatic calcifications develop after impaired calcium metabolism due to chronic renal failure or hyperparathyroidism. Dystrophic calcifications develop as a result of myocardial fibrosis, infections, sarcoidosis, and hemorrhagic events in the myocardium. The cell necrosis occurs in this pathology, resulting in myocardial damage. This type of calcification leads to local myocardial contraction disorder, diastolic dysfunction, arrhythmia, and eventually congestive heart failure [16].

Epidemiological studies have found a strong association between calcification and coronary artery-related event and mortality using coronary artery calcification scores. Cardiovascular prognosis and mortality can be predicted with these scoring. Calcifications have an important role in thrombotic complications of atherosclerosis. Progression in coronary artery calcification shows active atherosclerosis and high rupture risk in unstable plaques. On the other hand, calcifications in the coronary artery cause some problems in the invasive treatments. During percutaneous transluminal coronary angioplasty (PTCA), a high dilatation pressure is required due to calcific coronary artery structure. Technical difficulties also arise when adjusting the position of the stent. As a result, coronary artery calcifications cause dissection, thrombosis, and restenosis during PTCA [17]. Another issue is that long-term prognosis of patients who underwent PTCA for moderate and severe coronary artery calcification is also poor [18].

Calcifications also affect heart valves. The annulus of the mitral valve is affected from this calcification, especially in female, elder patients and in case of chronic renal failure, radiotherapy applications. The pathophysiology of mitral annular calcification (MAC) is similar to that of atherosclerosis. Excessive MAC makes it difficult to perform balloon valvuloplasty and valve-sparing surgical procedures. On the other hand, in patients with MAC who underwent valve replacement, paravalvular leakage, the circumflex coronary artery injury, arrhythmia, and patient artificial valve mismatch (because of the condition of small-size valve usage) may be observed [19]. During transcatheter mitral valve replacements, calcifications may lead to left ventricle outflow obstruction and paravalvular leakage [20].

Calcific aortic valve disease is the most common form of calcific valvular pathology. When we look at the pathogenesis of this disease, the ectopic calcium nodules are located on the aortic surface of the aortic valve and in the aortic annulus. The incidence of calcific aortic valve increases with age. However, calcification of bicuspid valves may be seen at an early age. Risk factors are similar to other cardiovascular diseases. Calcifications can reduce the success of prosthetic aortic valve surgery [21]. In the late stages of valve replacement for calcific aortic valve stenosis, fistulas may develop between the left ventricle and the right atrium [22]. In transcatheter aortic valve implantations (TAVI), the degree of valve calcification is routinely evaluated by preoperative multi-slice CT. In this way, the information about the presence of asymmetric calcification is obtained before the procedure [23]. As a complication, cerebral emboli originating from calcific aortic valve stenosis may occur [24]. In addition, valve degeneration may occur secondary to calcification in patients undergoing valve replacement with bioprosthetic valve [25].

Excessive aortic valve calcification and metastatic calcifications due to chronic renal failure and hyperparathyroidism may affect the conduction system of the heart. Many arrhythmia types, from nodal rhythm to branch blocks, may be observed due to these calcifications [26–28].

Calcifications in the arcus and thoracic aorta cause aneurysm development, aortic occlusions, and distal embolization. These calcifications in the aortic wall also affect the success of endovascular stenting and surgical interventions [29]. It has been observed that the possibility of developing intermittent claudication is increased in the follow-up of patients with abdominal aortic calcification [30].

İntracranial artery calcification has been demonstrated to be correlated with ischemic stroke, cognitive decline, and other vascular events by accumulating evidence from both Western and Asian populations [31]. As atherosclerotic vasculopathy is a systemic process, vascular calcification may play a role in cerebrovascular events in both qualitative and quantitative calcium scoring with intracranial atherosclerosis and ischemic events [32]. On the other hand, some studies showed that ruptured intracranial aneurysms had a lower calcification fraction and lacked macrocalcifications than unruptured intracranial aneurysms [33]. Another study showed that arterial calcification correlated with white matter hyperintensities and lacunes [34].

Calcification is rarely seen in the venous system. Venous calcifications in the literature are mostly associated with the portal vein [35].

## 6. Treatment

Treatment of vascular calcifications is distributed over a wide range. Developing new medications and technical devices reconstruct our treatment modalities with that disease. As is known, vascular calcifications are the major factor limiting endovascular treatment methods. One of the methods developed to overcome this problem is the peripheral intravascular lithotripsy (IVL) system. With this method, calcific lesions can be eliminated by applying pulsatile mechanical energy under fluoroscopy [36].

Obstructive disease of infra-inguinal arteries is treated with atherectomy methods. Various atherectomy devices have been developed for this method. Some of these are rotational, phoenix, directional, orbital, etc. The B-Laser atherectomy system is one of the new generation devices. This device is equipped with an optical fiber and circumferential designed blades for transmitting laser energy. Calcifications, fibrotic atherosclerotic plaques, and re-stenotic tissues are removed with the aspiration catheter added to the system [37].

There are several studies to improve medical treatment. Experimental animal studies have shown that angiotensin II receptor inhibitors prevent the vascular calcification due to hyperphosphatemia [38]. In another experimental animal study, the use of teniposide which inhibits DNA topoisomerase II in the treatment of cancer has been shown to prevent the development of vascular calcification [39]. Vitamin K II, added to the diet in chronic renal failure, acts on calcium hemostasis by preventing bone loss. Thus, it is shown that vitamin K II can prevent vascular calcification by adding it to the treatment regimen [40]. Another treatment modality is parathyroidectomy which is applied especially in vascular calcifications as a result of calcium and phosphate metabolism-related disorders [41].

## Author details

Mehmet Erin Tüysüz[1*] and Mehmet Dedemoğlu[2]

1 Department of Cardiovascular Surgery, Mersin City Training and Research Hospital, Mersin, Turkey

2 Department of Pediatric Cardiovascular Surgery, Mersin City Training and Research Hospital, Mersin, Turkey

*Address all correspondence to: drmehmeterin@yahoo.com

## References

[1] Boström K. Insight into the mechanism of vascular calcification. The American Journal of Cardiology. 2001;**88**:29E-22E

[2] Giachelli CM. Vascular calcification: In vitro evidence for the role of inorganic phosphate. Journal of the American Society of Nephrology. 2003;**14**(Suppl 4):s300-s304

[3] Thomson C. Vascular calcification in chronic renal failure. Nephron. Clinical Practice. 2003;**93**(4):c124-c130

[4] Grenom S, Lachepelle K, Marcil M, Omeroğlu A, Genest J, Varenes B. Surgical strategies for severe calcification of the aorta (porcelain aorta) in two patients with homozygous familial hypercholesterolemia. The Canadian Journal of Cardiology. 2007;**23**:1159-1161

[5] Schoen F, Cotran R. Blood vessels. In: Cotran R, Kumar V, Collins T, editors. Robbins Pathological Basis of Disesase. 6th ed. London: W.B. Saunders; 1999. pp. 493-541

[6] Allison M, Criquii M, Wriht C. Patterns and risk factors for systemic calcified atherosclerosis. Arteriosclerosis, Thrombosis, and Vascular Biology. 2004;**24**(2):331-336

[7] Reaven P, Saks J. Reduced coronary artery and abdominal calcification in Hispanics with type 2 diabetes. Diabetes Care. 2004;**27**(5):1115-1120

[8] Lee D, Joo H, Jung H, Lim D. Investigating potential mediator between statin and coronary artery calcification. PLoS One. 2018;**13**(9):e0203702

[9] Belay T. Involvement of vitamin k-dependent proteins in vascular calcification. Journal of Cardiovascular Pharmacology and Therapeutics. 2019;**24**(4):323-333

[10] Li N, Sanyour H, Remund T, Kelly P, et al. Vascular extracellular matrix and fibroblasts-coculture directed differentiation of human mesenchymal stem cells toward smooth muscle-like cells for vascular tissue engineering. Materials Science and Engineering: C. 2018;**93**:61-69. DOI: 10.1016/j.msec.2018.07.061

[11] Huang H, Sun Z, Hill M, et al. A calcium medicated mechanism coordinating vascular smooth muscle cell adhesion during KCI activation. Frontiers in Physiology. 2018;**9**:a1810. DOI: 10.3389 phys.2018.01810

[12] Tani E. Molecular mechanisms involved in development of cerebral vasospasm. Neurosurgical Focus. 2002;**12**:ECP1. DOI: 10.3171/foc.2002.12.3.8

[13] Hop J, Rinkel G, Algra A, et al. Case-fatality rates and functional outcome after subarachnoid hemorrhage: A systematic review. Stroke. 1997;**28**:660-664

[14] Barret H, Van der Heiden K, Farel E, et al. Calcifications in atherosclerotic plaques and impact on plaques biomechanics. Journal of Biomechanics. 2019;**87**:1-12

[15] Khalid N, Ahmad SA, Shlofmitz E. Pericardial Calcification. [Updated 2019 Nov 14]. In: StatPearls [Internet]. Treasure Island (FL): StatPearls Publishing; Jan 2019. Available from: https://www.ncbi.nlm.nih.gov/books/NBK538342/

[16] Yuki K, Osamu J, Atsushi K, Manabu M, Yuto K, et al. Massive bioventricular myocardial calcification in a patient with fulminant myocarditis requiring ventricular assist device support. Internal Medicine. 2019;**58**(9):1283-1286

[17] Loich P, Olivier L, Jean R, Michel G, Didier C, Jean F. Coronary

artery calcification: From crystal to plaque rupture. Archives of Cardiovascular Diseases. 2017;**110**(10):550-561

[18] Zhang Y, Song L, Song Y, Xu L, Wang H, et al. Impact coronary artery lesion calcification on the long-term outcome of patients with coronary heart disease after percutaneous coronary intervention. Zhonghua Xin Xue Guan Bing Za Zhi. 2019;**47**(1):33-41

[19] Philippe B, Christo M, Evin Y. Mitral annular calcification mitral stenosis: Therapeutic challenges and considerations. Current Treatment Options in Cardiovascular Medicine. 2019;**21**(4):19

[20] Mohammed H, Abdallah S, Mayra G, Charanjit R, Mackram E. Paravalvular leak repair after balloon-expandable transcatheter mitral valve implantation in mitral annular calcification: Early experience and lessons learned. Catheterization and Cardiovascular Interventions. 2019;**94**(5):764-772

[21] Viral M, Soy L. The genetic regulation of aortic valve development and calcific disease. Frontiers in Cardiovascular Medicine. 2018;**5**:162

[22] Anderson C, Rodriguez E, Kupson A. Delayed left ventricle-to-right atrial fistula following aortic valve replacement. The Journal of Heart Valve Disease. 2012;**21**(3):364-365

[23] Christian B, Maki O, Gerhard S, Cladius J, Jurgen R, Hendrick T, et al. Degree of valve calcification in patients undergoing transfemoral transcatheter aortic valve implantation with and without balloon aortic valvuloplasty: Findings from the multicenter EASE-IT TF registry. Catheterization and Cardiovascular Interventions. 2019;**94**(3):469-478

[24] Vernhet H, Torres G, Laharotte S, Tournut P, Bierme T, Froment S, et al. Spontaneous calcific cerebral emboli from calcified aortic valve stenosis. Journal of Neuroradiology. 1993;**20**(1):19-23

[25] Rutkovskaya N, Kagan E, Kondyukova N, Kuzmina O, Barborash L. Prediction of risk of calcification of heart valve bioprostheses on the basis of comprehensive assessment of recipients clinical factors and their compliance with therapy. Kardiologiia. 2018;**10**:27-33

[26] Mauntner R, Phillips J. Atrioventricular and intraventricular conduction disturbance in aortic valvular disease. Southern Medical Journal. 1980;**73**(5):572-578

[27] Vosnakidis A, Polymeropoulos K, Zarogoulidis P, Zarifis I. Atrioventricular nodal dysfunction secondary to hyperparathyroidism. Journal of Thoracic Disease. 2013;**5**(3):E 90-E 92

[28] Isotalo P, Halil A, Green M, Tang A, Lach B, Veinot J. Metastatic calcification of the cardiac conduction system with heart block: An under-reported entity in chronic renal failure patients. Journal of Forensic Sciences. 2000;**45**(6):1335-1338

[29] Jayalath R, Mangan S, Golledge J. Aortic calcification. European Journal of Vascular and Endovascular Surgery. 2005;**30**:476-488

[30] Nıskanen L, Suhonen M, Sııtonen O, Lehtınen J. Aortic and lower limb artery calcification in type 2 (non-insulin-dependent) diabetic patients and non-diabetic control subject. A five-year follow-up study. Atherosclerosis. 1990;**84**(1):61-71

[31] Wu X, Wang L, Zhong J, et al. Impact of intracranial artery calcification on cerebral hemodynamic changes. Neuroradiology. 2018;**60**:357-363

[32] Erbay S, Han R, Baccei S, et al. İntracranial carotid artery calcification on head CT and its association with ischemic changes on brain MRI in patients presenting with stroke-like symptoms: Retrospective analysis. Neuroradiology. 2007;**49**:27-33

[33] Gade P, Tulamo R, Lee K, et al. Calcification in human intracranial aneurysms is highly prevalent and displays both atherosclerotic and nonatherosclerotic types. Arteriosclerosis, Thrombosis, and Vascular Biology. 2019;**39**:2157-2167. DOI: 10.1161//ATVBAHA.119.312922

[34] Chen Y, Wei X, Lu J, et al. Correlation between intracranial arterial calcification and imaging of cerebral small vessel disease. Frontiers in Neurology. 2019;**10**:426. DOI: 10.3389/fneur.2019.00426

[35] Shammas NW, Chandra P, Brodmann M, Weinstock B, Sedillo G, Cawich I, et al. Acute and 30-day safety and effectiveness evaluation of Eximo Medical's B-Laser™, a novel atherectomy device, in subjects affected with infrainguinal peripheral arterial disease: Results of the EX-PAD-03 trial. Cardiovascular Revascularization Medicine. 29 Nov 2018. pii: S1553-8389(18)30565-7. DOI: 10.1016/j.carrev.2018.11.022. [Epub ahead of print]

[36] Price L, Faries P, Mckinsey J, Prakash K, Tang G, Kovacic J, et al. The epidemiology, pathophysiology, and novel treatment of calcific arterial disease. Surgical Technology International. 2019;**34**:351-358

[37] Shammas N, Chanda P, Brodman M, Weinstock B, Sedillo G, Cawich I, et al. Acute and 30-day safety and effectiveness evaluation of Eximo medical's B-Laser™, a novel atherectomy device, in subjects affected with infrainguinal peripheral arterial disease. Result of the EX-PAD-03 trial. Cardiovascular Revascularization Medicine. 2018. PII: S1553-8389(18)30565-7

[38] Kukida M, Mogi M, Ken-No H, Tsukada K, Bai H, Shan B, et al. AT2 receptor stimulation inhibits phosphate-induced vascular calcification. Kidney International. 2019;**95**(1):138-148

[39] Liu L, Zeng P, Yang X, Duan Y, Zhang W, Ma C, et al. Inhibition of vascular calcification. Arteriosclerosis, Thrombosis, and Vascular Biology. 2018;**38**(10):2382-2395

[40] Wasilewski G, Verloet M, Schurgers L. The bone-vasculature axis: Calcium supplementation and the role of vitamin K. Frontiers in Cardiovascular Medicine. 2019;**6**:6

[41] Gao Z, Li X, Miao S, Lun L. Impacts of parathyroidectomy on calcium and phosphorus metabolism disorder, arterial calcification and arterial stiffness in haemodialysis patients. Asian Journal of Surgery. 2019;**42**(1):6-10

# Section 3

# Hemodynamic

Chapter 5

# Normal Pressure Hydrocephalus

*Ravish Rajiv Keni, Harsh Deora and Amit Agrawal*


## Abstract

Normal pressure hydrocephalus (NPH) is characterized by dilated ventricles and a combination of gait impairment, cognition impairment, and loss of urinary control (urgency and incontinence). The only effective treatment for NPH is a CSF shunt; however, only a small percentage of patients ever receive it. The features of gait impairment in patients with NPH are difficult to distinguish from patients of neurodegenerative disorders with motor involvement, such as parkinsonism or dementia with Lewy bodies. CT or MRI imaging is required for the diagnosis of idiopathic normal pressure hydrocephalus. An Evans ratio of more than 0.3 indicates large ventricles, and a ratio of more than 0.33 indicates very large ventricles, but is not specific for idiopathic normal pressure hydrocephalus. The international and Japanese guidelines support shunt surgery as effective treatment of idiopathic normal pressure hydrocephalus, as does the American Academy of Neurology practice guideline. There is a need to provide longitudinal care of patients with idiopathic normal pressure hydrocephalus after shunt surgery as all symptoms respond well to shunt surgery.


**Keywords:** normal pressure hydrocephalus, shunts surgery

## 1. Introduction

Normal-pressure hydrocephalus (NPH) is the earliest identified cause of dementia which can be potentially treated [1, 2]. NPH was described by Hakim and Adams in 1965, and the entity was characterized by gait disturbances, impaired cognition, and urinary incontinence that is associated with ventricular enlargement without rise in cerebrospinal fluid (CSF) pressure [3, 4]. NPH may be primary or idiopathic NPH (without known precipitating factors) or secondary (due to trauma, hemorrhage, infection, mass lesions, or delayed aqueductal stenosis) [5–7].

## 2. Epidemiology

The exact incidence and prevalence of INPH is difficult to determine; however, the incidence of INPH is between 1.8 and 2.2 cases per 1,000,000 individuals [8, 9]. In a door to door survey from two German villages, the 0.41% prevalence of NPH was reported [10]. In patients with dementia, the reported incidence of NPH ranges between 1.6 and 5.4% [11, 12].

## 3. Pathophysiology

There are two main mechanisms involved in the pathogenesis of NPH [13, 14], that is, increased venous resistance and altered production and absorption of CSF. Studies have found that in patients with NPH, there is reduction in vascular compliance particularly involving superior sagittal sinus. Hakim and Adam's hypothesized [4] that in NPH reduced CSF absorption leads to raised intracranial pressure and over a period leading to compensatory ventricular enlargement. This new intracranial pressure state directs more CSF flow toward the Virchow-Robin spaces and thus into the brain parenchyma [15]. These metabolic and mechanical changes further leads to periventricular damage and raised myelin basic protein (a possible biomarker) elevated in these patients [16]. This leads to tissue compression, white matter ischemia and parenchymal changes characterized by myelin pallor. These changes further lead to periventricular damage, reduced cellular metabolism, clearance of toxins, and their sequel [15, 17]. Studies have shown that following CSF diversion, there is normalization in global brain stiffness and elasticity on magnetic resonance studies [18].

## 4. Clinical features

The classical clinical triad of INPH includes gait disturbance, dementia, and urinary incontinence [3–6, 8]. These symptoms are typically insidious in onset, and the patients are in their sixth and eighth decades. These changes occur in presence of ventriculomegaly without much evidence of cortical atrophy on brain imaging [2].

## 5. Gait disturbances

Gait disturbances are the most common initial symptom (present in 90% of the patients) and initially characterized by unsteadiness, frequent falls, slowness of gait, with difficulty initiating and turning, as the disease advances, these transform into magnetic, slow, broad based, and short steps (with preserved arm swing). These gait disturbances are not usually associated with increase in tone, exaggerated reflexes or weakness and usually there is absence of primary sensorimotor deficits, cerebellar dysfunction, or involuntary movements, involving difficulty integrating sensory information about the position of the body in relation to its environment. The impairment should be symmetric unless coexisting musculoskeletal disorders (e.g., knees, hips, and spine) cause asymmetry.

## 6. Dementia

INPH patients have subcortical frontal dysexecutive syndrome, manifesting as memory impairment, decreased attention, impaired planning, slowness of thought, and apathy. The cognitive findings of NPH reflect involvement of the prefrontal brain structures, similar to a subcortical dementia, with executive dysfunction (e.g., slow processing, and difficulty with problem solving) and memory deficits with poor retrieval and relatively intact recognition memory. Delirium is not typical in NPH and implies the presence of a concomitant disorder or medication side effect.

## 7. Urinary incontinence

The urological manifestations include frequency, urgency, and urge incontinence. In a series of 41 patients with possible iNPH, 95% patients had urodynamic evidence of detrusor overactivity [12]. Bladder manifestations in NPH have been attributed to the involvement of sacral fibers of corticospinal pathway. Patients are usually aware of the urinary urge and are concerned about their incontinence. Incontinence without awareness of urinary urge or that one's clothes are wet is not a feature of NPH. Patients or family should be asked about the use of incontinence pads or undergarments, as occasionally they do not consider the patient to be incontinent if the urine is contained by the pads or undergarments. As bladder symptoms are common in elderly patients, other causes are frequently present in patients with suspected NPH.

## 8. Imaging

The differential diagnosis of NPH other non-treatable causes of dementias and degenerative disorders is extremely for proper selection of potential candidates for CSF diversion. No brain imaging studies are sufficient to diagnose INPH; however ventricular enlargement with appropriate symptoms is necessary to establish a diagnosis of NPH. Combination of imaging modalities and correlation with clinical findings shall help to make a diagnosis of NPH [2]. Evans' index 0.3 or greater suggests significant ventriculomegaly (**Figures 1** and **2**) [19]. Other imaging features include:

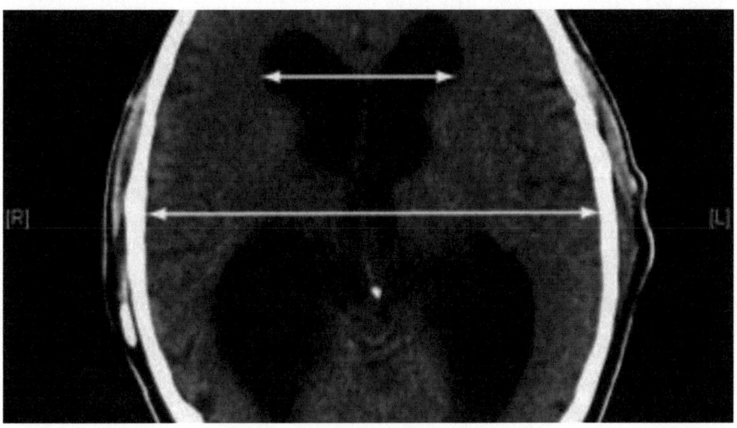


**Figure 1.**
*CT brain of a patient with INPH showing ventriculomegaly without significant cortical atrophy (Evan's index > 0.3).*

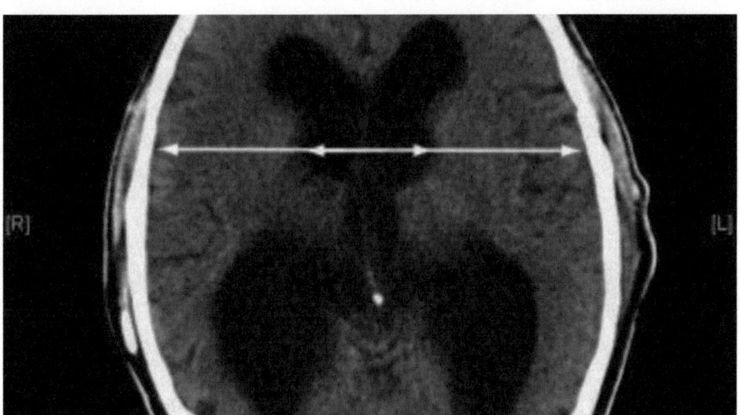


**Figure 2.**
*CT brain of a patient with INPH showing increased bicaudate ratio > 0.25.*

- Bicaudate ratio > 0.25
- Enlargement of temporal horn
- Periventricular abnormal signals
- Flow void in aqueduct or fourth ventricle

## 9. Supportive radiological investigations include

- Radionuclide cisternogram may show delayed clearance.
- Cine MRI can show increased ventricular flow rate
- SPECT-acetazolamide will demonstrate decreased periventricular perfusion which is not reversed with acetazolamide

Distinguishing dilated ventricles due to cerebral atrophy from NPH is difficult [19–22]. Focal atrophy is often indicative of a degenerative dementia, particularly if it is asymmetric (e.g., frontotemporal dementia) or is stereotypical, such as hippocampal atrophy in Alzheimer dementia. In NPH, the Sylvain fissures are disproportionately widened in comparison to the cortical sulci, which are flattened ("high tight" convexity). The appearance of a pulsation artifact in the cerebral aqueduct, or measurements of CSF stroke volume or velocity in the aqueduct using phase – contrast methods cannot be used alone to recommend shunt surgery, but can support the diagnosis of NPH and the need for further testing.

## 10. Classification of INPH

Based on clinical and radiological features, INPH can be classified into probable, possible, and unlikely categories [19]. Probable criteria include age > 40, symptoms > 3 months, gait disorder, urinary incontinence or dementia, Evan's index > 0.3, temporal horn enlargement, aqueductal/Fourth ventricle flow void, and callosal angle > 40 [19]. If there is papilloedema, or absence of triad or no ventriculomegaly, the diagnosis of NPH is unlikely [19].

## 11. Prognostic tests

The tests which are done to ascertain the benefit of surgical intervention in INPH include: lumbar puncture which has a sensitivity of 26%, and specificity of 100%, extended lumbar drainage (sensitivity of 50–80% and specificity of 80%), measurement of CSF outflow resistance measurement (if >18 mm Hg/ml/min than 46% sensitive and 87% specific) and cine phase-contrast MRI (has insufficient evidence).

## 12. Tap test

In this, 40-50 ml of CSF is removed, and pre- and post-tap with the Gait Scale (walking score + step score + time score) is assessed. The step score is based on the number of steps required for the patient to walk 10 m. Similarly, pre- and post-tap cognitive function assessed Folstein Mini Mental State Exam and within 2–4 hours after the CSF tap post-tap assessments are conducted. A significant response to the tap test indicates responsiveness to shunt surgery [23]. However, lack of significant response does not exclude shunt responsiveness because the tap test is specific, rather than sensitive. External lumbar drainage can be considered if iNPH is still clinically suspected after a patient has failed to improve after the tap test.

## 13. External lumbar drainage

In this test, CSF is drained (10 to 15 cc per hour) for 72 hours and patient is assessed before and after the drainage (positive predictive value 90% and negative predictive value 78%). Positive ELD indicates good benefit with shunt. Negative ELD indicates low risk-benefit ratio. Neuropsychological testing before and after external lumbar drainage may also be helpful. Most publications have cited 72 hours of CSF drainage, although some centers drain CSF for shorter periods [19, 20]. This test has the risk of headache, lumbar radiculopathy, and risk of meningitis.

## 14. CSF infusion testing

Infusion testing for assessment of CSF hydrodynamics is commonly used in Europe to diagnose NPH, but is rarely used in the United States or Canada. In CSF infusion test, Ringer lactate is infused via one spinal needle and a second needle simultaneously records CSF pressure. One of the most consistent findings in NPH research is that patients have an increased resistance to outflow.

## 15. ICP monitoring

The recordings in NPH reveal wave-form abnormalities similar to those originally described for brain tumor or acute injury, (i.e., B waves and A waves). The presence of unstable ICP (predominantly B waves) in NPH is well known, and the correlation with NPH shunt responsiveness ranges from 50 to 90%. Recently, analysis of the amplitudes of the ICP pulse pressure has been pro-posed as a predictive test in NPH.

## 16. Practice guidelines

If the CSF pressure is high, the patient should be investigated for other causes of obstructive hydrocephalus. If there is improvement of the patient after a 40 to 50-mL (high-volume) lumbar tap that the patient will likely respond well to shunting. An external ventricular drainage may be used in patients who fail to respond to a high-volume tap. Currently, there is no substantial evidence to support predictiveness to MRI CSF flow studies [19, 20].

## 17. Treatment

Treatment includes conservative measures and surgery for patients with favorable risk benefit ratio. Temporizing measures include acetazolamide and high volume tap. As per practice guidelines, surgery is considered for patients with favorable risk benefit ratio. Age alone is not an exclusionary criterion unless there are other surgical risk factors. Surgical options for the management of INPH include ventriculoperitoneal shunt and endoscopic third ventriculostomy. Literature favors low pressure programmable ventriculo peritoneal shunt as both over and under drainage can be managed in non-invasive manner. Endoscopic third ventriculostomy is indicated in patients with relative aqueduct stenosis and when there is triventricular hydrocephalus. Gangemi et al. reported 72% improvement with 4% complications rate [24].

## 18. Follow up after shunt surgery

Patients who have had shunt surgery should have periodic follow-up visits. The follow-up of patients with a shunt is similar to the follow-up of patients with parkinsonism or other chronic neurologic disorders. The interval history should cover all three NPH symptoms of gait impairment, incontinence, and dementia. The neurologic examination should include cognitive screening (e.g., MMSE), gait evaluation, and a general neurologic examination. Imaging may be done to rule out over-drainage, such as subdural effusion or hematoma, particularly in the first 6–12 months after shunt surgery until it is determined that the patient's condition and the appearance of the scan are stable. In most instances, a CT scan without contrast suffices. The setting of adjustable shunts should be confirmed during the follow-up visit, provided the neurologist has the device appropriate for the patient's shunt. Depending on the degree of symptomatic recovery and presence or absence of low-pressure signs and symptoms, the shunt setting can be raised or lowered in increments [25]. If there is suspicion regarding patency of the shunt radionucleotide, shunt patency test can determine the flow of radionuclide in the peritoneal cavity or the venous system (for ventriculoatrial shunts) [25].

## 19. Conclusion

NPH common, treatable disorder can be reliably diagnosed with an organized approach by most neurosurgeons and neurologists. Evidence supports the use of shunt surgery to treat patients with NPH, and when patients are properly selected, the benefit-to-risk ratio is favorable. Neurologists have a role in the longitudinal care of patients with NPH who have undergone shunt surgery, particularly in considering the differential diagnosis of any symptoms that may worsen after shunt surgery. Regular follow up and high index of suspicion is paramount.

## Author details

Ravish Rajiv Keni[1], Harsh Deora[2] and Amit Agrawal[3]*

1 Department of Neurology, Narayana Medical College and Hospital, Nellore, Andhra Pradesh, India

2 Department of Neurosurgery, NIMHANS, Bangalore, India

3 Department of Neurosurgery, All India Institute of Medical Sciences, Bhopal, Madhya Pradesh, India

*Address all correspondence to: dramitagrawal@gmail.com

## References

[1] Conn HO. Normal pressure hydrocephalus: New complications and concepts. Practical Neurology. 2007;7(4):252-258

[2] Kiefer M, Unterberg A. The differential diagnosis and treatment of normal-pressure hydrocephalus. Deutsches Ärzteblatt International. 2012;**109**(1-2):15-25

[3] Adams RD, Fisher CM, Hakim S, Ojemann RG, Sweet WH. Symptomatic occult hydrocephalus with normal cerebrospinal-fluid pressure. The New England Journal of Medicine. 1965;**273**(3):117-126

[4] Hakim S, Adams RD. The special clinical problem of symptomatic hydrocephalus with normal cerebrospinal fluid pressure. Observations on cerebrospinal fluid hydrodynamics. Journal of the Neurological Sciences. 1965;**2**(4):307-327

[5] Beyerl B, Black PM. Posttraumatic hydrocephalus. Neurosurgery. 1984;**15**(2):257-261

[6] Hebb AO, Cusimano MD. Idiopathic normal pressure hydrocephalus: A systematic review of diagnosis and outcome. Neurosurgery. 2001;**49**(5):1166-1184

[7] Shprecher D, Schwalb J, Kurlan R. Normal pressure hydrocephalus: Diagnosis and treatment. Current Neurology and Neuroscience Reports. 2008;**8**(5):371-376

[8] Krauss JK, Halve B. Normal pressure hydrocephalus: Survey on contemporary diagnostic algorithms and therapeutic decision-making in clinical practice. Acta Neurochirurgica. 2004;**146**(4):379-388

[9] Vanneste J, Augustijn P, Dirven C, Tan WF, Goedhart ZD. Shunting normal-pressure hydrocephalus: Do the benefits outweigh the risks? A multicenter study and literature review. Neurology. 1992;**42**(1):54-59

[10] Trenkwalder C, Schwarz J, Gebhard J, Ruland D, Trenkwalder P, Hense HW, et al. Starnberg trial on epidemiology of Parkinsonism and hypertension in the elderly. Prevalence of Parkinson's disease and related disorders assessed by a door-to-door survey of inhabitants older than 65 years. Archives of Neurology. 1995;**52**(10):1017-1022

[11] Beck JC, Benson DF, Scheibel AB, Spar JE, Rubenstein LZ. Dementia in the elderly: The silent epidemic. Annals of Internal Medicine. 1982;**97**(2):231-241

[12] Clarfield AM. The reversible dementias: Do they reverse? Annals of Internal Medicine. 1988;**109**(6):476-486

[13] Tarkowski E, Tullberg M, Fredman P, Wikkelso C. Normal pressure hydrocephalus triggers intrathecal production of TNF-alpha. Neurobiology of Aging. 2003;**24**(5):707-714

[14] Bateman GA. Vascular compliance in normal pressure hydrocephalus. AJNR. American Journal of Neuroradiology. 2000;**21**(9):1574-1585

[15] Nassar BR, Lippa CF. Idiopathic normal pressure hydrocephalus: A review for general practitioners. Gerontology and Geriatric Medicine. 2016;**2**:2333721416643702

[16] Pyykko OT, Lumela M, Rummukainen J, Nerg O, Seppala TT, Herukka SK, et al. Cerebrospinal fluid biomarker and brain biopsy findings in idiopathic normal pressure hydrocephalus. PLoS One. 2014;**9**(3):e91974

[17] Silverberg GD, Mayo M, Saul T, Rubenstein E, McGuire D. Alzheimer's disease, normal-pressure hydrocephalus,

and senescent changes in CSF circulatory physiology: A hypothesis. The Lancet Neurology. 2003;**2**(8):506-511

[18] Freimann FB, Streitberger K-J, Klatt D, Lin K, McLaughlin J, Braun J, et al. Alteration of brain viscoelasticity after shunt treatment in normal pressure hydrocephalus. Neuroradiology. 2012;**54**(3):189-196

[19] Relkin N, Marmarou A, Klinge P, Bergsneider M, Black PM. Diagnosing idiopathic normal-pressure hydrocephalus. Neurosurgery. 2005;**57**(3 Suppl):S4-S16

[20] Marmarou A, Bergsneider M, Klinge P, Relkin N, Black PM. The value of supplemental prognostic tests for the preoperative assessment of idiopathic normal-pressure hydrocephalus. Neurosurgery. 2005;**57**(3 Suppl):S17-S28

[21] Silverberg GD. Normal pressure hydrocephalus (NPH): Ischaemia, CSF stagnation or both. Brain. 2004;**127** (Pt 5):947-948

[22] Ishikawa M, Hashimoto M, Kuwana N, Mori E, Miyake H, Wachi A, et al. Guidelines for management of idiopathic normal pressure hydrocephalus. Neurologia Medico-Chirurgica. 2008;**48**:S1-S23

[23] Boon AJ, Tans JT, Delwel EJ, Egeler-Peerdeman SM, Hanlo PW, Wurzer HA, et al. Dutch Normal-Pressure Hydrocephalus Study: randomized comparison of low- and medium-pressure shunts. Journal of Neurosurgery. 1998;**88**(3):490-495

[24] Gangemi M, Maiuri F, Buonamassa S, Colella G, de Divitiis E. Endoscopic third ventriculostomy in idiopathic normal pressure hydrocephalus. Neurosurgery. 2004;**55**(1):129-134

[25] Williams MA, Malm J. Diagnosis and treatment of idiopathic normal pressure hydrocephalus. Continuum. 2016;**22**(2 Dementia):579-599

Chapter 6

# Neuronavigated and Laparoscopic-Assisted Ventriculoperitoneal Shunt Placement

*Sarah Wilson, Michael Crozier and Antonios El Helou*


## Abstract

Hydrocephalus is an abnormal accumulation of excess cerebrospinal fluid (CSF) in the brain causing increased intracranial pressure, which can arise from a variety of causes, including congenital, acquired, or idiopathic pathologies. Ventriculoperitoneal (VP) shunting is most commonly used to treat hydrocephalic patients, relieving the increased intracranial pressure by draining excess CSF from the ventricles to the peritoneal cavity. VP shunts are primarily completed using either an open or a more minimally invasive neuronavigated laparoscopic-assisted surgical technique. There is a high level of surgical complications, shunt failures and revision rates following VP shunting. It is suggested that different surgical techniques are associated with varying degrees of patient outcomes, surgical complications, and revision rates, with the less invasive laparoscopic-assisted approach producing improved results. We present our results on 14 consecutive hydrocephalic patients, analyzed retrospectively between 2017 and 2019, investigating the benefits offered by the neuronavigated laparoscopic-assisted insertion of VP shunts. Additionally, we explain our workflow and procedural technique. By investigating these differences, changes can be implemented in current routine procedures to ameliorate patient safety, surgical complications, and revision rates.


**Keywords:** hydrocephalus, ventriculoperitoneal shunt, laparoscopy, neuronavigation, complications, shunt failure, revision rates

## 1. Introduction

Hydrocephalus is a pathological accumulation of cerebrospinal fluid (CSF) in the ventricular system due to abnormal production, flow, or absorption of CSF [1]. The buildup of CSF increases the intracranial pressure (ICP), producing a variety of neurological defects concurrent with ventriculomegaly [2]. Arising from multiple congenital, acquired and idiopathic pathologies, hydrocephalus can ultimately lead to brain damage in the compressed tissues if left untreated [3, 4].

Hydrocephalus is primarily treated using a shunt system, draining the excess CSF from the cerebral ventricles into another region of the body where it can be absorbed. The peritoneal cavity remains the preferred drainage site in both pediatric and adult populations, accessed using a ventriculoperitoneal (VP) shunt [5].

Other surgical treatment options include third ventriculostomies and alternative shunt types [6] such as ventriculoatrial (VA), ventriculopleural, ventriculocisternal, and lumboperitoneal [7].

## 2. Ventriculoperitoneal shunt

VP shunts are comprised of a proximal inflow catheter, reservoir, valve mechanism, and a distal outflow catheter. The proximal catheter generally lies in the trigone of the lateral ventricle; however it can be inserted in the frontal horn if it follows an internalization of an external ventricular drain. The proximal catheter leads into the reservoir, which contains a small collection of CSF used for samples or to obtain pressure measurements. A retro-auricular unidirectional valve follows the reservoir and is responsible for controlling the flow of CSF into the distal catheter. The distal catheter then travels subcutaneously from the valve into the right upper abdominal quadrant where the excess CSF can freely drain into the peritoneal cavity [4, 8].

Although a commonly relied upon procedure to treat hydrocephalus, VP shunts are not without complications and failures. VP shunts are subject to a variety of complications of mechanical, functional, and infectious nature [6]. Mechanical complications consist of complications inhibiting the shunt from functioning, including shunt migration, obstruction, malpositioning, disconnection, and fracture. Contrarily, functional complications involve improperly functioning shunts such as overdrainage or underdrainage [6]. Finally, shunts are subject to various infections, the majority arising from normal skin flora and occurring within 30 days of surgery [3]. Current studies suggest an overall infection rate of 8.4% and a shunt failure rate, defined as a catheter-related problem necessitating surgical intervention [9], of 51.4% [10]. It has been shown that patients require 2–3 surgical revisions on average due to shunt failures in the 20 years after the original shunt placement [8], with the majority of shunt revisions occurring in the first 6–12 months [4, 8]. Specifically, 25–30% of all shunt revisions result from distal peritoneal catheter failure [5, 11, 12], such as preperitoneal placement, obstruction due to adhesions or pseudocysts, and malabsorption with secondary ascites [12].

## 3. Ventriculoperitoneal shunt: challenges

With time, the frequent revision rates and complications have provoked multiple changes and advancements in both VP shunt equipment, including the catheters and valve mechanisms [9, 13], as well as the surgical procedure itself [9]. Traditionally, VP shunts have been inserted using mini-laparotomy, although recently, a neuronavigated laparoscopically assisted approach has become a more commonly accepted surgical technique [9, 14]. Multiple studies have demonstrated that relative to the mini-laparotomy technique, a laparoscopically assisted approach has a shorter operative time and length of stay in the hospital, a decreased distal shunt failure rate [4, 9, 14], and a decreased risk of visceral injury [10]. Laparoscopy has also been shown to offer favorable outcomes with smaller incisions leading to reduced post-operative pain [11], faster mobilization and a preferred cosmetic appearance [5]. Many of the proposed benefits associated with laparoscopic-assisted VP shunts are a direct result of the increased visualization offered by laparoscopy. Laparoscopy allows for the verification of accurate peritoneal placement of the distal catheter as well as the proper functioning of the shunt by observing CSF outflow [5]. Laparoscopy can also be used to perform adhesiolysis, useful in the presence of excess adhesions, often found in patients who have undergone previous abdominal surgeries [11]. As shunt obstruction can commonly result from the distal catheter becoming lodged in a collection of adhesions, adhesiolysis offers a potential solution to prevent this from occurring, reducing complications and future shunts failures. Additionally, the mini-laparotomy approach has been associated with increased risks of post-operative hernia formation and adhesion formation [4]. Neuronavigation has also been shown to increase the accuracy of ventricular placement of the proximal catheter resulting in a decrease in proximal shunt revisions [15, 16]. However, as most neurosurgeons do not possess the necessary laparoscopy skill, collaboration with a general surgeon is required for the laparoscopic-assisted approach [4]. Incorporating a second surgeon may elicit difficulties in scheduling, requiring that both surgeons be available at given times [17].

Due to the high revision rates for VP shunts as well as the personal and medical burden of the complications and associated revisions, current practices must be assessed for alterations to improve these outcomes. Neuronavigated laparoscopic-assisted VP shunt placement is being regarded as a minimally invasive alternative to an open technique to improve surgical complications and patient outcomes.

## 4. Surgical technique

The procedure is done under general anesthesia, in the supine position with the head turned 30–45° toward the left, as right trigone is favored for the insertion of the ventricular catheter. The left upper limb is in abduction with the shoulder at 90°, and the right upper limb is tucked against the body. First generation cephalosporin is administered 30–60 minutes before incision. The neuronavigation magnetic system (Axiem, on Stealth by Medtronic) is used with 3D reconstruction of preoperative brain CT scan. Entry point, trajectory and length of insertion are defined on the navigation system. A Foley catheter is not used, as the risk of bladder injury is lowered by laparoscopic approach, which in turn reduces the post-operative UTI risk. A retro-auricular shaving for horizontal 2 cm incision or question mark incision is done. Scrubbing with chlorhexedine 2% is done at the cranial level and over the neck, chest and abdomen. Draping from the scalp to the pubic level is done in sterile fashion.

### 4.1 Tunneling of the peritoneal catheter

Starting at the scalp, an incision is made, dissection of the galea until reaching the entry point. Dissection of the subcutaneous cranio-cervical tissue is done.

A 60–90 cm passer is used from the scalp to the right upper quadrant (RUQ). The peritoneal catheter is tunneled through the passer and 5 mm incision is done at the RUQ. An anti-siphon programmable or pre-fixed pressure valve is connected to the peritoneal catheter.

### 4.2 Placement of ventricular catheter

The ventricular catheter is inserted using the navigation stylet until reaching the body of the right lateral ventricle. CSF is drained and a sample for culture is routinely sent. Ventricular catheter is connected to the valve and CSF flow through the valve to the peritoneal catheter is observed before peritoneal insertion of the catheter.

### 4.3 Placement of abdominal catheter

Laparoscopic approach to the peritoneum is done by the general surgeon. A supra-umbilical, longitudinal incision is incised through skin with the scalpel blade.

The incision may be altered due to previous surgery and concern for adhesions. Generally, we will go through old incisions using the supra-umbilical technique, but an infra-umbilical or epigastric open technique can be used as well. The fascia is elevated between two Kocher instruments and divided with scalpel blade. The peritoneum is divided between two snap instruments with scalpel blade. A finger is inserted into the abdomen to ensure adhesions are clear of the undersurface of the abdominal wall. Previous surgery and/or adhesions are not a contra-indication to this technique. Adhesions may be taken down carefully from the undersurface of the abdominal wall to allow placement of the laparoscopic balloon port. A 5–10 mm laparoscopic balloon port is placed intra-abdominally and the abdomen insufflated.

We maintain medium flow (20–30 L/min) and pressures (15 mmHg) for all cases. A 5 mm, 30-degree camera is inserted into the abdomen and used to visualize the undersurface of the abdominal wall. Placement of the catheter was generally in the RUQ but was also placed in left upper quadrant (LUQ) depending on adhesions from previous surgeries or due to the presence of previously placed shunts. At times we did navigate through heavy adhesions to guide the catheter placement but did not ever need to take down adhesions laparoscopically or add additional trocars for the catheter placement.

After the laparoscopic approach to the peritoneum is done, we approach the abdomen by a puncture using an introducer sheath and dilator (Arrow®). The catheter and CSF flow is observed in the peritoneal cavity. Once the shunt is placed the sheath is removed and skin closed with 4-0 subcuticular monocryl stitch.

After final satisfactory inspection of the abdomen is desufflated and the camera and laparoscopic balloon port removed. Fascia is closed with a purse-string 0-PDS suture. Skin is closed with a 4-0 subcuticular monocryl stitch. Incisions are infiltrated with 0.5% Marcaine with epinephrine. Steristrips and dry dressings are applied.

Following the completion of the laparoscopic portion of the procedure, the scalp closure is done in 2 layers and the entry point to the abdomen is closed in 1 layer.

Patient is awakened extubated and transferred to recovery room. Once fully awake, patient is transferred to the floor; diet is started at 6 hours post operatively in addition to increasing activity.

## 5. Methods

Fourteen consecutive hydrocephalic patients were treated with neuronavigated laparoscopically assisted VP shunts to explore the benefits offered by this surgical technique. Patient charts were collected retrospectively from February 2017 to March 2019. Collected charts were analyzed to obtain sex, age, BMI, indication for surgery, and whether the patient had a prior shunt placement or previous abdominal surgeries. Additionally, to assess the advantages of the neuronavigated laparoscopically assisted technique the variables collected were length of stay in hospital after surgery, operative time, intra- and post-operative complications, infection, and whether the shunt failed. No patients were excluded from this study. All surgeries were performed at the same institution by the same neurosurgeon and general surgeon. Clinical and radiological follow-up is done at 6-weeks post-operatively. The shunt series is used to evaluate the position of the shunt system and a brain CT is done to rule out over drainage (**Figure 1**).

The shunt series X-rays includes skull with an antero-posterior and lateral view, an antero-posterior chest x-ray and an antero-posterior abdominal x-ray.

The abdominal x-ray is repeated at 60 minutes to evaluate the peritoneal part of the shunt and its mobility (**Figure 2**).

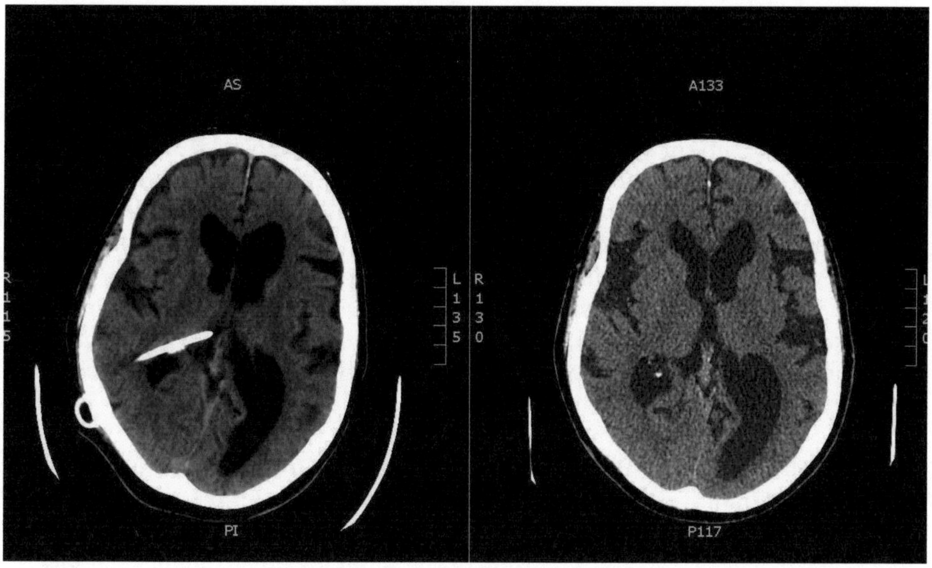


**Figure 1.**
*Pre (left) and post (right) operative brain Ct scan with ventricular catheter in the body of the right lateral ventricule.*

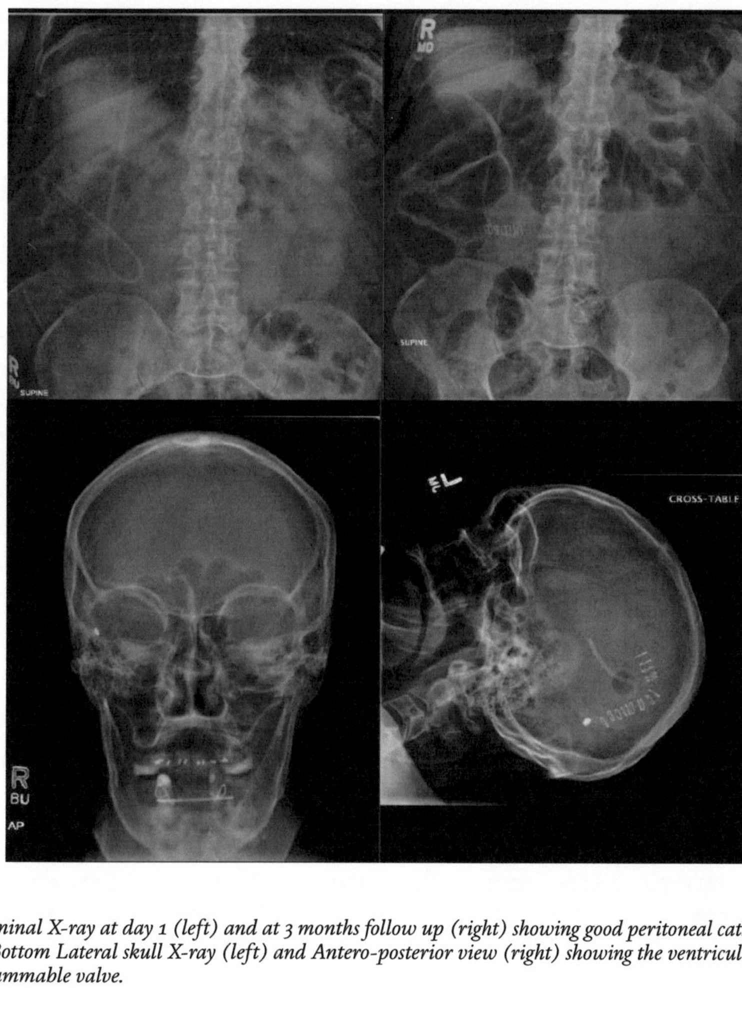


**Figure 2.**
*Top Abdominal X-ray at day 1 (left) and at 3 months follow up (right) showing good peritoneal catheter mobility. Bottom Lateral skull X-ray (left) and Antero-posterior view (right) showing the ventricular catheter and programmable valve.*

## 6. Results

There were 14 patients in total who received a ventriculoperitoneal shunt placement using a neuronavigated laparoscopic-assisted approach. The mean age of patients at the time of surgery was 56.8 years, although ranged from 31 to 78. There were 11 females and three males in the group. Eleven patients received a new VP shunt placement, whereas three patients were undergoing shunt revision. All patients except for one had undergone at least one previous abdominal surgery, with many of the patients having experienced multiple abdominal surgeries. Of note is the average BMI of the group being 31.2. Only one patient was within the normal range with a BMI of 24.6, one patient was classified as underweight at 14.6, four patients were considered overweight, and the remaining eight patients were obese with a BMI above 30.

Patients required a VP shunt for a variety of indications, with idiopathic normal pressure hydrocephalus (NPH) being the most common, occurring in half of the patients. Other indications included obstructive hydrocephalus secondary to a ventricular tumor, NPH secondary to subarachnoid hemorrhage (SAH), idiopathic intracranial hypertension, and a revision of the shunt for subependymal hemorrhage at birth. Average operative time for the VP shunt placements was approximately 45 minutes but ranged from 35 to 90 minutes. Patients on average stayed in the hospital for 2.25 days after the surgery, however, over 40% of patients were discharged after a single day in the hospital, 2/3 had left by 2 days, and all but one patient had left the hospital at 3 days. Two patients were not discharged from the hospital due to other medical conditions unrelated to the VP shunt placement and were therefore excluded from this calculation. There were no intraoperative complications that occurred, however it is worth noting that there were many patients with extensive abdominal adhesions due to previous abdominal surgeries, as well as the extra difficulty presented by the increased rate of obesity in the patient group.

Three patients experienced post-operative complications. One patient's shunt became infected with *Staph epidermis*, another patient experienced a functional complication of overdrainage with symptomatic bilateral subdural hematomas, requiring the removal of the shunt and drainage of the subdural hematomas. The remaining patient experienced mechanical dysfunction of the shunt. Each patient with a post-operative complication led to a shunt failure necessitating a shunt revision. The latter patient first underwent a proximal revision to replace both the ventricular catheter and the valve, due to valve malfunction. This same patient eventually experienced peritoneal complications requiring two distal shunt revisions on separate occasions. Following the second peritoneal complication, the patient decided to obtain a VA shunt insertion, which continues to offer successful treatment.

## 7. Discussion

VP shunts are one of the most common neurosurgical procedures performed [3]. Despite its widespread use and successes in the treatment of hydrocephalus, there are often complications and failures. This has encouraged the ongoing development of alternative procedural techniques producing better outcomes [5]. The cost associated with VP shunts produces a significant medical burden, which is only furthered by the numerous complications and shunts revisions following the initial surgery. Shunt revisions account for approximately 50% of all shunt-related costs and admissions [5, 12]. By decreasing the amount of shunt revisions and complications, both the medical and personal burden of VP shunts will greatly improve. The neuronavigated laparoscopic-assisted VP shunt placement performed in this study offers a safe and effective technique, bringing numerous benefits not seen with the traditional mini-laparotomy method.

The length of stay in the hospital followed a similar trend to other studies with most patients being discharged in the first 24 hours [18]. The more minimally invasive technique decreases the length of stay in the hospital as well as prompts a faster recovery rate [9, 14]. This allows for less resource use by individual patients and increased patient satisfaction by leaving the hospital soon after surgery and returning to regular activities faster than with the mini-laparotomy technique [9, 11, 14].

Of the most noteworthy benefits of a laparoscopic-assisted neuronavigated technique is the decreased proximal and distal revision rates. The decreased revision rates are largely due to the avoidance of catheter malposition during placement. The accuracy of ventricular [16, 17] and peritoneal [4, 14, 17] catheter placement has increased as a result of clear visualization of the placement in the proper anatomical locations. Once properly positioned, the laparoscopic approach helps prevent migration of the distal catheter because of the fewer abdominal incisions and the smaller peritoneal wall defect [10]. The decreased revision rates can be seen in our patient population, as only a single patient required a distal revision for shunt malposition as a result of peritoneal adhesions, as well as a ventricular repositioning due to a valve dysfunction. Additionally, the increased visualization offered by this technique can be used to confirm CSF outflow through the VP shunt, indicating a properly functioning shunt, before finishing surgery.

This technique should also be heavily considered for obese individuals as well as those who have undergone previous abdominal surgeries [12], the two patient populations demonstrating the highest number of distal complications with VP shunt placements [5]. Both obesity and peritoneal adhesions resulting from abdominal surgeries pose difficulties with visualization during surgery, which leads to improper placement of shunts and increased complications and shunt failures. Further advantages come with adhesiolysis that can be performed during laparoscopy, creating a clearer visualization for those with previous abdominal surgeries as well as preventing obstruction of the distal catheter by placing it within the peritoneal adhesions [4, 9].

There have been concerns over the laparoscopic-assisted approach to VP shunts in that they require two surgical teams and specific instrumentation, increasing the cost of the surgery [5, 9] as well as the difficulty of scheduling, especially for emergent cases [17]. However, with the countless benefits being demonstrated by laparoscopy and neuronavigation, it should be considered that the mentioned concerns are outweighed.

Our study has limitations, specifically in the small sample size and the surgeries all being performed by the same surgeons. It is possible that results could differ based on the level of expertise of a surgeon. General surgeons performing laparoscopy often will have more experience with adhesions and distorted anatomy as well as neurosurgeons using neuronavigation more often will gain more expertise. It has been suggested that neurosurgeons should be trained on laparoscopy in the future to both avoid the influence of the general surgeon's expertise and to prevent potential scheduling conflicts when organizing two surgical teams [9].

Advancements are continuing to be made in VP shunts technology and procedures. All advancements are aimed at continuing the improvement of patient outcomes and lifting the imposed medical and personal burden of VP shunts. Recently, there have been some new advancements in techniques including a percutaneous minimal access insertion without the use of laparoscopy, as well as a single-port laparoscopic surgery that show further promise in optimizing patient care and routine practices [19, 20].

## 8. Conclusion

Surgical management of hydrocephalus using neuronavigated laparoscopic-assisted VP shunt placements is becoming a widely accepted alternative to the traditional mini-laparotomy approach. This technique offers a safe, effective, and minimally invasive approach for VP placements in hydrocephalic patients. It provides accurate insertion of both the ventricular and peritoneal catheter, resulting in decreased complications of mechanical, functional, and infectious origin, as well as revision rates. As much of VP shunt-related costs result from shunt revisions, any technical advancements made to reduce revision rates will help alleviate the medical and financial burden associated with this common neurosurgical procedure. This technique should also be considered in more difficult patient cases involving obesity and extensive peritoneal adhesions from previous abdominal surgeries. The benefits offered by the neuronavigated laparoscopic-assisted approach are numerous and seem to outweigh any concerns surrounding this technique. This particular surgical approach should be considered in adjusting current routine practices, resulting in optimal care for hydrocephalic patients and decreasing VP shunt-related medical costs.

## Acknowledgements

We would like to acknowledge the Dalhousie Medical Research Foundation (DMRF) Lalia B. Chase Studentship that allowed for the medical student to participate in this research.

## Conflict of interest

All authors have no conflict of interest.

## Author details

Sarah Wilson[1], Michael Crozier[2] and Antonios El Helou[3]*

1 Dalhousie Medical School, New Brunswick, Canada

2 Department of General Surgery, The Moncton Hospital, Horizon Health Network, Moncton, New Brunswick, Canada

3 Department of Neurosurgery, The Moncton Hospital, Horizon Health Network, Moncton, New Brunswick, Canada

*Address all correspondence to: dr.antonios.elhelou@horizonnb.ca

## References

[1] Rekate HL. A contemporary definition and classification of hydrocephalus. Seminars in Pediatric Neurology. 2009;**16**(1):9-15

[2] Shaw R, Everingham E, Mahant N, Jacobson E, Owler B. Clinical outcomes in the surgical treatment of idiopathic normal pressure hydrocephalus. Journal of Clinical Neuroscience. 2016;**29**:81-86

[3] Gutierrez-Murgas Y, Snowden JN. Ventricular shunt infections: Immunopathogenesis and clinical management. Journal of Neuroimmunology. 2014;**276**(1-2):1-8

[4] Phan S, Liao J, Jia F, Maharaj M, Reddy R, Mobbs RJ, et al. Laparotomy vs minimally invasive laparoscopic ventriculoperitoneal shunt placement for hydrocephalus: A systematic review and meta-analysis. Clinical Neurology and Neurosurgery. 2016;**140**:26-32

[5] Dehcordi SR, De Tommasi C, Ricci A, Marzi S, Ruscitti C, Amicucci G, et al. Laparoscopy-assistedventriculoperitoneal shunt surgery: Personal experience and review of the literature. Neurosurgical Review. 2011;**34**(3):363-371

[6] Nguyen TA, Cohen PR. Scalp necrosis overlying a ventriculoperitoneal shunt: a case report and literature review. Dermatology Online Journal. 2015;**21**(10). Retrieved from: https://escholarship.org/uc/item/2rs544f9

[7] Hung CC, Chuang HY, Lin HL, Chu YT, Cheng CH. Intramuscular migration of venous catheter as a rare complication of Ventriculoatrial shunt: Case report and literature review. Journal of Neurological Surgery Part A: Central European Neurosurgery. 2017;**78**(04):412-416

[8] Bates P, Rajderkar D. Common and uncommon causes of ventriculoperitoneal shunt malfunction diagnosed on plain radiographs. Current Problems in Diagnostic Radiology. 2018;**47**(5):317-323

[9] He M, Ouyang L, Wang S, Zheng M, Liu A. Laparoscopy versus mini-laparotomy peritoneal catheter insertion of ventriculoperitoneal shunts: A systematic review and meta-analysis. Neurosurgical Focus. 2016;**41**(3):E7

[10] Rigante L, Navarro R, Roser F. Minimal exposure maximal precision ventriculoperitoneal shunt: How I do it. Acta Neurochirurgica. 2019;**161**(8):1619-1622

[11] Hanna RS, Essa AA, Makhlouf GA, Helmy AA. Comparative study between laparoscopic and open techniques for insertion of Ventriculperitoneal shunt for treatment of congenital hydrocephalus. Journal of Laparoendoscopic & Advanced Surgical Techniques. 2019;**29**(1):109-113

[12] Roth J, Sagie B, Szold A, Elran H. Laparoscopic versus non–laparoscopic-assisted ventriculoperitoneal shunt placement in adults. A retrospective analysis. Surgical Neurology. 2007;**68**(2):177-184

[13] Ros B, Iglesias S, Martín Á, Carrasco A, Ibáñez G, Arráez MA. Shunt overdrainage syndrome: Review of the literature. Neurosurgical Review. 2018;**41**(4):969-981

[14] Naftel RP, Argo JL, Shannon CN, Taylor TH, Tubbs RS, Clements RH, et al. Laparoscopic versus open insertion of the peritoneal catheter in ventriculoperitoneal shunt placement: Review of 810 consecutive cases. Journal of Neurosurgery. 2011;**115**(1):151-158

[15] Gilard V, Magne N, Gerardin E, Curey S, Pelletier V, Hannequin P, et al. Comparison of electromagnetic neuronavigation system and free-hand

method for ventricular catheter placement in internal shunt. Clinical Neurology and Neurosurgery. 2017;**158**:93-97

[16] Wilson TJ, McCoy KE, Al-Holou WN, Molina SL, Smyth MD, Sullivan SE. Comparison of the accuracy and proximal shunt failure rate of freehand placement versus intraoperative guidance in parietooccipital ventricular catheter placement. Neurosurgical Focus. 2016;**41**(3):E10

[17] Fahy AS, Tung S, Lamberti-Pasculli M, Drake J, Kulkarni A, Gerstle JT. Laparoscopic revision of Ventriculoperitoneal shunts in pediatric patients may result in fewer subsequent peritoneal revisions. Journal of Laparoendoscopic & Advanced Surgical Techniques. 2019;**29**(1):82-87

[18] Turner RD, Rosenblatt SM, Chand B, Luciano MG. Laparoscopic peritoneal catheter placement: Results of a new method in 111 patients. Operative Neurosurgery. 2007;**61**(3):161-167

[19] Hong WC, Lai PS, Chien YH, Tu YK, Tsai JC. Single-incision laparoscopic surgery (SILS) for ventriculoperitoneal shunt placement. Journal of Neurological Surgery Part A: Central European Neurosurgery. 2013;**74**(06):351-356

[20] Ochalski PG, Horowitz MB, Mintz AH, Hughes SJ, Okonkwo DO, Kassam AB, et al. Minimal-access technique for distal catheter insertion during ventricular peritoneal shunt procedures: A review of 100 cases. Journal of Neurosurgery. 2009;**111**(3):623-627

Section 4

# Diagnosis

Chapter 7

# Diagnosis of Symptomatic Intracranial Atherosclerotic Disease

*Dragoș Cătălin Jianu, Silviana Nina Jianu, Georgiana Munteanu, Traian Flavius Dan and Claudia Birsan*

## Abstract

Intracranial atherosclerotic stroke differs from extracranial atherosclerotic stroke in many aspects, including risk factors and stroke patterns. It occurs in association with in situ thrombotic occlusion, artery-to-artery embolism, branch occlusion, and hemodynamic insufficiency. Intracranial atherosclerotic stenosis (ICAS) could have only been diagnosed by transcranial Doppler (TCD) and transcranial color-coded sonography (TCCS), which are burdened by a risk of bias, or catheter angiography (DSA), which, on the contrary, is very precise, but rarely it is done in clinical practice due to its invasiveness. Computed tomography angiography (CT-A) and magnetic resonance imaging angiography (MR-A) have increased the identification of ICAS in a wider stroke population.

**Keywords:** intracranial atherosclerotic stenosis (ICAS), transcranial Doppler (TCD), transcranial color-coded sonography (TCCS), catheter digital subtraction angiography (DSA), computed tomography angiography (CT-A), magnetic resonance imaging angiography (MR-A)

## 1. Epidemiology, natural history, and risk factors of intracranial atherosclerotic disease

### 1.1 The incidence of intracranial atherosclerotic disease (ICAD)

Intracranial atherosclerosis is one of the most important causes of stroke worldwide [1]. All major intracranial arteries are affected by atherosclerotic disease, and between 6 and 50% of all world ischemic strokes are the result of ICAD [2]. Intracranial arterial atherosclerotic stenosis (ICAS) represents the most advanced stage of ICAD, and thus nonstenotic ICAD is much more common than stenotic ICAD [3].

Regarding the incidence of ICAD, it varies especially by ethnicity. Population groups which are at high risk for ICAS include: Asians (30–50% of all new ischemic strokes) [4], Hispanics, and population of African descent; conversely, the risk is lower in Caucasians (8–10% of all new ischemic strokes) [5]. The reason for racial differences is still unclear. The main hypotheses include: low lipid levels and high blood pressure (susceptibility to intracranial and intracerebral vascular disease);

high lipids and high blood pressure (susceptibility to extracranial occlusive vascular lesions); and diabetes mellitus and metabolic syndrome (for ICAS) [2, 6, 7]. Other studies include inherited susceptibility of intracranial vessels to atherosclerosis [8], acquired differences in the prevalence of risk factors [5], differential responses to the same risk factors [9], and different genetic susceptibility [7]. It is also possible that misclassifying patients with adult-onset Moya-Moya disease (MMD) as having ICAD may partly explain the high prevalence of ICAD in Asians [10]. A genome-wide linkage analysis and an exome analysis identified the strongest susceptibility gene for MMD in East Asian people: ring finger 213 (RNF213) [10]. An important role in the emergence of these ethnic differences can be represented by the lifestyle: the pattern of ischemic stroke is changing in Asian patients; due to the westernized lifestyle, the number of extracranial cervical disease is rising [11].

### 1.2 Prognosis of asymptomatic intracranial atherosclerotic disease (ICAD)

Regarding the prevalence of asymptomatic ICAD in general population, information is still limited, in the absence of large clinical trials [12]. The atherosclerotic process develops silently over years, until its lesions suddenly become symptomatic. Accordingly, early diagnosis of ICAD may improve the therapeutic strategy, while the disease is still asymptomatic. However, the natural history of asymptomatic ICAD is not fully known, especially in Caucasians [3].

The natural history of asymptomatic versus symptomatic ICAD differs from that of extracranial carotid disease (ECAD). Patients with symptomatic ICAD have a low risk of stroke in the stenotic arterial territory, compared to patients with asymptomatic ECAD, while patients with symptomatic ICAD have a higher risk, especially those with clinically significant hemodynamic stenosis, early after stroke [13]. Therefore, recent studies suggest that the annual risk of stroke in asymptomatic patients with at least 50% stenosis of a major intracranial artery is less than 10% [14]. Furthermore, patients with severe intracranial stenosis (70–99%) have a higher risk of stroke than do patients with moderate intracranial stenosis (50–69%) [14].

Arenillas designed a population-based study [3], which comes to clarify the natural history and the prevalence of asymptomatic ICAD in Caucasians. Study subjects (1503) were randomly selected from a population of 600 000 inhabitants, from March 2007 until June 2010. The primary enrollment criteria were: age over 50 years, no past history of cerebrovascular or ischemic heart disease, and moderate-to-high vascular risk. Presence and severity of ICAS were determined through the medium of transcranial color-coded duplex (TCCS) and subsequent MR angiography (MRA) confirmation. Preliminary results showed a prevalence of asymptomatic ICAD of 9% in the first 157 studied subjects [3].

Several transcranial Doppler (TCD) studies in an asymptomatic Asian population have also been conducted. They have come to the conclusion that the prevalence of asymptomatic ICAS ranged from 5.9 to 24.5% [15].

### 1.3 Risk factors for intracranial atherosclerotic disease (ICAD)

Oh Young Bang reported various conditions and risk factors for ICAD, from risk factors associated with asymptomatic ICAD to risk factors for stroke recurrence [16]. ICAD risk could not be fully related to conventional risk factors for stroke; therefore, specialists are still investigating specific risk factors for ICAD [3].

## 2. The mechanisms of ischemia in intracranial atherosclerotic disease (ICAD)

According to Arenillas [3], our traditional understanding of ICAD is based on the detection of hemodynamically relevant intracranial arterial stenosis (ICAS).

The main limitations of this classical approach are as follows:

1. It may be restricted to the most advanced stage of ICAD alone [3].

2. It is unable to differentiate atherosclerosis from stenosis caused by other entities. The etiological differential diagnosis of the arterial stenosis includes atherosclerotic disease, embolus with partial recanalization, arterial dissection, vasculitis, and vasospasm. Thus, it is important to note that while anatomic diagnosis of arterial narrowing can be made with appropriate accuracy using conventional imaging techniques, identifying the cause of stenosis involves iterative or multimodal imaging [3].

3. It may not be able to provide information about the histopathologic composition and activity of the intracranial atherosclerotic plaque. The importance of this last point is based on the fact that symptomatic intracranial atherosclerotic plaques are characterized not only by a higher degree of luminal stenosis but also by a richer content in lipid, intraplaque hemorrhage, and inflammatory cell infiltration, all of which are well-known determinants of plaque instability in the extracranial vasculature [3, 17].

Stroke associated with ICAD occurs in association with four mechanisms:

a. In situ thrombotic occlusion (with impaired anterograde flow). Plaque rupture reveals its thrombogenic core to clotting factors resulting a thrombus that can locally occlude the artery or even embolize distally. The term of "vulnerable plaques" refers to those ones with a large lipid core, the presence of intraplaque hemorrhage, or a thin or ruptured fibrous cap; this kind of plaques are liable to suffer anytime a rupture. Patients with unstable intracranial plaques may show large territorial lesions via sudden thrombotic occlusion [16].

b. Artery-to-artery embolism. This mechanism commonly causes multiple cortico-subcortical infarcts [16].

c. Hemodynamic insufficiency/failure (with impaired collateral flow and cerebrovascular reserve). Severe narrowing or occlusion of the lumen may lead to hypoperfusion of the distal brain territory, especially in patients with inadequate collateral flow. The hypoperfusion through a stenotic intracranial artery causes watershed or border-zone strokes [16].

d. Branch occlusion disease (BOD) is one of the main stroke mechanisms of ICAD. This mechanism, specific to ICAD, consists in growing of the plaque over the ostia of penetrating arteries. It is defined by a milder degree of stenosis and comma-shaped infarcts extending to the basal surface of the parent artery. BOD has been related to cryptogenic strokes [16, 18].

Thus, even mild stenosis of intracranial atherosclerotic arteries (<50%) may be clinically relevant, and high-resolution magnetic resonance imaging (HR-MRI) studies are needed to identify and determine the degree and location of stenosis in this patient group [19]. Oh Young Bang and others asserted that these mechanisms can coexist and interact in the same patient [16, 18, 20, 21].

### 2.1 Clinical recurrence rate

As we mentioned before, the annual recurrence rates for any ischemic stroke reported in the WASID trial were as high as 15 and 14% in the aspirin and warfarin arms, respectively [16].

It has been shown that symptomatic ICAD is particularly burdened with a high clinical recurrence rate [3]. Moreover, Famakin and coworkers reported that most subsequent strokes in patients with symptomatic ICAS occurred in the same arterial territory were nonlacunar, and nearly half of them were disabling [19]. Their results were similar to the findings in NASCET, which showed that 95% of strokes were ipsilateral in patients with 70–99% carotid stenosis, and 71% of strokes were ipsilateral in patients with 50–69% carotid stenosis [22].

It is also important to mention that Famakin and coworkers observed that patients with ICAS have a propensity for atherosclerotic stenosis at different sites within the intracranial circulation [19]. Supporting this idea, they reported that among the 27% of the strokes occurring outside the territory of the symptomatic intracranial artery, almost half (48%) could have been caused by previously asymptomatic or newly developed ICAS in a different vascular territory. However, in the same study, it was suggested that it is also possible that some of these strokes may have been caused by an embolus which partially recanalized leaving a residual stenosis [19]. Supporting this theory is data from another WASID analysis, which showed that asymptomatic ICAS that was present at study entry (coexistent with the symptomatic stenosis) was associated with a low rate of stroke (3.5% after 1 year of follow-up) [23].

Identifying whether ICAS is actually the cause of the present stroke (determining whether the stenosis is symptomatic or asymptomatic), it is however still a challenge, knowing that, according to Famakin, in up to 20% of the patients with stroke and IACS, there is another cause for its occurrence (extracranial large artery stenosis, cardiac embolism, and small artery occlusion can co-exist with ICAS) [19]. Nowadays, different noninvasive imaging techniques can provide physiological data on the mechanisms associated with ICAD-linked stroke and their forms of coexistence, including markers of anterograde and collateral flow, dynamic cerebrovascular reserve, static tissue perfusion, characteristics and morphological details of plaques with embolic potential, etc. [16, 18, 24].

All these data may improve stroke risk stratification, adding to clinical and anatomic (i.e., percent stenosis) predictors of stroke risk, developing mechanism-specific prevention and treatment strategies, and also serve in patients' selection for endovascular therapies [16, 18, 24].

## 3. Catheter-based digital substraction angiography (DSA)—diagnostic test for intracranial arterial stenosis (ICAS)

Catheter-based digital subtraction angiography (DSA) is the gold standard in the diagnosis of ICAS. ICAS is considered as symptomatic, if there are obvious radiological signs of acute ischemia in the supplying vascular area and if no other obvious cause (e.g., acute occlusion) is present.

Regarding the advantages of DSA, it allows [12]: the visualization of vessel contour—at a high resolution (microns); the localization of stenosis; and the estimation of degree and length of stenosis (DSA measures stenosis precisely); 3D reconstruction provides even greater detail, highlighting of collateral circulation (measure anterograde and collateral flow). Prabhakaran and coworkers suggested that DSA can identify the mechanisms of stroke in symptomatic ICAS by using surrogate imaging markers of stroke risk [12]: for the mechanism of *decreased antegrade flow*—the surrogate imaging marker of TICI (thrombolysis in cerebral infarction) flow grade; for the mechanism of *progression of stenosis*—the surrogate imaging marker of TICI (thrombolysis in cerebral infarction) flow grade; and for the mechanism of *poor collateral flow*—the surrogate imaging marker of collateral flow grade. However, being an invasive method that can generate periprocedural complications (periprocedural neurologic injury, access site injury, radiation risks, contrast risks, low availability, and great costs), DSA cannot be used in everyday routine clinical practice, in all patients [25].

### 3.1 DSA allows an excellent visualization of intracranial arterial contour, at a high resolution (microns)

Monitoring the natural history of stenosis due to ICAD may be a useful method in finding new possible treatments. Long-term angiographic progress of ICAS has not received much attention before WASID trial; Bauer et al. [26] reported the progression of atherosclerotic stenoses by location, including extracranial and intracranial sites. Overall, 35.3% of intracranial sites progressed. Craig et al. [27] noted that intracranial ICA stenoses progressed in 5 of 5 patients on follow-up angiography. Akins and coworkers retrospectively reviewed records over a 7-year period to identify patients with ICAS and serial angiograms. The most common location for an ICAS of 50% or greater was the intracranial portion of the ICA (49% of lesions), followed by the MCA (20%), PCA (11%), distal VA and BA (11%), and ACA (9%) [28].

Angiography is an excellent method for monitoring intracranial atherosclerosis, but this method defines the vessel lumen only; the disease process leading to luminal narrowing being inferred [28]. If the patient has widespread atherosclerosis, the stenosis is usually ascribed to this. The arterial narrowing is generally caused by local atherosclerosis, but associated thrombus may also contribute. Emboli also cause luminal narrowing. In this situation, the follow-up study may show the complete resolution of the stenosis due to spontaneous clot lysis. This pattern was encountered in 3 of the 45 sites studied by Akins. He noted that there are also other pathological conditions that can cause vessel narrowing, such as vasculitis, vasospasm, or malignancies. He concluded that ICAS is dynamic lesions [28].

### 3.2 DSA allows an excellent localization and evaluation of the degree and length of intracranial arterial stenosis (ICAS)

Angiographic measurement methods are routinely used nowadays in clinical practice to identify patients who may benefit from carotid endarterectomy [29]. Samuels affirmed that the established methods for measuring extracranial ICA stenosis are unsuitable for measuring the stenosis of a major intracranial artery because the intracranial arteries are often tortuous, have several branches, and are narrowing gradually in their distal portions [29].

If the prognosis of ICAS and the choice of therapy for these patients was clearly shown by WASID trial [2] to be based on the severity of ICAS, a repeatable method for measuring percent stenosis of the major intracranial arteries was required: standard WASID criteria for grading of ICAS [29].

All patients enrolled in the WASID trial have been subjected to DSA, to confirm a symptomatic ICAS (50–99%) of the ICA, MCA, VA, or BA. All major intracranial vessels were screened for stenosis stratified into three categories of lumen reduction (30–50, 50–70, and >70%). The percentage of stenosis of an intracranial artery was defined by Samuels [29].

$$\text{WASID method } [1 - (D_{stenosis}/D_{normal})] \times 100 = \% \text{ Stenosis.} \quad (1)$$

Rules applied for measuring a stenosis of the carotid siphon and basilar artery.

$D_{stenosis}$ is the residual diameter of the artery at the site of the most severe stenosis, and $D_{normal}$ is the diameter of the proximal normal artery.

- If the proximal segment is diseased, contingency sites are chosen to measure D normal: distal artery (second choice) or feeding artery (third choice).
- If tandem intracranial lesions are present (e.g., distal vertebral and mid-basilar), percent stenosis of both sites is measured and the more severe stenosis is selected.

When a "gap sign" is present (i.e., the lumen of the vessel cannot be visualized at the site of severe stenosis), D stenosis cannot be measured with calipers. In these cases, percent stenosis is defined as 99% luminal stenosis [29].

### 3.3 DSA is an excellent assessor of collateral intracranial arterial circulation

Cerebral collateral circulation is a supplementary vascular channels network that plays an important role in stabilizing the cerebral blood flow when the main arterial supplying systems fail (Liebeskind and coworkers) [30, 31]. Arterial insufficiency due to thromboembolism, hemodynamic compromise, or a combination of these factors may lead to the recruitment of collaterals [30, 31].

Impaired cerebral hemodynamics is a well-established predictor in large artery stroke [32]. Cerebral perfusion pressure distal to a high-grade stenosis or occlusion depends on collateral sources of blood flow. The anterior and posterior communicating arteries (ACoA, PCoA) provide most collateral flow in ICA and BA stenosis (primary collaterals), while distal pial and leptomeningeal anastomoses (secondary collaterals) are important in MCA stenosis [32]. DSA is the most valuable investigation that provides the assessment of collateral cerebral flow; Liebeskind and coworkers reporting that collateral flow on DSA was found to be absent in 69% of patients with symptomatic ICAS and it was also considered an independent predictor of recurrent ipsilateral stroke [30, 31].

Stroke risk, due to ICAD, increases with the arterial stenosis degree. Liebeskind and coworkers conducted a retrospective analysis of the baseline DSA acquired in the WASID trial, and they provided the first comprehensive evaluation of collaterals in modifying stroke risk in patients diagnosed with ICAD and its impact on subsequent stroke characteristics. They observed that the collateral circulation was adequately available for analysis in 287/569 patients from WASID (50%) subjects with proximal arterial stenoses ranging from 50 to 99% [30, 31].

According to Liebeskind, collateral brain circulation is one of the most significant factors that mediates the potentially devastating effects of cerebral ischemia. He asserted that patho-physiological recruitment of these collateral vessels (potential anastomotic connections) depends on the temporal course of numerous compensatory (hemodynamic, metabolic, and neural) mechanisms and on the caliber and patency of primary pathways that may rapidly compensate for decreased blood flow and the adequacy of secondary collateral routes [30, 31]. He asserted that collaterals maintain perfusion downstream from arterial occlusions in acute stroke, determining the hemodynamic characteristics of the ischemic penumbra, the evolution of infarct, and susceptibility for hemorrhagic transformation [30]. He suggested that focal neurologic symptoms manifest only when collaterals fail. Regarding the therapeutic point of view, robust collaterals are an effective predictor of arterial recanalization and good clinical outcomes in acute stroke [31]. It is also well known that arterial occlusion secondary to progressive atherosclerotic stenosis of an intracranial segment allows the development of robust collaterals over time, unlike the cardioembolic or abrupt thrombotic occlusion. Collaterals and functional demonstration of flow impairment may be more informative than isolated anatomic measures of maximal stenosis or length [30].

Liebeskind concluded that collateral circulation is a powerful determinant of stroke risk in ICAD, demonstrating a protective role with severe stenoses and perhaps distinguishing milder stenoses that are relatively unstable [30, 31].

## 4. Transcranian Doppler (TCD) and transcranian color—coded sonography (TCCS)—diagnostic tests for intracranial arterial stenosis (ICAS)

Intracranial circulation can be examined by transcranial Doppler ultrasonography (TCD) or transcranial color-coded duplex sonography (TCCS) through different bone windows (transtemporal, transforaminal, and transorbital). The signal can be enhanced by using ultrasound contrast agents [33–38]. TCD combines in real-time intracranial blood flow patterns and velocities modifications with arterial diameter in the stenotic vessels. The most important data are: depth, blood flow direction, different velocities (peak systolic-PSV, end diastolic-EDV, and mean blood flow velocity-MFV), pulsatility index-PI, and resistance index-RI. The physiological data assessed from TCD are complementary to the anatomical data analyzed from other neuroimaging techniques (DSA, CTA, and MRA) [33–38].

TCD has some advantages: inexpensive, noninvasive, portable test than can be performed bedside, serial examination, emboli detection, and vasomotor reactivity testing. TCD has high specificity, sensitivity, and negative predictive value (NPV) [33–38]. In the same time, TCD has some disadvantages: low reliability, technical limits (inadequate or absent windows, the tortuous course of the basilar artery, etc.), and operator-dependent results. TCD presents a modest positive predictive value (PPV) (36–75%). Therefore, it is useful to exclude significant ICAS with high certainty but requires confirmation by other imaging methods when stenosis is suggested [33–41]. The circle of Willis is complete in only 20% of cases; in other cases, one or several vascular segments may be hypoplastic or aplastic. Visualization of the intracranial vessels and assessment of cerebral hemodynamics are only possible with TCCS, but this technique still requires further certification in larger studies [33–41].

Prabhakaran and coworkers suggested that TCD can specify the mechanisms of stroke in symptomatic ICAS by using surrogate imaging markers of stroke risk: for the mechanism of decreased antegrade flow—the surrogate imaging marker of flow velocity; for the progression of stenosis—the flow velocity; for the poor collateral flow—the circle of Willis collaterals; for the artery-to-artery embolism—the microembolic signal; and for the impaired vasomotor reactivity—the cerebrovascular reactivity [33–41]. Serial monitoring of flow velocities by TCD can detect the evolution of ICAS and therapeutic effects [22, 41].

Transcranial ultrasound is used for multiple aims: TCD/TCCS can detect, localize, and grade the severity of ICAS; can detect and localize the intracranial arterial occlusion; can realize the real-time monitoring of recanalization in patients treated with systemic thrombolysis and of rescue reperfusion techniques (identification of reocclusion, hyper-perfusion syndrome, etc.); can detect clinically silent emboli: microembolic signals (MES), which recognizes patients at higher risk of embolic stroke; can recognize patients with extracranial internal carotid artery (ICA) stenosis at a higher stroke risk; can assess both collateral pathways and the vasomotor reactivity (VMR), which detects the risk stratification of hemodynamic stroke [22, 33, 37, 41]; and can identify intracranial arterial blood flow steals.

### 4.1 TCD/TCCS can detect, localize, and grade the severity of ICAS

In clinical practice, interpretation of TCD data should be individualized, with various parameters (velocities values, spectrum, waveform patterns, flow pulsatility, collateral flows, status of extracranial arteries, systemic conditions: anemia, etc.) (**Tables 1** and **2**) [35]. TCD presents higher precision for identification of ICAS in the MCA and BA than in other intracranial arteries, due to the tortuosity in the latter [33].

ICAS criteria are direct and indirect.

| Artery | Stenosis >50% (MFV, SPR) | Stenosis >70% (MFV, SPR) | Diffuse disease or near occlusion (MFV, SPR) |
|---|---|---|---|
| MCA | >100 cm/s, >2 | >120 cm/s, >3 | <30 cm/s, <1 |
| ACA | >80 cm/s, >2 | n.a., >3 | <30 cm/s, <1 |
| PCA | >80 cm/s, >2 | n.a., >3 | <30 cm/s, <1 |
| BA | >90 cm/s, >2 | >110 cm/s, >3 | <20 cm/s, <1 |
| VA | >90 cm/s, >2 | >110 cm/s, >3 | <20 cm/s, <1 |

*MCA, middle cerebral artery; ACA, anterior cerebral artery; PCA, posterior cerebral artery; BA, basilar artery; VA, vertebral artery; MFV, mean flow velocity; n.a., not available; and SPR, stenotic/prestenotic MFV ratio.*

**Table 1.**
*TCD criteria for intracranial stenosis (ICAS) [33].*

| Artery | Mild stenosis | Moderate stenosis | Severe stenosis |
|---|---|---|---|
| | Stenosis <50% (PSV) | Stenosis >50% (PSV) | Stenosis >80% |
| MCA | >155 cm/s | >220 cm/s | +Indirect signs |
| ACA | >120 cm/s | >155 cm/s | +Indirect signs |
| PCA | >100 cm/s | >145 cm/s | +Indirect signs |
| BA | >100 cm/s | >140 cm/s | +Indirect signs |
| VA | >90 cm/s | >120 cm/s | +Indirect signs |

*MCA, middle cerebral artery; ACA, anterior cerebral artery; PCA, posterior cerebral artery; BA, basilar artery; VA, vertebral artery; and PSV, peak systolic velocity.*

**Table 2.**
*TCCS criteria for intracranial stenosis (ICAS) [42].*

**A.** Direct criteria (modifications observed at the stenosis level) include:

a. A color aliasing phenomenon (only in TCCS exam), which may indicate augmented flow velocities, caused by a stenosis or other etiologies (tortuosity, etc.) [35].

b. A progressive focal increase of blood flow velocities in ≥50% stenosis or paradoxical velocity decrease with very severe stenosis, near-occlusion or diffuse intracranial disease (**Figures 1, 2**).

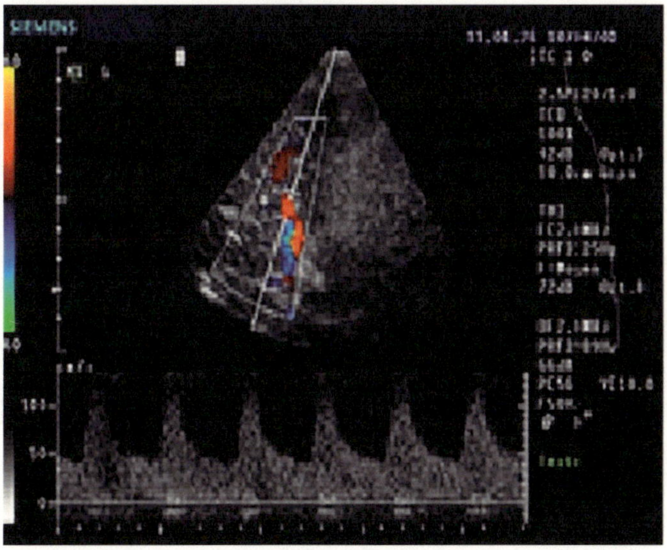

**Figure 1.**
*TCDS, transtemporal approach, axial midbrain plane, color mode (left M1 higher grade stenosis).*

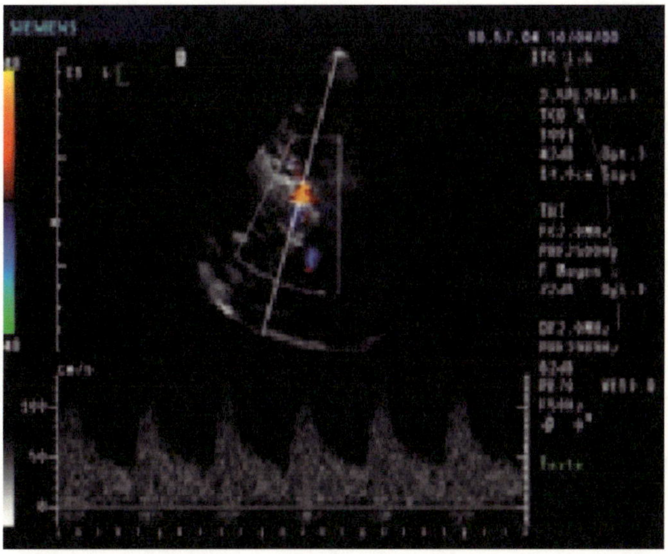

**Figure 2.**
*TCDS transtemporal approach, axial, midbrain plane, color mode (left C1 stenosis).*

Baracchini noted that, as a rule for a vessel with straight walls, a 50% diameter reduction double the velocity, and a 70% stenosis may triple the velocity at the end of the stenosis compared with a prestenotic segment or with the contralateral no affected side. The velocity values detected by TCCS are higher than those by TCD (due to angle correction) [35].

c. A significant (>30%) side-to-side difference of velocity (for symmetrical vessel segments after angle correction) [35].

**B.** Indirect criteria (changes observed in other arteries):

a. Only observed in very severe stenosis (>80%).

b. Are the same as for occlusion—proximal or distal flow alterations: a diastolic velocity drop; high RI in the feeding vessel or in the proximal segment of the stenotic vessel; a delayed systolic flow augmentation and velocity drop downstream; and flow diversion and signs of collateralization [35, 41–43].

TCD criteria for ICAS in anterior as well as posterior circulation have been validated against DSA, MRA, and CTA, and serve as reliable tools for their diagnosis (**Table 1**) [33].

The velocity criteria for ≥50% ICAS were detected by Feldmann and coworkers in (SONIA) trial [39], which standardized the data of TCD, MRA, and DSA. The cut points were the measures of continuous variables such as the percentage of stenosis on MRA or velocity on TCD for each intracranial arterial vessel:

a. MRA ≥50% stenosis, without occlusion, or the presence of a flow gap defined a positive test. Stenosis ≥50% on TCD was identified using an MFV >100 cm/s in MCA, >90 cm/s in the intracranial ICA, or >80 cm/s in the BA or VAs [39].

b. For 80% stenosis on MRA, the SONIA TCD-MFV (cm/s) cut points for 70–99% DSA stenosis of different arteries were: MCA 240, ICA 130, BA 130, and VA 130 [39].

SONIA trial established that both TCD and MRA could reliably exclude the presence of ICAS, rather than identifying them; abnormal findings on TCD or MRA requiring a confirmatory test such as DSA to diagnose ICAS [39].

The correlation between TCD and DSA for the identification of ≥50% ICAS at laboratories with (SONIA) TCD scanning protocol was established by Limin Zhao and coworkers [40]. Stenosis ≥50% on TCD was detected using an MFV >100 cm/s in the MCA, >90 cm/s in the intracranial ICA, or >80 cm/s in the VAs/BA. For ≥70% ICAS, they used expanded criteria (MFV-MCA >120 cm/s, MFV-VAs/BA >110 cm/s, stenotic/prestenotic velocity/ratio-SPR ≥3, and low velocity). These criteria demonstrated excellent-to-good sensitivity of TCD and indicated good agreement with DSA [40].

Baumgartner and coworkers conducted a TCCS study that evaluated PSV cutoff values for the assessment of >50 and <50% stenosis of the intracranial arteries (**Table 2**) [42].

### 4.2 TCD/TCCS can detect and localize the intracranial arterial occlusion

Intracranial occlusion can be directly or indirectly detected by ultrasound examination.

a. Direct criteria for intracranial arterial proximal occlusion are diagnosed using the thrombolysis in brain ischemia (TIBI) flow-grading system. They include: no flow signal (TIBI 0) and minimal flow signal (TIBI 1), while blunted flow signal (TIBI 2) and dampened flow signal (TIBI 3) are criteria for distal occlusion (**Figure 3**). A missing flow signal could be occlusion or hypoplasia/aplasia (it is essential to use ultrasound contrast agents and to verify for indirect criteria of intracranial arterial occlusion) [35, 36, 43, 44].

b. Indirect criteria for intracranial arterial occlusion comprise proximal or distal flow alterations: a diastolic velocity drop; high RI in the feeding vessel or in the proximal segment of the stenotic vessel; a delayed systolic flow augmentation and velocity drop downstream; and flow diversion and signs of collateralization (**Figure 4**) [33–38].

### 4.3 TCD/TCCS can realize the real-time monitoring of recanalization in acute ischemic stroke patients treated with systemic thrombolysis and of rescue reperfusion techniques (identification of reocclusion, hyperperfusion syndrome, etc.)

TCD/TCCS can detect the residual flow at thrombus-blood interface.

The TIBI flow grading system, TIBI: 0–5, was elaborated to identify residual flow and to monitor thrombus dissolution in real time [37, 43–45].

Absent flow (TIBI 0): no flow signals; or lack of regular pulsatile flow signals (using lowest pulse repetition frequency-PRF and increased color-gain settings).

Minimal (TIBI I): systolic spikes of variable velocity and duration; and absent diastolic flow during all cardiac cycles.

Blunted (TIBI II): flattened or delayed systolic flow acceleration compared with control side; positive end-diastolic velocity (EDV); and pulsatility index (PI) <1.2.

Dampened (TIBI III): normal systolic flow acceleration; positive EDV; and >30% decrease in mean flow volume (MFV) compared with control side.

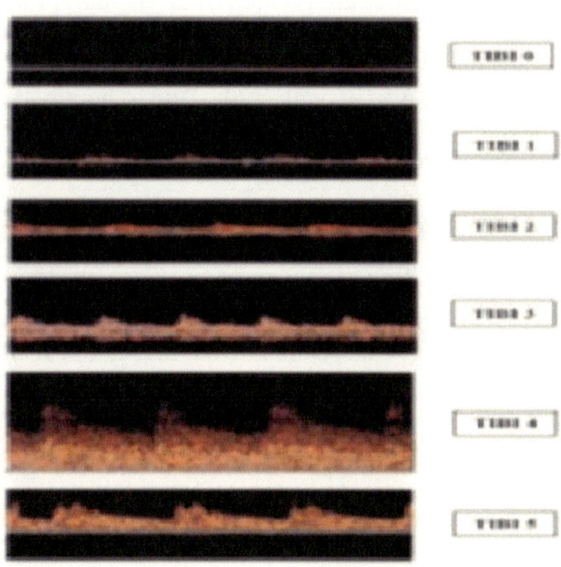

**Figure 3.**
*Thrombolysis in brain ischemia (TIBI) flow-grading system.*

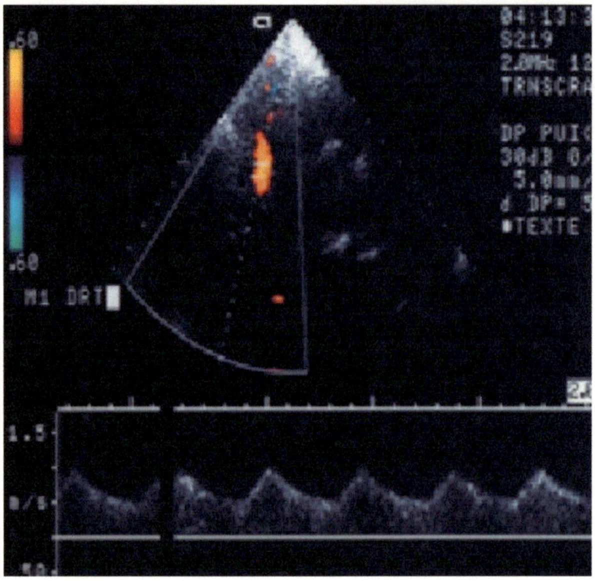

**Figure 4.**
*TCDS, transtemporal approach, axial midbrain plane, color mode (right proximal ICA occlusion, with right M1-MCA poststenotic flow pattern).*

Stenotic (TIBI IV): MFV >80 cm/s and velocity difference >30% compared with control side; if the velocity difference is <30%, look for additional signs of stenosis; and affected and comparison sides have MFV <80cm/s.

Normal (TIBI V): <30% MFV difference compared with control side; and similar wave form shapes compared with control side [37, 43–45].

TIBI flow grades I–III correspond to acute proximal intracranial artery occlusion, while a TIBI flow grade of IV is an indicative of proximal artery hemodynamically significant (>50%) stenosis.

The assessment of the diagnostic value of transcranial power motion-mode Doppler (PMD-TCD) against computed tomography angiography (CTA) in patients with acute ischemic stroke was evaluated by Tsivgoulis and coworkers. They asserted that PMD-TCD detected a substantial proportion of ICAS or occlusions, in concordance with CTA in patients with acute ischemic stroke. PMD-TCD identified data supplementary to the CTA: collateralization of flow with extracranial ICA stenosis/occlusion; real-time embolization-MES; and arterial blood flow steal [45].

The evaluation of the diagnostic value of PMD-TCD against DSA in the detection of acute posterior circulation steno-occlusive disease was realized by Tsivgoulis and coworkers. They showed that the higher value of PMD-TCD compared with single-gate TCD may be associated with its ability to observe flow on the PMD display along tortuous and long arterial segments that may not be readily identified by sonographers during a single-gate TCD exam. In conclusion, PMD-TCD can exclude vertebro-basilar artery occlusion and can select patients for DSA and endovascular interventions if the sonographers are confirmed by DSA [46].

An acute arterial occlusion differs from chronic as it is often partial and incomplete and exhibits dynamic processes (partial obstruction to flow, thrombus propagation, reocclusion, and sometimes spontaneous recanalization). TCD can rapidly identify patients with these lesions and detect not only the flow-limiting lesion but also the ongoing embolization, the collateralization, and the failure of the vasomotor reserve [37].

### 4.4 TCD can identify clinically silent emboli: microembolic signals (MES), which recognizes patients at higher risk of embolic stroke

MES detection in different interventional procedures (cerebral and coronary angiography, angioplasty, carotid endarterectomy, etc.) and in patients with extra and intracranial large artery atherosclerotic stenosis is useful in risk stratification, thus enabling to select those patients who could benefit from a more aggressive treatment [33, 41, 47]. MES detection requires continuous monitoring (at least 1 hour) of the major intracranial arteries. Most MES can be detected several days after the embolic event. The origin of emboli is important; the detection of an embolic signal in the distal MCA might represent an atherosclerotic plaque in the ipsilateral MCA or ICA. On the other hand, the identification of MES in multiple bilateral arteries indicates a cardiac origin [33, 41, 47].

### 4.5 TCD can recognize patients with extracranial ICA stenosis at a higher stroke risk, can assess both collateral pathways, and the vasomotor reactivity (VMR), which detects patients at higher risk of hemodynamic stroke

Severe extracranial ICA stenosis may produce embolic or hemodynamic hemispheric infarct [48]. While the risk of an embolic ischemic stroke increases with the severity of ICA's stenosis, the hemodynamic risk correlates less well with the degree of stenosis because of the functional capacity of the collateral pathways [48]. A complete circle of Willis and the possibility to activate primary collaterals (anterior communicating artery-ACoA, posterior communicating artery-PCoA) or secondary collaterals (ophthalmic artery-OA, lepto-meningeal arteries) reduce the risk of hemodynamic infarct ipsilateral to the extracranial ICA disease [33, 36, 38]. In patients with collateral flow signals (reversed OA, anterior cross-filling, and PCoA flow) identified by TCD, proximal ICA occlusion is confirmed by subsequent neck CTA, MRA, or DSA [33, 36, 38].

Vasomotor reactivity (VMR) defines the autoregulatory vasodilation of cerebral vessels in response to a vasodilatory challenge, such as hypercapnia or acetazolamide (apnea test, breath-holding test, and Diamox test). VMR represents a measure of dynamic cerebrovascular reserve capacity. Its study recognizes patients at higher risk of hemodynamic stroke, in both intra and extracranial large vessel disease, thus allowing to select those patients who could benefit from a more aggressive treatment [38, 48]. According to Prabhakaran, the presence of MES, poor collateral flow, and impaired VMR predict the high risk of recurrence in intracranial atherosclerosis [41].

TCD can identify intracranial arterial blood flow steals (reversed Robin Hood syndrome).

Intracranial arterial blood flow steals can be detected in chronic disease (e.g., subclavian artery stenoses, arterio-venous malformations, and fistulas) but also in patients with acute ischemic stroke. Flow diversion is the hallmark of a steal and can appear at any level of the intracranial arteries (large proximal vessels and small distal vessels) [33–35].

## 5. Magnetic resonance angiography (MRA) and high-resolution magnetic resonance imaging (HR-MRI) for the diagnosis of intracranial atherosclerotic disease (ICAD)

ICAD includes two major features: (a) atherosis caused by lipid deposits in the intima of the arteries and inflammation; and (b) sclerosis, as a result of endothelial dysfunction, leading to arterial stiffness [49].

Strokes associated with ICAD occur in association with four major stroke mechanisms: in situ thrombotic occlusion; branch occlusion; artery-to-artery embolism; and hemodynamic insufficiency [50, 51]. Unstable intracranial plaques can suddenly lead to thrombotic occlusion. Using transcranial duplex monitoring, artery-to-artery embolism can be discovered, which commonly causes multiple cortico-subcortical infarcts. Branch occlusive disease (BOD) is one of the main stroke mechanisms of ICAD, which can be characterized by a milder degree of stenosis [19] and comma-shaped infarcts extending to the basal surface of the parent artery [52].

The first two mechanisms are the consequences of plaque rupture, which reveals the thrombogenic core to clotting factors, resulting a thrombus that occludes the artery locally or embolizes distally [50].

The third mechanism, specific to ICAD, is the growth of plaque over the ostia of penetrating arteries resulting in occlusion, which was described by Caplan [53] as branch atheromatous disease. Lastly, high-grade narrowing or occlusion of the lumen may lead to the fourth mechanism: hypoperfusion of the distal brain territory, particularly in cases with inadequate collateral flow [31, 50].

MRA, CTA, DSA, TCD, and TCCS can detect ICAS of different histopathological nature (including partially recanalized emboli) and can assess ICAS progression and in-stent restenosis. Unfortunately, these methods are unable to directly exam plaque instability, with the exception of microembolic signals (MES) detection by TCD as a surrogate marker [3].

Arenillas suggested that for the detection of intracranial plaque morphology, the imaging techniques used include high-resolution MRI (HR-MRI), high magnetic field (3T) preferable, and intravascular ultrasound. This new concept allows the detection and characterization of nonstenotic intracranial atheroma, establishing its role in stroke of undetermined origin, and may have the power to confirm the atherosclerotic nature of ICAS [3].

### 5.1 Magnetic resonance angiography (MRA)

Degnana noted that 3D time-of-flight (TOF)-MRA is a imaging technique that noninvasively explores the intracranial arteries. It takes the advantage of the contrast between nonsaturated spins in the blood entering the imaging plane and the stationary adjacent tissue, which remains saturated. 3D TOF-MRA allows the visualization of any variation in blood flow. It provides detailed information about the lumen status of the intracranial vessels (**Figure 5**) [54].

The following arterial segments are assessed: bilateral intracranial ICA, ACA-A1/A2, MCA-M1/M2, PCA-P1/P2, BA, and VA. According to the severity of stenosis, there are four groups in which patients are classified: <50% or no stenosis, 50–69% stenosis, 70–99% stenosis, and occlusion groups. Focal flow void found on MRA with distal filling is considered as severe stenosis (70–99%) [55].

Other MR sequences, such as T2-/T1-weighted imaging, fluid-attenuated inversion recovery sequences, and diffusion-weighted imaging (DWI), are also performed on a conventional MRI on a 3.0 or 1.5T MR scanner [56].

Degnana asserted that MRA offers good equivalency with DSA for the detection of >50% stenosis with the reported sensitivity, specificity, and accuracy of 92, 91, and 91%, respectively [54].

Higher field strength scanners may carry additional benefits in improving signal intensity-to-noise ratio and background suppression; other sequences, such as novel sensitivity encoding (SENSE) TOF-MRA protocols, also have substantially abbreviated acquisition times [57].

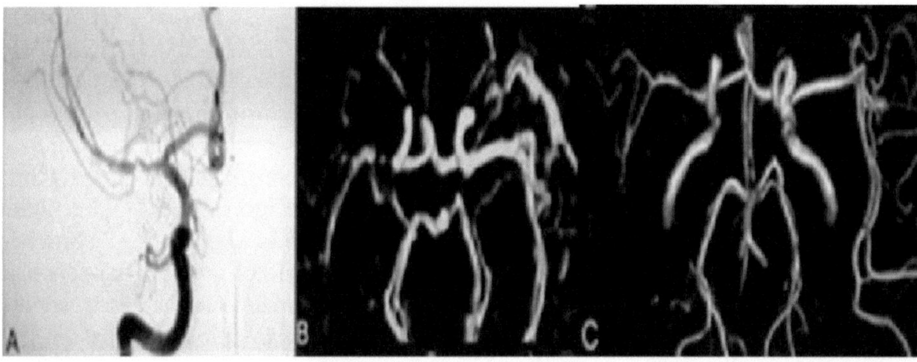


**Figure 5.**
*Comprehensive imaging of a patient with recent stroke depicting left MCA stenosis. A–C, DSA (A) confirms stenosis, but contrast – enhanced MRA (B) and volume-reduced TOF MRA (C) overestimate the degree of stenosis in this particular case [54].*

MRA has some advantages: noninvasive, no radiation, low cost, and widely available, but for the detection of ICAS requires confirmation by another imaging modality [51, 54]. The main disadvantage is that it overestimates stenosis. MRA can render ambiguous or erroneous results. The inability to distinguish between high-grade stenosis and occlusion is another major disadvantage [58].

In addition, MRA has magnet contraindications: limited to no use in morbidly obese and claustrophobic patients and those with implanted metallic objects [51]. Although CTA performs better overall compared with MRA for the purpose of determining the degree of stenosis (CTA can better visualize high-grade stenoses than MRA since the latter tends to overestimate the degree of stenosis), MRA is better than CTA at evaluating the petrous and cavernous ICA as bony artifacts affect CTA [51, 54].

Degnana noted that MRA can be superior in the evaluation of MCA stenosis compared with DSA but still only provides information about vessel patency alone. MRA can be an effective screening technique for patients with suspected MCA syndromes to detect stenosis within the intracranial vessels and to indicate the need for HR-MRI to accurately image the stenotic region [54, 59].

### 5.2 Contrast-enhanced (CE) MRA

It provides better anatomic visualization, particularly in the regions of changing blood flow directions; however, the visualization of smaller arteries remains limited [54, 60].

### 5.3 Quantitative MRA (QMRA)

Prabhakaran noted that QMRA, utilizing phase-contrast techniques, quantifies anterograde blood flow at distal site of stenosis; it exploits the phase shift in the signal of flowing blood, which is proportional to flow velocity, to quantify flow rate in medium and large vessels [51].

### 5.4 High-resolution MRI (HR-MRI)

The conventional imaging such as DSA, MRA, CTA, and TCD fall short in characterizing the presence of no occlusive atherosclerotic disease, because it focuses on the vessel lumen estimate luminal stenosis by measuring blood flow velocity [2, 54].

HR-MRI can be used to assess intracranial arterial disease, both atherosclerotic and nonatherosclerotic [50].

According to Bodle, HR-MRI represents MR acquisitions using clinically available 1.5–3.0 Tesla magnetic field strength targeted to intracranial arterial pathology that are of sufficient quality to visualize the arterial wall, separate from the lumen of the proximal circle of Willis vessels. HR-MRI can be accomplished at 1.5 T by limiting the field of view to focus on a single vessel or point of interest, but higher field strength at 3 T has many advantages over conventional MRI (1.5 T). Image quality in MRI depends on several factors (e.g., slice thickness, field of view, signal-to-noise ratio, matrix size, and magnetic field strength) [50, 61]. Image acquisition is faster and there are increased signal-to-noise and contrast-to-noise ratios, with better image quality for black-blood imaging. The increased signal and contrast that 3 T provides improves the detection of complex atherosclerotic plaque and can identify plaque components in larger arteries [50, 62].

HR-MRI allows the direct assessment of intracranial atherosclerotic plaques; it is capable of characterizing plaque location, severity, and morphology, and discriminating from other nonatherosclerotic etiologies [3, 50, 51].

Bodle also suggested that an intracranial plaque with HR-MRI features of intraplaque hemorrhage and a ruptured fibrous cap in a patient with downstream ischemia is likely associated with artery-to-artery embolism, whereas a stable plaque with a large amount of fibrous tissue and small lipid core resulting in high-grade stenosis may cause hypoperfusion [50]. Thus, HR-MRI may directly determine stroke mechanism and play a role in selecting secondary prevention therapies (e.g., patients with hypoperfusion may benefit from intracranial revascularization procedures that patients with artery-to-artery embolism may not benefit) [50].

The simplest use of HR-MRI of the MCA is the calculation of the degree of MCA stenosis, which may be stated as:

$$\%\text{Stenosis} = (1 - \text{Lumen area}/\text{Reference lumen area}) \times 100, \qquad (2)$$

where the reference lumen area is the area of the nonoccluded lumen, preferably at a proximal segment [2].

Bodle mentioned that ICAS can be caused by diverse pathologies (e.g., atherosclerosis, inflammation, and vasospasm), with diverse treatment implications. HR-MRI may noninvasively differentiate between the etiologies of ICAS by identifying plaque components or unique enhancement patterns [50].

Patients with symptomatic (versus asymptomatic) and non-BOD type (versus BOD) ICAD had characteristic changes in: (a) the wall area (larger plaques); (b) plaque signals (eco-centric enhancement and heterogeneous signal intensity suggesting unstable plaque); and (c) remodeling patterns (positive remodeling suggesting outward expansion of the vessel wall) [63].

On the contrary, superiorly located MCA plaques (near to the orifices of penetrating arteries) are associated with BOD-type ICAD [64].

Bodle asserted that, in other vascular beds, the determination of atherosclerotic plaque constituents has helped in risk-stratify patients and select treatments. Using clinical, imaging, and pathological correlations, studies of coronary and carotid artery disease have detected characteristics that indicate plaque vulnerability: lipid core size, intraplaque hemorrhage, and fibrous cap thickness. These vulnerable plaque characteristics are also present in ICAD [50, 65] but are less well studied (**Table 3**). Bodle also noted that intraplaque hemorrhage (IPH) from rupture of plaque microvessels causing the accumulation of erythrocyte membranes, deposition of cholesterol, macrophage infiltration and enlargement of the necrotic core

| Plaque characteristic | TOF-MRA | T1-weighted | PD-weighted | T2-weighted |
|---|---|---|---|---|
| Fibrous cap | Isointense/ hypointense | Isointense | Isointense/ hyperintense | Hyperintense |
| Lipid-rich necrotic core | Isointense | Isointense/ hyperintense | Hyperintense | Hypointense |
| Hemorrhage | Hyperintense | Hyperintense to hypointense (with age of hemorrhage) | Hypointense to hyperintense | Hypointense to hyperintense |
| Calcification | Hypointense | Hypointense | Hypointense | Hypointense |

**Table 3.**
*Plaque characteristics on multiple contrast weightings based on carotid imaging literature [50, 65]*

results in atheroma growth, and plaque destabilization. A large amount of lipid within the necrotic core of a plaque is another sign of plaque vulnerability HR-MRI measurement of lipid-necrotic core area in extracranial ICA plaques correlates well with pathology [50].

HR-MRI can identify fibrous cap characteristics (thin, thick, or ruptured) in extracranial ICAs. The fibrous cap is a layer of connective tissue covering the lipid-necrotic core. Thick fibrous caps are less prone to rupture [50].

HR-MRI is noninvasive, but less available, still with limited clinical value, requiring extensive postprocessing. Bodle asserted that imaging characteristics in ICAD have not yet been correlated with pathological specimens because, while the HR-MRI of the extracranial ICAs can be correlated with endarterectomy specimens, intracranial vessels are not accessible to pathology sampling in live patients. Therefore, the signal characteristics of intracranial plaque components can only be extrapolated from extracranial ICAs HR-MRI [50].

Another disadvantage is the small size (2.0–5.0 mm) and the depth of the intracranial vessels, which require relatively long acquisition times, making HR-MRI imaging difficult because of patient motion artifact and limitations in resolution.

According to Bodle, HR-MRI can help to identify stroke mechanisms, determine the degree and etiology of stenoses, identify nonstenotic plaques, and identify potentially high-risk plaque components. These plaque characteristics are not visualized with conventional luminal imaging and may be important predictors of stroke [50].

## 6. Multidetector computed tomography and multidetector computed tomography angiography for the diagnosis of intracranial atherosclerotic disease (ICAS)

### 6.1 Nonenhanced multidetector computed tomography (MDCT)

The study of the prevalence, and of the risk factors for intracranial internal carotid artery calcification (ICAC), as a marker of intracranial atherosclerosis was determined by Bos and coworkers. They assessed a white population (2495 persons) from the population-based Rotterdam Study with a no enhanced multidetector (16-slice or 64-slice) computed tomography (MDCT) of the intracranial ICAs. A calcified plaque had >130 Hounsfield units. They concluded that ICAC was highly prevalent and occurred in over 80% of older, white persons [66].

### 6.2 Multidetector computed tomography angiography (MCTA)

A comprehensive high-resolution intracranial vessel assessment is possible by the introducing of multislice CT (MSCT: multiple row scanning: 4, 16, 64, up to 320 rows, associated with an increased rotational speed: 0.5 s/rotation). MSCT represents the first-line imaging modality in stroke patients [67]. CTA calculates the degree of stenosis using the published method for the Warfarin-Aspirin Symptomatic Intracranial Disease Study (WASID) (vide supra) [2].

According to Arenillas, CTA detects the degree of stenosis for each of 15 large intracranial arterial segments assessed: bilateral supraclinoid ICAs, A1-ACA, M1-ACM, M2-ACM, P1-PCA, proximal, mid, and distal BA, and intracranial VA. CTA identifies and characterizes the ICAS of different histopathological nature (including partially recanalized emboli), being unable to directly assess plaque instability. It allows the examination of ICAS progression and in-stent restenosis [3, 68]. The stenotic lesions are considered to be atherosclerotic in nature, if no cases with subarachnoid hemorrhage or intracerebral hemorrhage are detected by CT head (in consequence, vasospasm is unlikely the cause of these ICAS). Arterial segments are excluded from the analyses of stenosis, if they are identified to be congenitally hypoplastic or seen only through collaterals or cross-filling [69].

The prevalence, distribution, calcification, and the risk factors predisposing ICAS in a white stroke population were investigated by Homburg and coworkers. All patients underwent MDCT of the brain and MDCTA (with a 16-slice MDCT scanner or a 64-slice MDCT scanner with a standardized protocol) of the extracranial and intracranial arteries in a single session [70]. They concluded that the majority of ICAS was observed in the posterior circulation. ICAS in the proximal intracranial arteries was mainly classified, but in distal arteries, it was frequently nonclassified, indicating a different pathophysiology of atherosclerotic disease in the two segments. The absence of calcification on CT of the brain does not exclude the presence of ICAS in the distal arteries. Association of nonclassified ICAS and ESR may indicate a prominent role for inflammatory factors in intracranial arteries disease (ICAD) [71].

### 6.3 CTA versus DSA

CTA was compared with DSA for the detection and measurement of stenosis/ occlusions in large intracranial arteries by Nguyen and coworkers [69]. They reported high sensitivity and a high PPV for CTA for the detection of occlusion and stenosis of greater than 50%. CTA has relatively fewer risks, costs less, is more readily available, and appears to have the same accuracy as DSA, to identify the exact site of arterial occlusion in acute ischemic stroke. Maximum intensity projections and volume rendering can help to quickly identify the occlusion. On the other hand, CTA does not appear to be as reliable as DSA for determining the presence of stenosis in small arteries distal to the first 1 cm of the artery [72].

### 6.4 CTA versus MRA

CTA has several advantages compared with MRA: better anatomic visualization of the circle of Willis and of the state of the arteries [73] and quite accurate in the evaluation of stenosis, since the latter tends to overestimate high-grade stenosis attributable to turbulent flow; CTA is more accurate for identifying occlusion (sensitivity, 100%; specificity, 99.4–100%) than for measuring the degree of stenosis [68]. CTA is minimally invasive, performed quickly, modest cost, scanner availability 24/7, operator-independent, less susceptible to motion artifacts than MRA, and less dependent on hemodynamic effects compared with MRA [68, 69, 74, 75].

Its disadvantages, besides radiation risk exposure, are patient movement, contrast risk reactions (allergy to iodine contrast agents), different contra-indications (nephron-toxicity-serum creatinine levels >1.2 mg/dL, etc.), and difficult evaluation of arteries within bone canals (particularly of the carotid siphon) due to bone artifacts. However, intracranial, with the proper examination and postprocessing techniques, is possible to use CTA to assess the petrous and cavernous portions of the ICA. Multiplanar reformation (MPR) can display 2D images in various planes without any loss of information. Maximum intensity projection (MIP) enhances high attenuation contrast tissues, including bone, wall calcification, or blood vessels. Since calcifications can interfere with the evaluation of the degree of stenosis, bone elimination is done during post-processing [68, 69].

### 6.5 CTA versus 3D-TOF-MRA and DSA

Bash et al. [76] retrospectively examined 28 subjects with ischemic stroke or TIA comparing CTA and MRA using DSA as the gold standard, among intracranial arteries with stenosis >30% (anterior circulation vessels 42 versus 58% posterior circulation arteries). They concluded that CTA demonstrated a higher sensitivity, specificity, and PPV than those of MRA for the evaluation of stenotic and occluded intracranial vessel segments. CTA has a high interoperator reliability for the quantitation of stenotic lesions when expert readers are used. Helical CTA is superior to DSA in the demonstration of arterial patency in posterior circulation arteries when very low- or balanced flow states are present due to a severe stenosis [76]. In the era of the mechanical thrombectomy with stent-retriever, when faster puncture time to endovascular therapy became very important, CTA became essential due to its shorter scan time and the evaluations of collaterals on multiphase imaging, which can contribute to faster recanalization and better evolution [68].

### 6.6 CTA versus DSA versus TCCS

Roubec and coworkers compared ICAS in 67 patients with stroke using three different methods: TCCS, CTA, and DSA in a common clinical practice. They found substantial agreement between CTA and DSA, and moderate agreement between TCCS and DSA as well as CTA and TCCS, for the evaluation of ICAS [77].

### 6.7 Intracranial nonocclusive thrombosis (iNOT)

The frequency and clinical course of patients with acute ischemic stroke or TIA who had intracranial nonocclusive thrombus (iNOT) on CTA of the circle of Willis were assessed by Puez and coworkers [78]. Before CTA, a noncontrast CT (NCCT) was accomplished in all cases. iNOT has been described first on DSA or MRA [79, 80]. Criteria to diagnose iNOT rather than occlusive thrombus or atherosclerotic stenosis were: (1) residual lumen present and eccentric; (2) nontapering thrombus; (3) smooth and well-defined thrombus margins; and (4) absence of vessel wall calcification [78]. Puez concluded that iNOT was relatively uncommon. Probably, iNOT may be more frequently diagnosed when performing early CTA in such patients. The majority of patients had a good clinical outcome. Clinical deterioration was associated with unchanged or enlarged iNOT in repeated vascular studies, whereas diminished or resolved iNOT was associated with a benign clinical course. Particularly, in patients with minor symptoms, iNOT may indicate increased risk for clinical deterioration. Puez's study supported the importance of urgent vascular imaging in these patients [78].

Clot length can be examined by thin-sliced noncontrast CT and CTA. A better visualization of collateral circulation (which is an important prognostic factor for favorable outcome) can be realized with multiphase CTA [81, 82].

## 7. Conclusions

This chapter focuses on key findings and recent approaches in diagnosis of intracranial arterial atherosclerotic stenosis (ICAS), with an emphasis on novel procedures to define the underlying mechanisms of stroke in intracranial atherosclerotic disease (ICAD). The importance of ICAS as a principal cause of ischemic stroke in Caucasians is undervalued as compared to that of extracranial atherosclerotic stenosis (ECAS) and nonvalvular atrial fibrillation (NVAF). On the other hand, intracranial arterial calcifications, stenosis, and occlusions represent the most frequent disturbance observed in intracranial arteries [83].

Intracranial arterial stenosis is caused by an atherosclerotic plaque in more than 90% of cases (ICAS). Intracranial atherosclerotic stroke differs from extracranial atherosclerotic stroke in many aspects, including risk factors and stroke patterns. Unlike in patients with ECAS or NVAF, stroke correlated to ICAD occurs in association with various stroke mechanisms such as in situ thrombotic occlusion, artery-to-artery embolism, branch occlusion, and hemodynamic insufficiency [83].

## Author details

Dragoş Cătălin Jianu[1,2*], Silviana Nina Jianu[3], Georgiana Munteanu[2], Traian Flavius Dan[2] and Claudia Birsan[2]

1 Department of Neurology, "Victor Babes" University of Medicine and Pharmacy, Timisoara, Romania

2 Department of Neurology, Clinical Emergency County Hospital, Timisoara, Romania

3 Department of Ophthalmology, Military Emergency Hospital, Timisoara, Romania

*Address all correspondence to: dcjianu@yahoo.com

## References

[1] Caplan LR, Gorelick PB, Hier DB. Race, sex and occlusive cerebrovascular disease: A review. Stroke. 1986;**17**:648-655

[2] Gorelick PB, Wong LK, Bae H, Pandey D. Large artery intracranial occlusive disease, a large worldwide burden but a relatively neglected frontier. Stroke. 2008;**39**:2396-2399

[3] Arenillas JF. Intracranial atherosclerosis: Current concepts. Stroke. 2011;**42**:S20-S23. DOI: 10.1161/STROKEAHA.110.597278

[4] Wong LK. Global burden of intracranial atherosclerosis. International Journal of Stroke. 2006;**1**:158-159

[5] Sacco RL, Kargman DE, Gu Q, Zamanillo MC. Race-ethnicity and determinants of intracranial atherosclerotic cerebral infarction. The Northern Manhattan Stroke Study. Stroke. 1995;**26**:14-20

[6] Bang OY, Kim JW, Lee JH, Lee MA, Lee PH, Joo IS, et al. Association of the metabolic syndrome with intracranial atherosclerotic stroke. Neurology. 2005;**65**:296-298

[7] Kim JS, Caplan LR, Wong KS. Intracranial atherosclerosis: Pathophysiology, diagnosis and treatment. Frontiers of Neurology and Neuroscience. 2016;**40**:34-43. DOI: 10.1159/000448309

[8] Mak W, Cheng TS, Chan KH, Cheung RT, Ho SL. A possible explanation for the racial difference in distribution of large-arterial cerebrovascular disease: Ancestral european settlers evolved genetic resistance to atherosclerosis, but confined to the intracranial arteries. Medical Hypotheses. 2005;**65**:637-648

[9] Bang OY, Saver JL, Liebeskind DS, Pineda S, Yun SW, Ovbiagele B. Impact of metabolic syndrome on distribution of cervicocephalic atherosclerosis: Data from a diverse race-ethnic group. Journal of the Neurological Sciences. 2009;**284**:40-45

[10] Kamada F, Aoki Y, Narisawa A, Abe Y, Komatsuzaki S, Kikuchi A, et al. A genome-wide association study identifies RNF213 as the first Moyamoya disease gene. Journal of Human Genetics. 2011;**56**:34-40

[11] Hachinski V. Stroke in Korean. Stroke. 2008;**39**:1067

[12] Prabhakaran S, Romano JG. Current diagnosis and management of symptomatic intracranial atherosclerotic disease. Current Opinion in Neurology. 2012;**25**(1):18-26. DOI: 10.1097/WCO.0b013e32834ec16b (Review)

[13] Chimowitz MI, Lynn MJ, Howlett-Smith H, Stern BJ, Hertzberg VS, Frankel MR, et al. Comparison of warfarin and aspirin for symptomatic intracranial arterial stenosis. New England Journal of Medicine. 2005;**352**:1305-1316

[14] Lopez-Cancio E, Dorado L, Millan L, Alzamora M, Reverte S, Sunol A, et al. Final results of the Barcelona-Asymptomatic Intracranial Atherosclerosis (ASIA) study: Prevalence and risk factors. Stroke. 2011;**42**:e87-e88

[15] Wong KS, Ng PW, Tang A, Liu R, Yeung V, Tomlinson B. Prevalence of asymptomatic intracranial atherosclerosis in high-risk patients. Neurology. 2007;**68**:2035-2038

[16] Bang OY. Intracranial atherosclerosis: Current understanding and perspectives. Journal of Stroke. 2014;**16**(1):27-35

[17] Chen XY, Wong KS, Lam WW, Zhao HL, Ng HK. Middle cerebral artery atherosclerosis: Histological comparison between plaques associated with and not associated with infarct in a postmortem study. Cerebrovascular Diseases. 2008;**25**:74-80

[18] Ryoo S, Park JH, Kim SJ, Kim GM, Chung CS, Lee KH, et al. Branch occlusive disease: clinical and magnetic resonance angiography findings. Neurology. 2012;**78**:888-896

[19] Famakin BM, Chimowitz MI, Lynn MJ, Stern BJ, George MG, WASID Trial Investigators. Causes and severity of ischemic stroke in patients with symptomatic intracranial arterial stenosis. Stroke. 2009;**40**:1999-2003. DOI: 10.1161/STROKEAHA.108. 546150

[20] Caplan LR, Hennerici M. Impaired clearance of emboli (washout) is an important link between hypoperfusion, embolism, and ischemic stroke. Archives of Neurology. 1998;**55**:1475-1482

[21] Wong KS, Li H, Lam WWM, Chan YL, Kay R. Progression of middle cerebral artery occlusive disease and its relationship with further vascular events after stroke. Stroke. 2002;**33**:532-536

[22] Barnett HJM, Taylor DW, Eliasziw M, Fox AJ, Ferguson GG, Haynes RB, et al. Benefit of carotid endarterectomy in patients with symptomatic moderate or severe stenosis. New England Journal of Medicine. 1998;**339**:1415-1425

[23] Nahab F, Cotsonis G, Lynn M, Feldmann E, Chaturvedi S, Hemphill JC, et al. Prevalence and prognosis of coexistent asymptomatic intracranial stenosis. Stroke. 2008;**39**:1039-1041

[24] Prabhakaran S, Soltanolkotabi M, Honarmand AR, Bernstein RA, Lee VH, Conners JJ, et al. Perfusion-based selection for endovascular reperfusion therapy in anterior circulation acute ischemic stroke. American Journal of Neuroradiology. 2014;**35**(7):1303-1308. DOI: 10.3174/ajnr.A3889

[25] Cloft HJ, Lynn MJ, Feldmann E, Chimowitz M. Risk of cerebral angiography in patients with symptomatic intracranial atherosclerotic stenosis. Cerebrovascular Diseases. 2011;**31**:588-591

[26] Bauer RB, Boulos RS, Meyer JS. Natural history and surgical treatment of occlusive cerebrovascular disease evaluated by serial arteriography. The American Journal of Roentgenology Radium Therapy and Nuclear Medicine. 1968;**104**:1-17

[27] Craig DR, Mageuro K, Watridge C, Robertson JT, Barnett HJM, Fox AJ. Intracranial internal carotid artery stenosis. Stroke. 1982;**13**:825-828

[28] Akins PT, Pilgram TK, Cross DT 3rd, Moran CJ. Natural history of stenosis from intracranial atherosclerosis by serial angiography. Stroke. 1998;**29**:433-438. DOI: 10.1161/01.STR.29.2.433

[29] Samuels OB, Joseph GJ, Lynn MJ, Smith HA, Chimowitz MI. A standardized method for measuring intracranial arterial stenosis. American Journal of Neuroradiology. 2000;**21**:643-646

[30] Liebeskind DS, Cotsonis GA, Saver JL, Lynn MJ, Cloft HJ, Chimowitz MI. Collateral circulation in symptomatic intracranial atherosclerosis. Journal of Cerebral Blood Flow & Metabolism. 2011;**31**:1293-1301

[31] Liebeskind DS, Cotsonis GA, Saver JL, Lynn MJ, Turan TN, Cloft HJ, et al. Collaterals dramatically alter stroke risk in intracranial

atherosclerosis. Annals of Neurology. 2011;**69**:963-974

[32] Derdeyn CP, Grubb RL, Powers WJ. Cerebral hemodynamic impairment: methods of measurement and association with stroke risk. Neurology. 1999;**53**:251-259

[33] Sharma VK, Wong KS, Alexandrov AV. Transcranial Doppler. In: Kim JS, Caplan LR, Wong KS, editors. Intracranial Atherosclerosis: Pathophysiology, Diagnosis and Treatment. Front Neurol Neurosci. Basel, Karger. Vol. 40. 2016. pp. 124-140. DOI: 10.1159/000448309

[34] Valdueza JM. Chapter 9B. Transcranial insonation-TCCS advanced arterial protocol. In: Csiba L, Baracchini C, editors. Manual of Neurosonology. Cambridge, UK: Cambridge University Press; 2016. pp. 130-139

[35] Baracchini C, Niederkorn K. Chapter 10. Intracranial stenosis/occlusion. In: Csiba L, Baracchini C, editors. Manual of Neurosonology. Cambridge, UK: Cambridge University Press; 2016. pp. 154-164

[36] Kaps M. Chapter 11. Extracranial and intracranial collateral pathways. In: Csiba L, Baracchini C, editors. Manual of Neurosonology. Cambridge, UK: Cambridge University Press; 2016. pp. 165-168

[37] Tsivgoulis G, Katsanos AH, Krogias C. Chapter 12. Acute ischemic stroke. In: Csiba L, Baracchini C, editors. Manual of Neurosonology. Cambridge, UK: Cambridge University Press; 2016. pp. 169-179

[38] Jianu DC, Chapter IV. Transcranial Doppler and transcranial color-coded duplex sonography-diagnostic tests for intracranial arterial stenosis. In: Jianu DC, editor. Diagnosis of Symptomatic Intracranial Atherosclerotic Disease. Saarbruken, Germany: Scholars'Press, OmniScriptum Gmbh & Co.KG; 2015. pp. 83-128

[39] Feldmann E, Wilterdink JL, Kosinski A, Lynn M, Chimowitz MI, Sarafin J, et al. The stroke outcomes and neuroimaging of intracranial atherosclerosis (SONIA) trial. Neurology. 2007;**68**:2099-2106

[40] Zhao L, Barlinn K, Sharma VK, Tsivgoulis G, Cava LF, Vasdekis SN, et al. Velocity criteria for intracranial stenosis revisited: An international multicenter study of transcranial Doppler and digital subtraction angiography. Stroke. 2011;**42**:1-6

[41] Prabhakaran S, Romano JG. Current diagnosis and management of symptomatic intra-cranial atherosclerotic disease. Current Opinion in Neurology. 2012;**25**(1):18-26. DOI: 10.1097/ WCO.0b013e3283 4ec16b

[42] Baumgartner RW, Mattle HP, Scroth G. Assessment of >50% and <50% intracranial stenosis by transcranial color-code duplex sonography. Stroke. 1999;**30**:87-92

[43] Demchuk AM, Christou I, Wein TH, et al. Accuracy and criteria for localizing arterial occlusion with transcranial Doppler. Journal of Neuroimaging. 2000;**10**:1-12

[44] Alexandrov AV, Demchuk AM, Wein TH, Grotta JC. Yield of transcranial Doppler in acute cerebral ischemia. Stroke. 1999;**30**:1604-1609.12

[45] Tsivgoulis G, Sharma VK, Lao AY, Malkoff MD, Alexandrov A. Validation of transcranial Doppler with computed tomography angiography in acute cerebral ischemia. Stroke. 2007;**38**:1245-1249

[46] Tsivgoulis G, Sharma VK, Hoover SL, Lao AY, Ardelt AA, Malkoff MD, et al.

Applications and advantages of power motion-mode Doppler in acute posterior circulation cerebral ischemia. Stroke. 2008;**39**:1197-1204

[47] Markus HS, Droste DW, Brown MM. Detection of asymptomatic cerebral embolic signals with Doppler ultrasound. Lancet. 1994;**343**:1011-1012

[48] Norris JW, Zhu CZ. Stroke risk and critical carotid stenosis. The Journal of Neurology, Neurosurgery, and Psychiatry. 1990;**53**:235-237

[49] Gomez CR, Qureshi AI. Medical treatment of patients with intracranial atherosclerotic disease. Journal of Neuroimaging. 2009;**19**(Suppl 1):25S-29S

[50] Bodle JD, Feldmann E, Swartz RH, Rumboldt Z, Brown T, Turan TN. High-resolution magnetic resonance imaging: An emerging tool for evaluating intracranial arterial disease, Stroke. 2013;**44**:287-292. DOI: 10.1161/STROKEAHA.112.664680

[51] Prabhakaran S, Warrior L, Wells KR, Jhaveri MD, Chen M, Lopes DK. The utility of quantitative magnetic resonance angiography in the assessment of intracranial in-stent stenosis. Stroke. 2009;**40**(3):991-993. DOI: 10.1161/STROKEAHA.108.522391

[52] Nah HW, Kang DW, Kwon SU, Kim JS. Diversity of single small subcortical infarctions according to infarct location and parent artery disease: analysis of indicators for small vessel disease and atherosclerosis. Stroke. 2010;**41**:2822-2827

[53] Caplan LR. Intracranial branch atheromatous disease: A neglected, understudied, and underused concept. Neurology. 1989;**39**:1246-1250

[54] Degnan AJ, Gallagher G, Teng Z, Lu J, Liu Q, Gillard JH. MR angiography and imaging for the evaluation of middle cerebral artery atherosclerotic disease. American Journal of Neuroradiology. 2012;**33**:1427-1435

[55] Nederkoorn PJ, van der Graaf Y, Eikelboom BC, van der Lugt A, Bartels LW, Mali WP. Time-of-flight MR angiography of carotid artery stenosis: does a flow void represent severe stenosis? The American Journal of Neuroradiology. 2002;**23**:1779-1784

[56] Pu Y, Liu L, Wang Y, Zou X, Pan Y, Soo Y, et al. Geographic and sex difference in the distribution of intracranial atherosclerosis in China. Stroke. 2013;**44**:2109-2114. DOI: 10.1161/STROKEAHA.113.001522

[57] Willinek WA, Gieseke J, von Falkenhausen M, Born M, Hadizadeh D, Manka C, et al. Sensitivity encoding (SENSE) for high spatial resolution time-of-flight MR angiography of the intracranial arteries at 3.0 T. Rofo. 2004;**176**:21-26

[58] Sadikin C, Teng MM, Chen TY, Luo CB, Chang FC, Lirng JF, et al. The current role of 1.5T non-contrast 3D time-of-flight magnetic resonance angiography to detect intracranial steno-occlusive disease. Journal of the Formosan Medical Association. 2007;**106**:691-699

[59] Man BL, Fu YP, Chan YY, Lam W, Hui CF, Leung WH, et al. Use of magnetic resonance angiography to predict long-term outcomes of ischemic stroke patients with concurrent stenoses in Hong Kong. Cerebrovascular Diseases. 2009;**28**:112-118

[60] Wright VL, Olan W, Dick B, Yu H, Alberts-Grill N, Latour LL, et al. Assessment of CE-MRA for the rapid detection of supra-aortic vascular disease. Neurology. 2005;**65**:27-32

[61] Bammer R, Hope TA, Aksoy M, Alley M. Time-resolved 3D quantitative flow MRI of the major intracranial

vessels: Initial experience and comparative evaluation at 1.5 T and 3.0 T in combination with parallel imaging. Magnetic Resonance in Medicine. 2007;**57**:127-140

[62] Hofmann LV, Liddell RP, Eng J, Wasserman BA, Arepally A, Lee DS, et al. Human peripheral arteries: Feasibility of transvenous intravascular MR imaging of the arterial wall. Radiology. 2005;**235**:617-622

[63] Kim JM, Jung KH, Sohn CH, Moon J, Han MH, Roh JK. Middle cerebral artery plaque and prediction of the infarction pattern. Archives of Neurology. 2012;**69**:1470-1475

[64] Yoon Y, Lee DH, Kang DW, Kwon SU, Kim JS. Single subcortical infarction and atherosclerotic plaques in the middle cerebral artery: High-resolution magnetic resonance imaging findings. Stroke. 2013;**44**:2462-2467

[65] Turan TN, Bonilha L, Morgan PS, Adams RJ, Chimowitz MI. Intraplaque hemorrhage in symptomatic intracranial atherosclerotic disease. Journal of Neuroimaging. 2011;**21**:159-161

[66] Bos D, van der Rijk MJM, Geeraedts TEA, Hofman A, Krestin GP, Witteman JCM, et al. Intracranial carotid artery atherosclerosis: Prevalence and risk factors in the general population. Stroke. 2012;**43**:1878-1884. DOI: 10.1161/STROKEAHA.111. 648667

[67] Klingebiel R, Busch M, Bohner G, et al. Multislice CT angiography in the evaluation of patients with acute cerebrovascular disease- a promising new diagnostic tool. Journal of Neurology. 2002;**249**(1):43-49

[68] Jung SC, Kang D-W, Turan TN. Vessel and vessel wall imaging. In: Kim JS, Caplan LR, Wong KS, editors. Intracranial Atherosclerosis: Pathophisiology, Diagnosis and Treatment. Front Neurol Neurosci. Basel, Switzerland: Karger. Vol. 40. 2016. pp. 109-123. DOI: 10.1159/000448308

[69] Nguyen-Huynh NM, Wintermark M, English J, Lam J, Vittinghoff E, Smith WS, et al. How accurate is CT angiography in evaluating intracranial atherosclerotic disease? Stroke. 2008;**39**:1184-1188. DOI: 10.1161/STROKEAHA.107.502906

[70] Homburg PJ, Rozie S, van Gils MJ, Jansen T, de Weert TT, Dippel DW, et al. Atherosclerotic plaque ulceration in the symptomatic internal carotid artery is associated with non-lacunar ischemic stroke. Stroke. 2010;**41**:1151-1156

[71] Homburg PJ, Rozie S, van Gils MJ, van den Bouwhuijsen QJA, Niessen WJ, DWJ D, et al. Association between carotid artery plaque ulceration and plaque composition evaluated with multidetector CT angiography. Stroke. 2011;**42**:367372. DOI: 10.1161/STROKEAHA.110.597369

[72] Villablanca JP, Rodriguez FJ, Stockman T, Dahliwal S, Omura M, Hazany S, et al. Mdct angiography for detection and quantification of small intracranial arteries: comparison with conventional catheter angiography. American Journal of Roentgenology. 2007;**188**:593-602

[73] Kwon BJ, Han MH, Lee SR, Hahm CK, Go JS, Chang KH. Measurement of normal intracranial artery diameter using three-dimensional reconstruction rotational angiogram. Journal of the Korean Society of Radiology. 2004;**50**:95-100

[74] Korogi Y, Takahashi M, Mabuchi N, Miki H, Shiga H, Watabe T, et al. Intracranial vascular stenosis and occlusion Diagnostic accuracy of three-dimensional, Fourier transform, time-of-flight MR angiography. Radiology. 1994;**193**:187-193

[75] Jianu DC, Chapter VI. Multidetector computed tomography and multidetector computed tomography angiography for the diagnosis of intracranial atherosclerotic disease. In: Jianu DC, editor. Diagnosis of Symptomatic Intracranial Atherosclerotic Disease. Saarbruken, Germany: Scholars' Press, Omni Scriptum Gmbh & Co.KG; 2015. pp. 161-188

[76] Bash S, Villablanca JP, Jahan R, Duckwiler G, Tillis M, Kidwell C, et al. Intracranial vascular stenosis and occlusive disease: Evaluation with CT angiography, MR angiography, and digital subtraction angiography. American Journal of Neuroradiology. 2005;**26**:1012-1021

[77] Roubec M, Kuliha M, Jonszta T, Prochazka V, Fadrna T, Filip M, et al. Detection of intracranial arterial stenosis using transcranial color-coded duplex sonography, computed tomographic angiography, and digital subtraction angiography. Journal of Ultrasound in Medicine. 2011;**30**:1069-1075

[78] Puetz V, Dzialowski I, Coutts SB, Hill MD, Krol A, O'Reilly C, et al. Frequency and clinical course of stroke and transient ischemic attack patients with intracranial nonocclusive thrombus on computed tomographic angiography. Stroke. 2009;**40**:193-199. DOI: 10.1161/STROKE AHA.108.526277

[79] Buchan A, Gates P, Pelz D, Barnett HJM. Intraluminal thrombus in the cerebral-circulation—Implications for surgical-management. Stroke. 1988;**19**:681-687

[80] Yamagami H, Kitagawa K, Ohtsuki T, Matsumoto M, Hori M. Embolic cerebral infarction caused by intraluminal thrombus in the carotid siphon successfully treated with combination of anticoagulant and antiplatelet drugs. Circulation Journal. 2005;**69**:1147-1149

[81] Goyal M, Demchuk AM, Menon BK, et al. Randomized assessment of rapid endovascular treatment of ischemic stroke. The New England Journal of Medicine. 2015;**372**:1019-1030

[82] Federau C, Wintermark MCT. CT-angiography, and perfusion-CT evaluation of stroke. In: Caplan LR et al., editors. Cerebrovascular Diseases. 2nd ed. London, UK: Academic Press; 2017. pp. 686-694

[83] Jianu DC. Diagnosis of Symptomatic Intracranial Atherosclerotic Disease. Saarbruken, Germany: Scholars' Press, Omni Scriptum Gmbh & Co.KG; 2015. pp. 5-188

Chapter 8

# Poor-Grade Aneurysmal Subarachnoid Hemorrhage: Diagnosis, Therapeutical Management, and Prognosis

*Bing Zhao, Haixia Xing, Shenghao Ding, Yaohua Pan and Jieqing Wan*


## Abstract

Aneurysmal subarachnoid hemorrhage (aSAH) is a devastating neurological condition and these patients often have unfavorable outcomes at the long-term follow-up. Poor-grade aSAH is a severe subtype of aSAH and is defined as World Federation of Neurosurgical Surgeon (WFNS) grade IV or V. All patients should be treated by a multidisciplinary team that consists of vascular neurosurgeons, interventional neuroradiologists, neurologists, and anesthetists. Aneurysm rebleeding occurs in the poor-grade aSAH within the first 72 h after ictus. Timing of treatment for aSAH has shifted from delayed to early treatment of ruptured aneurysms, and there will be a trend toward early or ultra-early treatment for poor-grade aSAH. However, there is no consensus regarding the optimal timing of treatment for poor-grade aSAH. Endovascular coiling has provided a viable alternative to surgical clipping. An increasing number of patients have received endovascular treatment. There are limited data on high-level clinical trials focused on the treatment of poor-grade aSAH. An accurate prediction model remains challenging. Predicting long-term outcome is essential to support treatment decision-making. We reviewed the current therapeutical management and prognosis of poor-grade aSAH.


**Keywords:** intracranial aneurysms, subarachnoid hemorrhage, poor-grade, treatment, prognosis

## 1. Introduction

Aneurysmal subarachnoid hemorrhage (aSAH) is a devastating neurological condition and is associated with high morbidity and mortality. Poor-grade aSAH accounts for approximately 30% of all aSAH, and it is a severe subtype of aSAH. These patients more often present with acute hydrocephalus, severe intraventricular hemorrhage, microcirculatory disturbances, and even multi-organ failure after ictus [1, 2] . Traditionally, these patients are managed conservatively, and only those who show clinical improvement were selected for aggressive treatment [1, 3, 4]. However, aneurysm rebleeding occurs in patients with poor-grade aSAH, and about 50% of rebleeding is at the early stage after the hemorrhage [5]. Nowadays endovascular coiling, surgical clipping, and intensive neurocritical care have improved outcomes in patients with poor-grade aSAH [6–11]. However, more than 60% of patients have unfavorable outcomes with severe disability [12]. The treatment decision-making is still challenging. There are limited data on high-level clinical trials focusing on the treatment of poor-grade aSAH. Therefore, we review the current therapeutical management and prognosis of poor-grade aSAH.

## 2. Diagnosis

Several grading systems, including Glasgow coma score (GCS), WFNS grade (World Federation of Neurological Societies), Hunt & Hess scale, or modified Hunt & Hess scale, have been used for initial clinical assessment of aSAH. Patients with poor-grade aSAH often present with stupor or coma because of the primary brain injury. WFNS grade has better inter- and intraobserver reliability than Hunt & Hess scale and makes it more appropriate [13]. Poor-grade aSAH is defined as WFNS grade IV or V (a GCS score of 7–12 for grade IV and 3–6 for grade V) [14]. It is important to detect ruptured aneurysms in the setting of poor-grade aSAH. These patients are often unstable and require sedation or anesthesia during examination.

Traditionally, digital subtraction angiography (DSA) is the gold standard technique for detecting ruptured aneurysms [15–19]. CT angiography (CTA) is less invasive and less time-consuming in providing information on ruptured intracranial aneurysms as a primary examination tool for aSAH. Current studies have reported the sensitivity and specificity of CTA for detecting intracranial aneurysms [20]. Matsumoto et al. [21] reported that 27 patients underwent successful surgical clipping based on CTA alone. Our previous study reported that more than a third of patients underwent successful surgical treatment on the basis of CTA alone [22]. All ruptured aneurysms were detected and clipped. Complications and clinical outcomes did not significantly differ between CTA alone and DSA group. Therefore, CTA can provide fast and accurate diagnostic and anatomic information on ruptured aneurysms and it can be safely and effectively used in most patients with poor-grade aSAH requiring surgical treatment. Patients with smaller ruptured aneurysms or multiple aneurysms may be considered for additional DSA examination.

## 3. Aneurysm rebleeding and predictor of the rebleeding

Rebleeding more often occurs in patients with poor-grade aSAH [23–27]. Van Donkelaar et al. [28] reported that 41 (11.0%) of 374 patients experienced rebleeding. Of the 297 patients included in our previous study, 30 (10.1%) patients experienced rebleeding; 14 (46.7%) cases occurred within 24 h after ictus, 11 (36.7%) occurred between 1 and 7 days, and 5 (16.6%) occurred after 7 days [5]. High blood pressure, poor-grade clinical condition, modified Fisher grade, posterior circulation aneurysms, larger aneurysms (>10 mm), intracerebral or intraventricular hemorrhage are reported to be important predictors of rebleeding after aSAH [24, 28–30]. Van Donkelaar et al. [28] reported that a higher modified Fisher grade was a strong risk factor associated with a rebleeding probably because the amount of blood was a marker of stability of the ruptured aneurysm wall.

Many neurosurgeons use preoperative ventricular drainage in all patients with poor-grade aSAH to maintain adequate cerebral perfusion [15, 24, 31–33]; however, there is no guideline for the drainage after poor-grade aSAH. Laidlaw and Siu reported that 2 of 133 patients treated with surgery underwent ventricular drainage because of the concern of rebleeding [34]. On the other hand, several studies found no increased risk of rebleeding after the drainage [35, 36]. Our previous study showed that a lower Fisher grade, ruptured anterior cerebral artery aneurysms, and preoperative external ventricular drainage were independently associated with rebleeding after poor-grade aSAH [5]. Therefore, these patients may have increased risk of rebleeding after ventricle drainage without aneurysm repair, and early aneurysm treatment may be considered for patients who required emergency ventricle drainage.

## 4. Therapeutical management

Poor-grade aSAH should be treated with a multidisciplinary team that consists of neurologists, neurosurgeons, interventional neuroradiologists, and anesthetists. Emergency treatment should include aggressive resuscitation to keep the basic life support. Central venous catheters are first inserted for fluid and medicine administration and hemodynamic monitoring. Systolic blood pressure should be maintained below 160 mmHg to prevent the rebleeding. Oral or nasotracheal intubation should be performed if the patients require respiratory support.

### 4.1 Timing of treatment

There is no consensus regarding the optimal timing of treatment for poor-grade aSAH. Traditionally, these patients have been managed medically and only undergo the treatment of the ruptured aneurysm when clinically stabilized and improved. In the past decades, several studies have shown that early surgery (within 72 h of ictus) improved the outcome in selected patients with poor-grade aneurysms [15–17, 33, 37–39]. At more than 6 months of follow-up, 46% of patients had a good outcome after early surgical clipping [40]. Zentner et al. [41] reported that early surgery resulted in a good outcome of 22% of patients with the worst grade. A study of 103 patients with grade V showed a good outcome in 26% of patients at follow-up [42]. Despite the rates of morbidity and death remaining high in patients with WFNS grade V, these findings suggest that early aneurysm repair is feasible and safe for poor-grade aSAH. Early treatment for ruptured aneurysm may help reduce the risk of rebleeding and manage cerebral vasospasm and delayed ischemia. Patients with younger age, WFNS IV after emergency resuscitation, and middle cerebral artery aneurysms are more likely to have a favorable outcome after early surgery [43].

Aneurysm treatment as early as possible is recommended to prevent rebleeding after initial aSAH [44, 45]. Ultra-early treatment (within 24 h) reduces the risk of rebleeding and improves outcomes in most patients with good-grade aSAH [46–48]. However, there is no evidence to support ultra-early treatment of poor-grade aSAH because these patients experience more severe brain swelling than good-grade patients [42, 49]. With development in microsurgical techniques, there has been growing interest in ultra-early treatment of aSAH. A current series of 78 patients with poor-grade treated with surgical treatment showed 44 patients (56%) had a good outcome, including 26% of patients presenting with WFNS grade V, and surgery was performed within 24 h after admission [33]. In a multicenter and contemporary cohort of poor-grade aSAH, 47 (40%) of 118 patients underwent ultra-early surgery, 16 (34%) patients in ultra-early surgery group and 42 (59%) patients in delayed group had a good outcome [50]. Laidlaw et al. [17, 34]reported 40% of patients were independent after 3 months and 45% died. With coiling, there are few technical limitations to ultra-early treatment of aSAH as the limitations related to inflammation and brain swelling do not affect the technical aspects of the procedure [51].

A current meta-analysis and systemic review of poor-grade aSAH evaluated outcomes by timing of treatment modality and found that patients receiving ultra-early treatment (within 48 h of aSAH) had the highest rates of good neurological outcome (61% compared to 40% for early and 47% for delayed) [12]. Park et al. [47] reported that ultra-early surgery did not significantly decrease the incidence of rebleeding of poor-grade aSAH and also that it was not associated with outcomes [18, 47, 48]. Ultra-early aneurysm treatment of poor-grade aSAH still remains controversial.

### 4.2 Surgical treatment

Surgical treatment includes external ventricular drainage for hydrocephalus or intraventricular hemorrhage, surgical clipping of ruptured aneurysms, and decompressive craniectomy. Surgical selections are based on aneurysm morphology, patient's neurological condition, and treatment relative risk following multidisciplinary consultation. Patients with associated large intracerebral hemorrhage (more than 30 ml) are more often considered for surgical clipping. After surgery, patients are transferred to the intensive care unit, and they are treated with standard management for vasospasm. Illustrative case receiving surgical clipping is shown in **Figure 1**.

The international subarachnoid aneurysm trial (ISAT) demonstrated that for aSAH amenable to both treatments, patients treated with endovascular coiling had better outcomes than patients treated with surgical clipping [52]. Although endovascular treatment has been used as an available alternative to surgery for aSAH, surgical treatment is still an important treatment modality for poor-grade aSAH. In the contemporary multicenter cohorts of poor-grade aSAH, patients receiving clipping more often had a lower GCS score, a WFNS grade of V, a higher Fisher grade and modified Fisher grade, and a ruptured anterior circulation aneurysm than those receiving coiling [53]. Patients with WFNS grade V after emergency resuscitation, a better Fisher grade, brain herniation, the presence of ICH, or the absence of IVH more often underwent early surgical clipping [43]. Patients with brain herniation more commonly are treated with surgery. There are no significant differences in rebleeding, cerebral infarction, symptomatic vasospasm, seizure, pneumonia between coiling and clipping groups. There is also no significant difference in outcomes at 6 and 12 months between the two treatments [53].

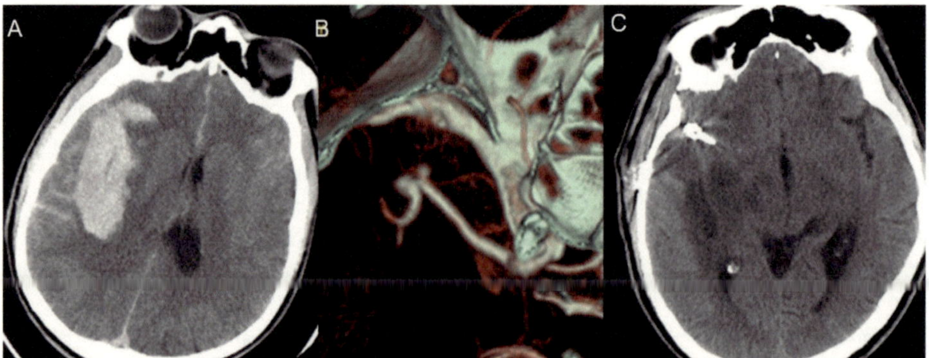


**Figure 1.**
*A 45-year-old male presented with unconsciousness for 2 h and had a Glasgow coma score of 6 and World Federation of Neurosurgical Surgeon grade of V at admission. He was treated with emergency surgical clipping of ruptured aneurysm and hematoma evacuation. He recovered well and had a modified Rankin scale of 1 at 12 months of follow-up. (A) Emergency CT scan shows a large frontotemporal parietal lobe hematoma and midline shift to left side. (B) CT angiography shows a right middle cerebral artery bifurcation aneurysm. (C) CT shows a slight edema of surgical field after 10 days of surgery.*

Decompressive craniectomy has been reported in the treatment for severe traumatic brain injury, massive ischemic stroke, and aSAH [54–60]. This procedure can reduce increased intracranial pressure and improve cerebral perfusion and outcomes in selected patients with ruptured aneurysms with associated intracerebral hemorrhage [61]. However, there are no studies focusing on the safety and efficacy of decompressive craniectomy for poor-grade aSAH compared with conventional craniotomy. Our previous study has shown that primary decompressive craniectomy does not increase postoperative complications and can be performed safely in poor-grade sSAH. More than one-half of patients benefit from primary decompressive craniectomy.

### 4.3 Endovascular treatment

Since the ISAT study, endovascular treatment is more commonly used than clipping for ruptured aneurysm. Aneurysms can be coiled though the minimally invasive endovascular approach to reduce the rate of rebleeding and avoid brain swelling and high intracranial pressure. Endovascular treatment is performed in continuity with the initial angiography and requires less treatment time. The current results at the 3- and 6-year follow-up in the ruptured aneurysm treatment study showed that there was no significant difference in outcome between the two treatments for ruptured aneurysms [62, 63]. A current systematic review of surgical and endovascular treatment of poor-grade aSAH has also shown that the proportion of patients with endovascular coiling increased from 10.0 to 62.0% between 1990 and 2000 and 2010 and 2014 [12]. Therefore, endovascular coiling is a feasible and reasonable option for poor-grade aSAH. Illustrative case receiving coiling is shown in **Figure 2**.

Mocco et al. [31] reported that 35 (35.7%) of 98 patients received coiling, and there was also similar outcome between coiling and clipping for poor-grade aSAH. In our prospective and multicenter registry of 262 patients with poor-grade ruptured aneurysm, 133 (50.8%) patients received endovascular coiling within 21 days after poor-grade aSAH [53]. An unadjusted analysis showed that the rate of outcome (mRS 0–2 or mRS 0–3) at discharge at 6 and 12 months in the coiled patients was higher than that in the clipped patients probably because of selection bias. In our exploratory analysis, there was no significant difference in clinical outcomes between the two groups. Patients receiving coiling had a higher risk of radiological

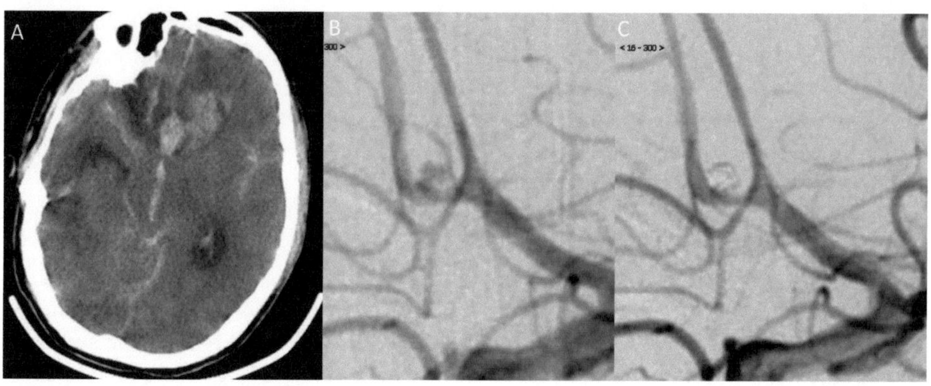


**Figure 2.**
*A 53-year-old male presented with unconsciousness for 1 h and had a Glasgow coma score of 5 and World Federation of Neurosurgical Surgeon grade of V at admission. He was treated with emergency coiling of ruptured aneurysm and external ventricle drainage. He had a modified Rankin scale of 3 at 12 months of follow-up. (A) Emergency CT scan shows severe subarachnoid hemorrhage and frontal lobe hematoma. (B) Preoperative angiography shows a very small anterior communicating artery aneurysm. (C) Immediate angiography shows complete occlusion of aneurysms using coils.*

hydrocephalus than clipped patients, and there was a trend toward clinical hydrocephalus after coiling. However, Zaidi et al. [64] found that there was no difference in hydrocephalus among patients treated by coiling or clipping.

With advances of endovascular technology, stent-assisted coiling has been used in the treatment of ruptured aneurysms. There is a main concern about the safety of stent-assisted coiling for poor-grade ruptured aneurysms. A review reported clinical outcomes in the stent-assisted coiling were worse than those in the coiling alone of acutely ruptured aneurysms [65]. Several studies showed that hemorrhagic complications often occurred in patients with acutely ruptured aneurysms after stent-assisted coiling and external ventricular drainage probably because of dual-antiplatelet therapy [66–68]. Using a multicenter poor-grade aneurysm study, we compared perioperative complications, and clinical outcomes between the stent-assisted coiling and the coiling-alone groups [69]. Twenty-three (17.6%) patients were treated with stent-assisted coiling compared with 108 (82.4%) patients treated with coiling alone. There were no statistically significant differences in intraprocedural rupture, procedure-related ischemic complication, ventricle drainage-related hemorrhagic complication, and symptomatic vasospasm between the stent-assisted coiling group and the coiling-alone group. However, there was a trend toward rebleeding after stent-assisted coiling. The hemorrhagic complication should be considered before the treatment decision-making. Therefore, treatment of wide-necked ruptured aneurysms remains challenging and we still require improvement of endovascular treatment of wide-neck ruptured aneurysms. A clinical trial focused on poor-grade ruptured aneurysms may be necessary to assess the efficacy of the treatment.

## 5. Outcomes and prognosis

The clinical outcomes of patients with aneurysm rebleeding remain very poor probably because of a severe secondary brain injury caused by a large cerebral hematoma or severe intraventricular hemorrhage. The rebleeding is independently associated with poor outcome (odds ratio [OR] 36.37, $p < 0.001$) and associated with mortality (OR 25.03, $p < 0.001$) at 12 months [5]. Tanno et al. [70] reported that 152 (84%) of 181 patients presented with semicoma to coma after rebleeding. Of the 30 patients with rebleeding in our previous study, 22 (73.3%) patients died at discharge. At 12 months, 2 (6.7%) patients had a modified Rankin Score (mRS) of 1, 1 (3.3%) had a mRS of 4, and 26 (86.7%) died [5]. A higher modified Fisher grade before rebleeding, larger aneurysms, and a lower GCS score after rebleeding were independently associated with increased mortality. A lower WFNS grade treated with aggressive treatment is more likely to have a good outcome [71].

Aggressive treatment and successful aneurysm repair can reduce the rebleeding and improve clinical outcomes in selected patients. In a current review of poor-grade aSAH, the rate of good outcome increased from 37.0 to 44.0% over the years. Good outcome was 38% (95% CI = 33–43%) in the endovascular group and 39% (95% CI = 34–44%) in the surgical group at the over 6 months of follow-up [12]. In our multicenter poor-grade aneurysm study [53], 52 (19.8%) patients had a mRS score of 0 or 1, 98 (29.8%) had a mRS score of 0–2, 112 (32.4%) had a mRS score of 0–3, and 51 (19.5%) had died at discharge. Ninety-five (36.3%) patients had a mRS score of 0 or 1, 115 (43.9%) had a mRS of 0–2, 126 (48.1%) had a mRS of 0–3, and 103 (39.3%) had died at 12 months. The outcome is improved after endovascular coiling or clipping over time of the follow-up [53]. In a prospective database of poor-grade aSAH patients, 40% of the 98 patients had a favorable outcome at 12 months [31]. In the 136 patients receiving endovascular coiling, 59 (43.3%) patients had a mRS of 0 or 1, and 64 (47.0%) had a poor outcome (mRS4-6) [72].

| Authors | Study design | Mean time of follow-up | Treatments | Predictors of poor outcome |
|---|---|---|---|---|
| Le Roux et al. | Retrospective | 6 months | Clipping | Hunt & Hess Grade V, blood glucose, fibrin degradation products, severity of ventricular hemorrhage, low density on CT, no clinical improvement |
| Huang et al. | Retrospective | 6 months | Clipping | Hunt-Hess grade, aneurysm size, rehemorrhage before surgery, acute hydrocephalus |
| Mocco et al. | Prospective | 12 months | Clipping and coiling | Older than 65 years, hyperglycernia preoperative Hunt & Hess Grade V, and aneurysm size of at least 13 mm |
| Zhao et al. | Prospective | 12 months | Clipping | Older age, WFNS grade V, brain herniation, intraventricular hemorrhage, non-middle cerebral artery aneurysms |
| Zhao et al. | Prospective | 12 months | Coiling | Older age, WFNS grade of V, higher modified Fisher grade, wider neck aneurysm |
| Zheng et al. | Prospective | 12 months | Clipping, coiling, and conservative treatment | Older age, lower Glasgow coma scale score (GCS), the absence of pupillary reactivity, higher modified Fisher grade, and conservative treatment |

**Table 1.**
*Summary of predictors of poor outcome at the long-term follow-up.*

About one-half of patients achieve a good outcome after the treatment, therefore predicting outcome after poor-grade aSAH is essential to support early treatment [73]. A few prognostic prediction models have been reported [3, 31, 74]. However, these studies are from a single center or have a limited sample size. Older age, lower GCS score, absence of pupil reactivity, higher modified Fisher grade, and conservative treatment are associated with poor outcome in most studies [3, 31, 74, 75]. These predictors of poor outcome are summarized in **Table 1**. We developed an integer-based outcome risk score (*WAP*) to predict the long-term outcomes [76]. The WAP score consists of three variables: *W*FNS grade, *A*ge (three categories), and *P*upillary reactivity. The sum of the weighted scores was used to assess the overall score and was ranged from 0 to 4. The predicted risk of poor outcome ranged from 25.5% for a WAP score of 0 to 96.2% for a score of 4. The risk score is easily measured and may complement treatment decision-making [76].

## 6. Conclusions

Poor-grade aSAH is a severe subtype of subarachnoid hemorrhage caused by ruptured aneurysms. Timing of treatment for the aSAH has shifted from delayed to early surgery, and there will be a trend toward ultra-early treatment for poor-grade aSAH. However, there is no consensus regarding the optimal timing of treatment for poor-grade aSAH. Although endovascular treatment has been used as an available alternative to surgical clipping for aSAH, surgical treatment is still an important treatment modality for poor-grade aSAH. Despite advancements in aneurysm treatment, the morbidity and mortality of poor-grade aSAH remain high. Many retrospective studies have reported the predictors of outcomes, but there is not appropriate prediction model for poor-grade aSAH. The treatment decision-making is still challenging. Further prospective cohort study or clinical trials focused on poor-grade aSAH are required to help guide treatment decisions for this devastating condition.

## Acknowledgements

This work was supported by Shanghai Municipal Education Commission—Gaofeng Clinical Medicine Grant Support (20171914), Shanghai Municipal Commission of Health and Family Planning (201740080), Shanghai Science and Technology Project (18411962700), and the Clinical Research Plan of SHDC (16CR3031A, 16CR2045B), the Shanghai Jiaotong University Medical Engineering and translational Cross-cutting Research Foundation (YG2017MS45, ZH2018ZDA07), Shanghai Jiaotong University School of Medicine Research Project (DLY201821).

## Author details

Bing Zhao[1], Haixia Xing[2], Shenghao Ding[1], Yaohua Pan[1] and Jieqing Wan[1]*

1 Department of Neurosurgery, Renji Hospital, Shanghai Jiao Tong University School of Medicine, Shanghai, China

2 Department of Pathology, Shanghai East Hospital, Tongji University School of Medicine, Shanghai, China

*Address all correspondence to: jieqingwan@126.com

## References

[1] Hutchinson PJ, Power DM, Tripathi P, Kirkpatrick PJ. Outcome from poor grade aneurysmal subarachnoid haemorrhage-which poor grade subarachnoid haemorrhage patients benefit from aneurysm clipping? British Journal of Neurosurgery. 2000;**14**:105-109

[2] Wartenberg KE, Sheth SJ, Michael Schmidt J, Frontera JA, Rincon F, Ostapkovich N, et al. Acute ischemic injury on diffusion-weighted magnetic resonance imaging after poor grade subarachnoid hemorrhage. Neurocritical Care. 2011;**14**:407-415

[3] Le Roux PD, Elliott JP, Newell DW, Grady MS, Winn HR. Predicting outcome in poor-grade patients with subarachnoid hemorrhage: A retrospective review of 159 aggressively managed cases. Journal of Neurosurgery. 1996;**85**:39-49

[4] Mitra D, Gregson B, Jayakrishnan V, Gholkar A, Vincent A, White P, et al. Treatment of poor-grade subarachnoid hemorrhage trial. AJNR. American Journal of Neuroradiology. 2015;**36**:116-120

[5] Zhao B, Fan Y, Xiong Y, Yin R, Zheng K, Li Z, et al. Aneurysm rebleeding after poor-grade aneurysmal subarachnoid hemorrhage: Predictors and impact on clinical outcomes. Journal of the Neurological Sciences. 2016;**371**:62-66

[6] Taylor CJ, Robertson F, Brealey D, O'Shea F, Stephen T, Brew S, et al. Outcome in poor grade subarachnoid hemorrhage patients treated with acute endovascular coiling of aneurysms and aggressive intensive care. Neurocritical Care. 2011;**14**:341-347

[7] Diaz RJ, Wong JH. Clinical outcomes after endovascular coiling in high-grade aneurysmal hemorrhage. Canadian Journal of Neurological Sciences. 2011;**38**:30-35

[8] Pereira AR, Sanchez-Pena P, Biondi A, Sourour N, Boch AL, Colonne C, et al. Predictors of 1-year outcome after coiling for poor-grade subarachnoid aneurysmal hemorrhage. Neurocritical Care. 2007;**7**:18-26

[9] Bracard S, Lebedinsky A, Anxionnat R, Neto JM, Audibert G, Long Y, et al. Endovascular treatment of Hunt and Hess grade IV and V aneurysm. AJNR - American Journal of Neuroradiology. 2002;**23**:953-957

[10] Suzuki S, Jahan R, Duckwiler GR, Frazee J, Martin N, Vinuela F. Contribution of endovascular therapy to the management of poor-grade aneurysmal subarachnoid hemorrhage: Clinical and angiographic outcomes. Journal of Neurosurgery. 2006;**105**:664-670

[11] Bergui M, Bradac GB. Acute endovascular treatment of ruptured aneurysms in poor-grade patients. Neuroradiology. 2004;**46**:161-164

[12] Zhao B, Rabinstein A, Murad MH, Lanzino G, Panni P, Brinjikji W. Surgical and endovascular treatment of poor-grade aneurysmal subarachnoid hemorrhage: A systematic review and meta-analysis. Journal of Neurosurgical Sciences. 2017;**61**:403-415

[13] Shirao S, Yoneda H, Kunitsugu I, Ishihara H, Koizumi H, Suehiro E, et al. Preoperative prediction of outcome in 283 poor-grade patients with subarachnoid hemorrhage: A project of the chugoku-shikoku division of the Japan neurosurgical society. Cerebrovascular Diseases. 2010;**30**:105-113

[14] Report of world federation of neurological surgeons committee on a universal subarachnoid hemorrhage grading scale. Journal of Neurosurgery. 1988;**68**:985-986. DOI:10.3171/jns.1988.68.6.0985. PMID: 3131498

[15] Bailes JE, Spetzler RF, Hadley MN, Baldwin HZ. Management morbidity and mortality of poor-grade aneurysm patients. Journal of Neurosurgery. 1990;**72**:559-566

[16] Oda S, Shimoda M, Sato O. Early aneurysm surgery and dehydration therapy in patients with severe subarachnoid haemorrhage without ich. Acta Neurochirurgica. 1996;**138**:1050-1056

[17] Laidlaw JD, Siu KH. Ultra-early surgery for aneurysmal subarachnoid hemorrhage: Outcomes for a consecutive series of 391 patients not selected by grade or age. Journal of Neurosurgery. 2002;**97**:250-258. Discussion 247-259

[18] Sandstrom N, Yan B, Dowling R, Laidlaw J, Mitchell P. Comparison of microsurgery and endovascular treatment on clinical outcome following poor-grade subarachnoid hemorrhage. Journal of Clinical Neuroscience. 2013;**20**:1213-1218

[19] Gupta SK, Ghanta RK, Chhabra R, Mohindra S, Mathuriya SN, Mukherjee KK, et al. Poor-grade subarachnoid hemorrhage: Is surgical clipping worthwhile? Neurology India. 2011;**59**:212-217

[20] Westerlaan HE, Van Dijk JM, Jansen-van der Weide MC, de Groot JC, Groen RJ, Mooij JJ, et al. Intracranial aneurysms in patients with subarachnoid hemorrhage: Ct angiography as a primary examination tool for diagnosis--systematic review and meta-analysis. Radiology. 2011;**258**:134-145

[21] Matsumoto M, Sato M, Nakano M, Endo Y, Watanabe Y, Sasaki T, et al. Three-dimensional computerized tomography angiography-guided surgery of acutely ruptured cerebral aneurysms. Journal of Neurosurgery. 2001;**94**:718-727

[22] Zhao B, Lin F, Wu J, Zheng K, Tan X, Cao Y, et al. A multicenter analysis of computed tomography angiography alone versus digital subtraction angiography for the surgical treatment of poor-grade aneurysmal subarachnoid hemorrhage. World Neurosurgery. 2016;**91**:106-111

[23] Inagawa T, Kamiya K, Ogasawara H, Yano T. Rebleeding of ruptured intracranial aneurysms in the acute stage. Surgical Neurology. 1987;**28**:93-99

[24] Naidech AM, Janjua N, Kreiter KT, Ostapkovich ND, Fitzsimmons BF, Parra A, et al. Predictors and impact of aneurysm rebleeding after subarachnoid hemorrhage. Archives of Neurology. 2005;**62**:410-416

[25] Rosenorn J, Eskesen V, Schmidt K, Ronde F. The risk of rebleeding from ruptured intracranial aneurysms. Journal of Neurosurgery. 1987;**67**:329-332

[26] Davies BM, Chung KH, Dulhanty L, Galea J, Patel HC. Pre-protection re-haemorrhage following aneurysmal subarachnoid haemorrhage: Where are we now? Clinical Neurology and Neurosurgery. 2015;**135**:22-26

[27] Starke RM, Connolly ES Jr. Rebleeding after aneurysmal subarachnoid hemorrhage. Neurocritical Care. 2011;**15**:241-246

[28] van Donkelaar CE, Bakker NA, Veeger NJ, Uyttenboogaart M, Metzemaekers JD, Luijckx GJ, et al. Predictive factors for rebleeding after aneurysmal subarachnoid hemorrhage: Rebleeding aneurysmal subarachnoid hemorrhage study. Stroke; a Journal of Cerebral Circulation. 2015;**46**:2100-2106

[29] Tang C, Zhang TS, Zhou LF. Risk factors for rebleeding of aneurysmal

subarachnoid hemorrhage: A meta-analysis. PLoS One. 2014;**9**:e99536

[30] Boogaarts HD, van Lieshout JH, van Amerongen MJ, de Vries J, Verbeek AL, Grotenhuis JA, et al. Aneurysm diameter as a risk factor for pretreatment rebleeding: A meta-analysis. Journal of Neurosurgery. 2015;**122**:921-928

[31] Mocco J, Ransom ER, Komotar RJ, Schmidt JM, Sciacca RR, Mayer SA, et al. Preoperative prediction of long-term outcome in poor-grade aneurysmal subarachnoid hemorrhage. Neurosurgery. 2006;**59**:529-538. Discussion 529-538

[32] Ransom ER, Mocco J, Komotar RJ, Sahni D, Chang J, Hahn DK, et al. External ventricular drainage response in poor grade aneurysmal subarachnoid hemorrhage: Effect on preoperative grading and prognosis. Neurocritical Care. 2007;**6**:174-180

[33] Huang AP, Arora S, Wintermark M, Ko N, Tu YK, Lawton MT. Perfusion computed tomographic imaging and surgical selection with patients after poor-grade aneurysmal subarachnoid hemorrhage. Neurosurgery. 2010;**67**:964-974. Discussion 975

[34] Laidlaw JD, Siu KH. Poor-grade aneurysmal subarachnoid hemorrhage: Outcome after treatment with urgent surgery. Neurosurgery. 2003;**53**:1275-1280. discussion 1280-1272

[35] McIver JI, Friedman JA, Wijdicks EF, Piepgras DG, Pichelmann MA, Toussaint LG 3rd, et al. Preoperative ventriculostomy and rebleeding after aneurysmal subarachnoid hemorrhage. Journal of Neurosurgery. 2002;**97**:1042-1044

[36] Hellingman CA, van den Bergh WM, Beijer IS, van Dijk GW, Algra A, van Gijn J, et al. Risk of rebleeding after treatment of acute hydrocephalus in patients with aneurysmal subarachnoid hemorrhage. Stroke; a Journal of Cerebral Circulation. 2007;**38**:96-99

[37] Nowak G, Schwachenwald R, Arnold H. Early management in poor grade aneurysm patients. Acta Neurochirurgica. 1994;**126**:33-37

[38] Versari PP, Talamonti G, D'Aliberti G, Villa F, Solaini C, Collice M. Surgical treatment of poor-grade aneurysm patients. Journal of Neurosurgical Sciences. 1998;**42**:43-46

[39] Chiang VL, Claus EB, Awad IA. Toward more rational prediction of outcome in patients with high-grade subarachnoid hemorrhage. Neurosurgery. 2000;**46**:28-35. discussion 35-26

[40] Zhao B, Cao Y, Tan X, Zhao Y, Wu J, Zhong M, et al. Complications and outcomes after early surgical treatment for poor-grade ruptured intracranial aneurysms: A multicenter retrospective cohort. International Journal of Surgery. 2015;**23**:57-61

[41] Zentner J, Hoffmann C, Schramm J. Results of early surgery in poor-grade aneurysm patients. Journal of Neurosurgical Sciences. 1996;**40**:183-188

[42] Wostrack M, Sandow N, Vajkoczy P, Schatlo B, Bijlenga P, Schaller K, et al. Subarachnoid haemorrhage WFNS grade V: Is maximal treatment worthwhile? Acta Neurochirurgica. 2013;**155**:579-586

[43] Zhao B, Tan X, Zhao Y, Cao Y, Wu J, Zhong M, et al. Variation in patient characteristics and outcomes between early and delayed surgery in poor-grade aneurysmal subarachnoid hemorrhage. Neurosurgery. 2016;**78**:224-231

[44] Connolly ES Jr, Rabinstein AA, Carhuapoma JR, Derdeyn CP, Dion J, Higashida RT, et al. Guidelines for the management of aneurysmal subarachnoid hemorrhage: A guideline for healthcare professionals from the American heart association/American stroke association. Stroke; a Journal of Cerebral Circulation. 2012;**43**:1711-1737

[45] Steiner T, Juvela S, Unterberg A, Jung C, Forsting M, Rinkel G. European stroke organization guidelines for the management of intracranial aneurysms and subarachnoid haemorrhage. Cerebrovascular Diseases. 2013;**35**:93-112

[46] Phillips TJ, Dowling RJ, Yan B, Laidlaw JD, Mitchell PJ. Does treatment of ruptured intracranial aneurysms within 24 hours improve clinical outcome? Stroke; a Journal of Cerebral Circulation. 2011;**42**:1936-1945

[47] Park J, Woo H, Kang DH, Kim YS, Kim MY, Shin IH, et al. Formal protocol for emergency treatment of ruptured intracranial aneurysms to reduce in-hospital rebleeding and improve clinical outcomes. Journal of Neurosurgery. 2015;**122**:383-391

[48] Wong GK, Boet R, Ng SC, Chan M, Gin T, Zee B, et al. Ultra-early (within 24 hours) aneurysm treatment after subarachnoid hemorrhage. World Neurosurgery. 2012;**77**:311-315

[49] Wilson DA, Nakaji P, Albuquerque FC, McDougall CG, Zabramski JM, Spetzler RF. Time course of recovery following poor-grade sah: The incidence of delayed improvement and implications for SAH outcome study design. Journal of Neurosurgery. 2013;**119**:606-612

[50] Zhao B, Zhao Y, Tan X, Cao Y, Wu J, Zhong M, et al. Factors and outcomes associated with ultra-early surgery for poor-grade aneurysmal subarachnoid haemorrhage: A multicentre retrospective analysis. BMJ Open. 2015;**e007410**:5

[51] Luo YC, Shen CS, Mao JL, Liang CY, Zhang Q, He ZJ. Ultra-early versus delayed coil treatment for ruptured poor-grade aneurysm. Neuroradiology. 2015;**57**:205-210

[52] Molyneux A, Kerr R, Stratton I, Sandercock P, Clarke M, Shrimpton J, et al. International subarachnoid aneurysm trial (ISAT) of neurosurgical clipping versus endovascular coiling in 2143 patients with ruptured intracranial aneurysms: A randomised trial. Lancet. 2002;**360**:1267-1274

[53] Zhao B, Tan X, Yang H, Li Z, Zheng K, Xiong Y, et al. Endovascular coiling versus surgical clipping for poor-grade ruptured intracranial aneurysms: Postoperative complications and clinical outcome in a multicenter poor-grade aneurysm study. AJNR. American Journal of Neuroradiology. 2016;**37**:873-878

[54] Smith ER, Carter BS, Ogilvy CS. Proposed use of prophylactic decompressive craniectomy in poor-grade aneurysmal subarachnoid hemorrhage patients presenting with associated large sylvian hematomas. Neurosurgery. 2002;**51**:117-124. Discussion 124

[55] Buschmann U, Yonekawa Y, Fortunati M, Cesnulis E, Keller E. Decompressive hemicraniectomy in patients with subarachnoid hemorrhage and intractable intracranial hypertension. Acta Neurochirurgica. 2007;**149**:59-65

[56] Schirmer CM, Hoit DA, Malek AM. Decompressive hemicraniectomy for the treatment of intractable intracranial hypertension after aneurysmal subarachnoid hemorrhage. Stroke. 2007;**38**:987-992

[57] Otani N, Takasato Y, Masaoka H, Hayakawa T, Yoshino Y, Yatsushige H, et al. Surgical outcome following decompressive craniectomy for poor-grade aneurysmal subarachnoid hemorrhage in patients with associated massive intracerebral or sylvian hematomas. Cerebrovascular Diseases. 2008;**26**:612-617

[58] Uozumi Y, Sakowitz O, Orakcioglu B, Santos E, Kentar M, Haux D, et al. Decompressive craniectomy in patients with aneurysmal subarachnoid hemorrhage: A single-center matched-pair analysis. Cerebrovascular Diseases. 2014;**37**:109-115

[59] Guresir E, Schuss P, Vatter H, Raabe A, Seifert V, Beck J. Decompressive craniectomy in subarachnoid hemorrhage. Neurosurgical Focus. 2009;**26**:E4

[60] Dorfer C, Frick A, Knosp E, Gruber A. Decompressive hemicraniectomy after aneurysmal subarachnoid hemorrhage. World Neurosurgery. 2010;**74**:465-471

[61] Zhao B, Zhao Y, Tan X, Cao Y, Wu J, Zhong M, et al. Primary decompressive craniectomy for poor-grade middle cerebral artery aneurysms with associated intracerebral hemorrhage. Clinical Neurology and Neurosurgery. 2015;**133**:1-5

[62] Spetzler RF, McDougall CG, Albuquerque FC, Zabramski JM, Hills NK, Partovi S, et al. The barrow ruptured aneurysm trial: 3-year results. Journal of Neurosurgery. 2013;**119**:146-157

[63] Spetzler RF, McDougall CG, Zabramski JM, Albuquerque FC, Hills NK, Russin JJ, et al. The barrow ruptured aneurysm trial: 6-year results. Journal of Neurosurgery. 2015:**123**:609-617

[64] Zaidi HA, Montoure A, Elhadi A, Nakaji P, McDougall CG, Albuquerque FC, et al. Long-term functional outcomes and predictors of shunt-dependent hydrocephalus after treatment of ruptured intracranial aneurysms in the brat trial: Revisiting the clip vs coil debate. Neurosurgery. 2015;**76**:608-613. Discussion 613-604; quiz 614

[65] Bodily KD, Cloft HJ, Lanzino G, Fiorella DJ, White PM, Kallmes DF. Stent-assisted coiling in acutely ruptured intracranial aneurysms: A qualitative, systematic review of the literature. AJNR - American Journal of Neuroradiology. 2011;**32**:1232-1236

[66] Chung J, Lim YC, Suh SH, Shim YS, Kim YB, Joo JY, et al. Stent-assisted coil embolization of ruptured wide-necked aneurysms in the acute period: Incidence of and risk factors for periprocedural complications. Journal of Neurosurgery. 2014;**121**:4-11

[67] Amenta PS, Dalyai RT, Kung D, Toporowski A, Chandela S, Hasan D, et al. Stent-assisted coiling of wide-necked aneurysms in the setting of acute subarachnoid hemorrhage: Experience. *Neurosurgery*. 2012;**70**:1415-1429. Discussion 1429

[68] Kim DJ, Suh SH, Kim BM, Kim DI, Huh SK, Lee JW. Hemorrhagic complications related to the stent-remodeled coil embolization of intracranial aneurysms. Neurosurgery. 2010;**67**:73-78. Discussion 78-79

[69] Zhao B, Tan X, Yang H, Zheng K, Li Z, Xiong Y, et al. Stent-assisted coiling versus coiling alone of poor-grade ruptured intracranial aneurysms: A multicenter study. Journal of NeuroInterventional Surgery. 2017;**9**:165-168

[70] Tanno Y, Homma M, Oinuma M, Kodama N, Ymamoto T. Rebleeding from ruptured intracranial aneurysms in north eastern province of

Japan. A cooperative study. Journal of the Neurological Sciences. 2007;**258**:11-16

[71] Zhao B, Yang H, Zheng K, Li Z, Xiong Y, Tan X, et al. Predictors of good functional outcomes and mortality in patients with severe rebleeding after aneurysmal subarachnoid hemorrhage. Clinical Neurology and Neurosurgery. 2016;**144**:28-32

[72] Zhao B, Yang H, Zheng K, Li Z, Xiong Y, Tan X, et al. Preoperative and postoperative predictors of long-term outcome after endovascular treatment of poor-grade aneurysmal subarachnoid hemorrhage. Journal of Neurosurgery. 2017;**126**:1764-1771

[73] Howard BM, Barrow DL, et al. Outcomes for patients with poor-grade subarachnoid hemorrhage: To treat or not to treat? *World Neurosurgery*. 2015

[74] Schuss P, Hadjiathanasiou A, Borger V, Wispel C, Vatter H, Guresir E. Poor-grade aneurysmal subarachnoid hemorrhage: Factors influencing functional outcome-a single-center series. World Neurosurgery. 2016;**85**:125-129

[75] Mack WJ, Hickman ZL, Ducruet AF, Kalyvas JT, Garrett MC, Starke RM, et al. Pupillary reactivity upon hospital admission predicts long-term outcome in poor grade aneurysmal subarachnoid hemorrhage patients. Neurocritical Care. 2008;**8**:374-379

[76] Zheng K, Zhong M, Zhao B, Chen SY, Tan XX, Li ZQ, et al. Poor-grade aneurysmal subarachnoid hemorrhage: Risk factors affecting clinical outcomes in intracranial aneurysm patients in a multi-center study. Frontiers in Neurology. 2019;**10**:123

Chapter 9

# Contrast-Induced Nephropathy

*Ahmed Shawky Elserafy and Tarek Abdelsalam*

## Abstract

With the worldwide increase in the incidence of atherosclerotic coronary artery disease, the rate of coronary interventions has increased. One of the serious complications of this procedure is contrast-induced nephropathy (CIN). This complication can lead to poor outcomes, with an increase in morbidity and mortality of patients. The pathophysiology and risk factors for the occurrence of contrast-induced nephropathy are several and interconnected. The most proposed management of this entity is prophylaxis and thus avoidance of its occurrence. We will take a deeper look on the pathophysiology, the mechanisms by which this complication is aggravated, and how to expect and manage such a problem.

**Keywords:** coronary intervention, contrast, nephropathy

## 1. Introduction

Contrast-induced nephropathy (CIN) is a grave complication of angiographic procedures and arises from administration of iodinated contrast media (CM) [1]. CIN is the third most common cause of hospital acquired acute renal injury representing about 12% of the cases. The incidence of CIN varies from 0 to 24% depending on the patient's risk factors [2]. It is generally a transient and reversible state of acute renal failure [3]. However, the development of CIN is linked to a more prolonged hospital stay, an increased morbidity and mortality, and a high healthcare cost. Treatment of CIN is predominantly of supportive nature, consisting of calculated fluid and electrolyte management; however, dialysis may be required in some cases [3].

## 2. Definition

Clinical and experimental studies have used different laboratory parameters to define CIN [4, 5]. Currently, CIN is most commonly defined when either of the following occur within 48 h after contrast administration and persisting for 2–5 days [6, 7]:

- A 25% increase in serum creatinine (SCr) concentration from baseline value

- An absolute increase in SCr of at least 0.5 mg/dL (44.2 μmol/L)



IntechOpen

## 3. Epidemiology

CIN is one of the most significant causes of hospital-acquired acute kidney injury (AKI) [8] and presents about 12% of the cases [9]. It represents the third most common cause after renal hypoperfusion (42%) and postoperative renal injury (18%). The reported incidence of CIN following percutaneous coronary intervention (PCI) lies between 0 and 24%. This depends on the associated risk factors, with the greatest incidence being reported after emergency PCI [10, 11]. A meta-analysis which included 40 studies showed a 6% incidence of CIN following contrast-enhanced computed tomography (CT) [12], 9% following peripheral angiography [3], and 4% following intravenous pyelography [13]. The incidence of CIN is low in patients with normal renal function (0–5%) [14]. However, there is an incidence of 12–27% in patients having preexisting renal impairment [15]. Moreover, in one study, an incidence as high as 50% was found in patients with diabetic nephropathy undergoing coronary angiography despite the use of low-osmolar CM (LOCM) and adequate hydration. Also, up to 15% of them needed dialysis [16]. Development of CIN is associated with a longer duration of hospital stay and an increased morbidity and mortality, in addition to more costs [1, 17]. Elevation of post-PCI serum creatinine may have prognostic significance regardless of the initial kidney functions. In fact, a slight elevation in serum creatinine (25–35 μmol/l) is associated with an increase in 30-day mortality [18]. Furthermore, post-PCI serum creatinine elevation has been reported to be linked to higher 1-year mortality than periprocedural myocardial necrosis [19].

## 4. Risk factors

Mild, transient decreases in GFR occur after contrast administration in nearly all patients. The development of clinically significant acute renal failure depends very much upon the presence or absence of certain risk factors (**Table 1**); factors that increase the incidence of development of CIN are linked to the patient's comorbid conditions, the procedure to be performed, and the nature of the contrast agents [21].

### 4.1 Preexisting renal disease

Preexisting renal disease with an elevated basal level of serum creatinine is the most important risk factor for the occurrence of CIN. The incidence of CIN in patients with preexisting chronic kidney disease is extremely high, ranging from

| Degree of risk | Nonmodifiable risk factors | Modifiable risk factors |
|---|---|---|
| Major | Preexisting renal disease<br>Diabetes mellitus | Osmolality and ionic content of contrast medium<br>Volume of contrast medium administered<br>Repeated exposure to contrast medium |
| Minor | Age<br>Gender<br>Reduced ejection fraction<br>Congestive heart failure<br>Hypertension | Dehydration<br>Myocardial infarction less than 24 h before angiography<br>Circulatory collapse<br>Anemia |

**Table 1.**
*Common risk factors for contrast nephropathy after coronary angiography [20].*

14.8 to 55% [20]. As depicted in a study, despite pre-procedure adequate hydration and the use of nonionic CM, CIN happened in one-third of the 439 patients who underwent PCI and had basal creatinine level more than or equal to 1.8 mg/dl [22]. The higher the basal serum creatinine level, the greater the risk of developing CIN. As seen in a study, if basal serum creatinine level is estimated to be ≤1.2 mg/dl, the risk of development of CIN is just 2% [23]. In patients with values of creatinine in the range of 1.4–1.9 mg/dl, the risk of CIN in comparison with that in the previous group increases fivefold (10.4%) [23]. Regarding patients with baseline serum creatinine more than or equal to 2.0 mg/dl, 62% of them developed CIN [24]. However, baseline creatinine is not reliable enough for the determination of patients who are at risk for CIN. This arises due to the variation on the basis of gender, age, and muscular mass. For instance, a normal serum creatinine value probably correlates with a moderate decrease in renal function. In order to properly evaluate renal function, assessment of creatinine clearance should be done. The direct measurement of the creatinine clearance is not practical to be done; however, its estimation based on the Cockcroft-Gault formula or Modification of Diet in Renal Disease equation can be easily performed. Multiple studies have proven that an estimated glomerular filtration rate (eGFR) of 60 mL/min/1.73 $m^2$ is a cutoff value for considering patients at high risk for the development of CIN. Thus, the estimation of GFR is crucial for CIN risk assessment [25].

### 4.2 Diabetes mellitus

Diabetic patients represent a very important proportion of those undergoing contrast exposures due not only to the prevalence of diabetes in the general population but also the ability of the disease to cause a wide spectrum of diseases which require radiological procedures using contrast media. The incidence of CIN in diabetic patients varies from 5.7 to 29.4% [26]. Importantly, in diabetic patients with preserved renal function and without other risk factors, the rates of CIN are approximately equal to those of a nondiabetic population [27], while clinically important CIN mostly happens in a group of diabetics with preexisting renal impairment [27].

### 4.3 Age

Several studies showed that older age is an independent predictor of CIN [28]. The reasons for higher risk are multifactorial, which encompasses age-related changes in renal function including decreased glomerular filtration rate, renal concentration ability, and tubular secretion. The presence of multi-vessel coronary artery disease, mandating complex more prolonged PCI, combined with more difficult vascular access that results from tortuosity and calcification of the vessels that frequently requires a greater amount of contrast, and therefore represent additional factors of elevated CIN risk in elderly.

### 4.4 Gender

Ovarian hormones can have an influence upon the renin-angiotensin system as well as the renal blood flow. In a retrospective study of 8628 patients who underwent PCI, female sex presented an independent risk predictor of CIN (OR = 1.4, $p < 0.0001$). One-year analyses of outcomes by gender demonstrated a higher mortality rate when compared to males in a cohort of CIN patients (14 vs 10%, $p = 0.05$) [29].

### 4.5 Heart failure

Advanced congestive heart failure (New York Heart Association class III or IV), reduced left ventricular ejection fraction, or any history of congestive heart failure are independent predictors of CIN and contribute to a greater risk in patients who have diabetes or renal disease. The risk arises as a result of decreased renal blood flow due to low cardiac output in those patients. Moreover, the risk is enhanced by this population's use of specific medications such as aspirin, diuretics, and angiotensin converting enzyme (ACE) inhibitors [30].

### 4.6 Anemia

Anemia can cause deterioration of renal ischemia which can be an acceptable explanation for the higher incidence of contrast-induced nephropathy in patients with a lower hematocrit level. A baseline hematocrit value of less than 39% for men and less than 36% for women is considered a risk that leads to a higher incidence of CIN. This relation was investigated in a prospective study of 6773 patients who underwent PCI [31]. A lower basal hematocrit value was an independent risk predictor of CIN; and every 3% decline in basal hematocrit resulted in a significant increase in the occurrence of CIN in patients with and without chronic kidney disease (11 and 23%, respectively). Dangas et al. showed that the basal hematocrit level is an independent risk factor for the occurrence of CIN among patients with chronic kidney disease ($OR = 0.95$, $p < 0.00001$) [17].

### 4.7 Hyperuricemia

Contrast media have a uricosuric effect, which is caused by increased renal tubular secretion of uric acid. Moreover, hyperuricemia is accompanied by an activated renin-angiotensin-aldosterone system, enhanced synthesis of reactive oxygen species, increased endothelin-1, tubular obstruction by uric acid, and an inhibited nitric oxide synthesis that provokes the development of CIN [32].

### 4.8 Hypercholesterolemia

Altered nitric oxide-dependent renal vasodilatation is common in hypercholesterolemia. Hypercholesterolemia enhanced the occurrence of CIN through the reduced production of nitric oxide [24].

### 4.9 Hypovolemia

Hypovolemia leads to active sodium reabsorption, which is an oxygen-dependent process, and increases neurohumoral vasoconstrictive stimuli that can diminish medullary oxygenation. The toxic actions of contrast media on the renal tubular lumen can be exaggerated in hypovolemia. Decreased circulatory volume and renal perfusion augment vasoconstriction of renal vasculature after administration of CM. Volume expansion decreases the activity of the renin-angiotensin system, increases the perfusion of the medulla, and minimizes the elevation in blood viscosity and osmolality. Currently, the most effective preventive measure against the development of CIN is proper hydration [33].

### 4.10 Hypertension

The alteration in intrarenal expression of vasoactive mediators, mainly renin-angiotensin system and nitric oxide, is a common cause that ranks hypertension as an important risk factor for CIN. Impaired nitric oxide-dependent renal vasodilatation is common in individuals who are hypertensive. In addition, a decreased nephron count could predispose hypertensive patients to CIN.

### 4.11 Nephrotoxic drugs

Nephrotoxic drugs that inhibit the vasodilatory effects of prostaglandins make the kidneys extremely vulnerable to the toxic effect of contrast media. Aminoglycosides, sulfonamides, and their combinations with furosemide are very risky. Cyclosporin A may intensify medullary hypoxia, and cisplatin can bind to sulfhydryl groups. Mannitol can increase the metabolic load and the oxygen consumption of the kidney, and amphotericin B can cause the combined effect of mannitol and cyclosporine A. It has been demonstrated that nonselective NSAIDs and selective COX-2 inhibitors decrease the availability of vasodilatory prostaglandins in the kidneys and enhance the vasoconstrictive effect of CM [34].

### 4.12 ACE inhibitors and angiotensin receptor blockers

ACE inhibitors have been identified as a risk factor for CIN because of their ability to reduce renal function. On the contrary, some small studies have shown that the inhibition of angiotensin II can decrease renal vasoconstriction following the injection of contrast media. In a randomized controlled study including 71 patients with diabetes who underwent coronary angiography and randomized to captopril (25 mg thrice daily) or control, there was a significant decrease in CIN in the patients who received captopril compared with the control group (6 vs 29%, respectively, $p < 0.02$) [35]. A randomized controlled study was performed on 80 patients with serum creatinine less than 2 mg/dl who underwent coronary angiography where captopril was administered in 48 patients preceding coronary angiography. CIN occurred in five patients (10.4%) in the captopril group, compared with only one patient (3.1%) in the control group ($p = 0.02$) [36]. We can say that holding ACE inhibitor or ARB use before coronary angiography is to be considered.

### 4.13 Acute myocardial infarction

A study by Rihal and his colleagues pointed that acute myocardial infarction occurring within 24 h before administration of the CM is a risk predictor to CIN ($OR = 1.85$, $p = 0.0006$). This study showed that CIN represents a frequent complication in acute myocardial infarction. This can occur, as well, in patients with a normal baseline renal function [30]. In 2082 percutaneous interventions for acute myocardial infarction, a more than sevenfold (3.2 vs 23.3%) elevation in 1-year mortality in patients who acquired CIN was acknowledged [37].

### 4.14 Contrast medium-related risk factors

#### *4.14.1 Increased dose of contrast medium*

Based upon multiple sources, the relatively unhazardous cutoff point of contrast amount ranges from 70 mL up to 220 mL. However, very small doses as much as 20–30 mL are capable of inducing CIN. In a study that included patients performing coro¬nary angiography, each 100 mL of contrast medium administered was linked to a significant increase of 12% in the risk of CIN ($OR = 1.12$, $p = 0.02$) [32]. A clear accepted dose is four times the creatinine clearance.

#### 4.14.2 High-osmolar and ionic CM

Most side effects attributable to contrast media are linked to its hypertonicity. Currently, four main types of contrast media are used in practice today, including nonionic low-osmolar, ionic low-osmolar, nonionic iso-osmolar, and ionic high-osmolar contrast media. In a large study which compared the nonionic low-osmolality agent iohexol to the ionic high-osmolality agent meglumine/sodium diatrizoate in patients with preexisting renal impairment undergoing angiography, patients with renal impairment who received diatrizoate were 3.3 times more liable to develop CIN in comparison with those receiving iohexol [38]. NEPHRIC trial is a randomized, prospective study that made a comparison between the nonionic iso-osmolar CM iodixanol with the nonionic low-osmolar CM iohexol in 129 patients with renal impairment and diabetes undergoing coronary or aortofemoral angiography. The incidence of CIN was 3% in the iodixanol group and 26% in the iohexol group ($p = 0.002$) [39]. In one other randomized study, the incidence of CIN provoked by iodixanol and iohexol was compared in 124 patients with basal creatinine level >1.7 mg/dl. The incidence of CIN was 3.7% in iodixanol group and 10% in iohexol group ($p > 0.05$) [17]. In addition, CM are classified as ionic and nonionic. A randomized trial of 1196 patients performing coronary angiography showed that nonionic CM lowered the incidence of CIN in patients with preexisting renal impairment [38]. In high-risk patients, it is better to avoid the use the high-osmolar and ionic CM to lower the risk of CIN.

## 5. Pathophysiology

No definitive causative has been defined as regards the pathogenesis of CIN in the literature. The most accepted theory for the development of CIN following contrast administration relies upon the vasoconstriction of the vessels in the renal medulla leading to reduced oxygen delivery [40]. Reduced oxygen delivery and prolonged vasoconstriction leads to enhanced production of oxygen-free radicals like hydrogen peroxide and superoxide leading to increased damage [41]. Other suggested causes of this condition are elevated blood viscosity, reperfusion injury, direct toxic damage to the cells, and the release of dopamine, angiotensin II, and vasopressin. These factors induce further vasoconstriction and damage the renal function [42]. The use of supportive therapy in critically ill patients, for instance, the mechanical ventilation and inotropic drugs, and the variable health risks this group of patients have as anemia and sepsis have been shown to increase additional kidney damage resulting from vasoconstriction and hypoxia [43].

### 5.1 Regional hypoxia as a cause of contrast-induced nephropathy (CIN)

Renal perfusion is very high in the cortex. The medullary portions are maintained at the border of hypoxia such that $pO2$ levels can be as low as 20 mmHg [44]. This is the price for maintaining the countercurrent mechanism used for the control of urine excretion. A vulnerable kidney region is the deeper part of the outer medulla, an area far from the vasa recta which supply the renal medulla with blood. It is there where the thick ascending limbs of the loop of Henle encounter hypoxic damage [45]. The cause for the vulnerability of the outer medullary portion of the nephron is the relatively higher oxygen needs due to salt reabsorption. The addition of contrast media to the medium augments the hypoxic injury imposed upon this region by increasing the renal vascular resistance, as seen in the rat model [46]. A second factor that has been postulated to mediate CIN is an elevated oxygen demand due to an enhanced workload in the tubular cells. First, there is a temporary increase in GFR that follows giving contrast media [47], and second, osmotic diuresis may reduce the para-cellular absorption of the proximal tubular cells, causing a greater load of NaCl that has to be absorbed in the distal tubules. Liss et al. [48] have shown that contrast media can enhance medullary blood flow to the kidney, although pO2 decreases, which is supported also by a study of Heyman et al. [49]. These two studies suggest that an increased oxygen demand has taken place following contrast media injection. Local kidney hypoxia can be augmented by the systemic effects of some contrast media, such as transiently diminished cardiac output [50] and abnormal pulmonary ventilation-perfusion relationship [51]. Also, the amount of oxygen delivered to the peripheral tissues might be impaired, since contrast media can increase oxygen affinity of hemoglobin [52]. If renal outer medullary hypoxia causes CIN, the blockade of the transporters in this portion of the nephron must have helpful effects on its prevention. The major part of the transport that occurs in the medullary thick ascending limb is the $Na-K^+-2Cl^-$ cotransporter, which, as mentioned above, is blocked by furosemide. Blocking this transport would significantly decrease the local oxygen consumption.

### 5.2 Radiocontrast-mediated changes in renal blood supply

Renal blood flow and intrarenal microcirculation are markedly altered by contrast medium (CM) [53]. The extent and distribution of renal hemodynamic changes depends on the species investigated as well as on the type, volume, and rate of contrast administration. Moreover, renal hemodynamic effects of CM gravely depend on the hydration state and on additional predisposing factors that may have an effect on the renal circulation and the tone of the renal vasculature, such as chronic renal disease, diabetes mellitus, senility, and inflammation. In an early study in dogs subjected to a high-osmolar CM, total renal blood flow was transiently enhanced for 5–15 min, followed by a decline by 25% below baseline, reaching beyond a couple of hours [54]. In healthy humans, renal blood flow fell 8% over 30 min after the intravenous administration of conventional doses of CM [53]. On the contrary, in patients with chronic kidney disease undergoing coronary angiography, a transient short augmentation of renal blood flow was followed by a dramatic 40% decline, lasting for more than 3 h [54].

### 5.3 Cytotoxic effects on renal tubular cells

Investigations performed in vitro on cell lines are used to assess the renal tubular cell function or damage. A porcine cell line of renal proximal tubules, LLC-PK1, was used by Hardiek et al. [55] to investigate the occurrence of CIN. An effect on apoptosis was not elucidated, even though proliferation was impaired. Diminished proliferation will have a hazardous effect on renal function with a delay of hours to days, which may help in explaining the course of CIN. Independent of the contrast media used, tubular cell damage can occur. A more specific distortion of proximal tubular function seems to be a perturbation of mitochondrial enzymatic activity and mitochondrial membrane potential [56]. The degree of mitochondrial enzymatic activity impairment depends mainly on two features of the contrast media: the ionic nature as well as the molecular structure. Remarkably, low-osmolar contrast media had the least observed effects, followed by the iso-osmolar contrast media. Ionic compounds showed the most deleterious effects [56]. In the distal tubule, contrast media may trigger apoptotic effects in the cells, as depicted in the Madin-Darby canine kidney (MDCK) cell line model [57].

### 5.4 Generation of oxygen-free radicals

Among the often-discussed mechanisms, superoxide and other reactive oxygen species (ROS) have been discussed to be an aggravating factor for CIN. Oxygen free radicals are endogenously produced, and levels can increase during oxidative stress. The commonest oxygen radicals are superoxide ($O_2^-$), hydrogen peroxide ($H_2O_2$), and hydroxyl radical ($OH^-$) [58]. $O_2^-$ and $OH^-$ are more reactive in comparison with $H_2O_2$, which is not a radical but shows greater membrane permeability. $O_2^-$ rapidly scavenges nitric oxide (NO) and could diminish NO activity in the renal vessels. Since NO decreases oxygen consumption, it is considerable to speculate that decreased (scavenged) NO levels in diabetes increases oxygen consumption, thus leading to reduced partial oxygen pressure values with consequences for endothelial-epithelial structure and function. ROS can play a role in the effects of various vasoconstrictors that are considered necessary for the development of CIN. Because ROS are extracellular signaling molecules, they can have a crucial role in mediating the effects of vasoconstrictors, such as thromboxane A2, angiotensin II, adenosine, endothelin (ET)-1, and norepinephrine. The adverse effects of CM on kidney function can therefore involve the generation of ROS, for example, via adenosine formation. This idea is supported by experiments in which the generation of ROS was inhibited by allopurinol or the amount of ROS was decreased by $O_2^-$ dismutase. In these models, CM-induced reductions in glomerular filtration rate are attenuated [59].

## 6. Preventive measures against contrast-induced nephropathy

### 6.1 Adequate hydration

#### *6.1.1 Intravenous hydration*

Adequate hydration for patients performing CM-enhanced imaging studies was suggested approximately 40 years ago [30]. The beneficial effects of hydration were initially reported in the early 1980s by studies that compared outcomes of hydrated patients with historical controls [60, 61]. These reports were supported by the first RCT in 1994, concluding that patients with chronic renal impairment benefit better from intravenous (0.45%) saline administration (for 12 h before and 12 h after angiography) in comparison with saline plus mannitol or furosemide [62]. Since then, multiple RCTs have assured the benefit of intravenous normal saline (0.9%) hydration that is started 12 h preceding to 12 h after CM injection [63–65] in the prevention against CIN over 0.45% saline [65] or a fluid bolus (300 mL) during CM administration only [66]. The rate of infusion was reported as 1 mL/kg/h [67]. CM safety committee endorse a regime of intravenous infusion of 1.0–1.5 mL/kg/h for at least 6 h before and after CM administration [68].

#### *6.1.2 Oral hydration*

In order to overcome the limitations of outpatient intravenous hydration, investigators have assessed the use of pre-procedure oral hydration followed by post-procedure intravenous hydration in patients who are admitted for catheterization on the day of procedure. In an RCT on patients with mild-to-moderate renal insufficiency, Taylor et al. reported an effective protocol which includes pre-angiography oral hydration (1000 mL clear fluids over 10 h) that is followed by 6 h of intravenous hydration (0.45% normal saline solution at 300 mL/h) that starts just before CM exposure [69]. The results were comparative with overnight intravenous hydration (0.45% normal saline solution at 75 mL/h for both 12 h before and after angiography). A limitation of this protocol can be high infusion rate (300 mL/h) post-procedure for the patients having left ventricular impairment. Trivedi and his colleagues demonstrated different results as they observed that patients with unrestricted oral hydration had more opportunities of acute renal impairment compared to those receiving normal saline for 24 h (at a rate of 1 mL/kg/h) beginning 12 h before the scheduled catheterization ($p = 0.005$) [68]. In this study, however, there was no set protocol for oral hydration for patients to follow that probably could have contributed to its ineffectiveness. Later, Dussol et al. randomized 312 patients with chronic kidney disease (CKD) to receive either per oral sodium chloride (NaCl) (dose: 1 g/10 kg bodyweight/day for 2 days before the procedure), intravenous normal saline 15 mL/kg for the 6 h preceding the procedure (control arm), theophylline, or furosemide in addition to the treatment given to patients in the control arm [70]. Oral saline hydration was found to have comparative effectiveness as intravenous saline hydration as regards preventing CI-AKI.

#### *6.1.3 Sodium bicarbonate-based hydration*

The acidic PH promotes free radical production (which is found in tubular urine) [71], while elevated pH of normal extracellular fluid inhibits it [72, 73]. Since CM administration escalates the oxidative stress and increases the generation of free radicals and reactive oxygen species (ROS), alkalinizing renal tubular fluid with bicarbonate appears to be a logical strategy to protect against renal injury [74]. As a result of active reabsorption, bicarbonate concentration in the renal tubules lowers (to about 6 mEq/L), and the tubular fluid pH is approximately 6.5 near the end of the proximal tubule in the renal medulla [75]. In the descending loop of Henle, water and chloride are passively reabsorbed. This elevates urine pH to ~7.4 at the tip of the papilla, and this part is spared from contrast nephropathy [76], which suggests that higher pH is protective. Also important is the observation that outer medulla is the most susceptible to CIN [62] and has acidic pH [72] that promotes activity of ROS. Superoxide, a ROS generated by ischemia, might react with medullary NO to produce the potent oxidant peroxynitrite [73]. At physiologic concentrations, bicarbonate scavenges peroxynitrite and other ROSs produced from NO [74]. Thus, several oxidant mechanisms of renal injury might be avoided using sodium bicarbonate. The useful effect of higher proximal tubular pH is approved by a report that acetazolamide, a carbonic-anhydrase inhibitor which blocks proximal tubular bicarbonate reabsorption, is protective in contrast-induced renal failure [77]. Merten et al. reported first study on the use of sodium bicarbonate in humans as a nephron-protective agent [78]. Patients received 154 mEq/l of either NaCl (in 5% dextrose $H_2O$) or sodium bicarbonate (in dextrose $H_2O$), as a bolus of 3 mL/kg/h for 1 h before iopamidol contrast, followed by an infusion of 1 mL/kg/h for 6 h after the procedure. CIN occurred in 8 patients (13.6%) infused with NaCl but in only 1 (1.7%) of those receiving sodium bicarbonate ($p = 0.02$). Afterwards, many RCTs have compared the efficacy of sodium bicarbonate with saline hydration regarding the prophylaxis against CIN. These have been reviewed in multiple meta-analysis [79–82], which concluded that sodium bicarbonate-based saline hydration is more efficacious to saline hydration only.

#### *6.1.4 Pharmacological prophylaxis*

Various drugs have been assessed as prophylactic nephroprotective agents against contrast-induced acute kidney injury (CI-AKI) such as N-acetylcysteine

(NAC) [36, 83], statins [84, 85], ascorbic acid [76, 86], and theophylline [87]. However, only statins have been approved for the prevention against the occurrence of CIN. Currently, the CM safety committee recommends the withdrawal of nephrotoxic drugs before CM administration [85].

### *6.1.5 N-Acetylcysteine (NAC)*

NAC gives protection against CIN by improving the body's antioxidant abilities [88]. In vitro, NAC does this efficiently by scavenging hypochlorous acid as well as reacting with hydroxyl radicals [89]. In vivo due to its extensive degradation, it is likely that any antioxidant effect it exerts would be indirect, most probably by inducing glutathione synthesis. Different studies have suggested that NAC guards against glutathione depletion [90, 91] and elevates renal glutathione levels [92]; the latter has been demonstrated to result in the reduction of renal injury in ischemia reperfusion models [93, 94] and recently in CIN [95, 96]. Glutathione cannot enter the cell; instead, it must be formed inside the cell from glycine, glutamate, and cysteine [97]. Cysteine offers the active HS group which is crucial for the glutathione synthesis and thus is the rate-limiting factor in this process. NAC after deacylation produces cysteine that passes to the renal cells and serves as a precursor for glutathione synthesis. It can also produce vasodilator effects [98]. By ameliorating contrast-induced vasoconstriction, NAC can produce its nephron-protective role [99]. Increase in the medullary blood flow with NAC has also been demonstrated [100, 101]. The first clinical use of NAC for CIN was reported by Tepel et al. [83]. Eighty-three patients who had chronic renal impairment were randomly planned either to take oral NAC (600 mg twice daily) and 0.45% saline intravenously, before and after administration of the CM, or to receive placebo and saline. NAC-receiving patients had lower incidence of CIN. Since then numerous studies have assessed the role of NAC against CIN. Those studies have been done mainly in patients undergoing coronary angiography [102]. Some 17 meta-analyses have been published as regards this subject [76, 86, 87, 103–116], 10 that approve its use (most of which were published early on). Most of these meta-analyses reported vast heterogeneity that makes it difficult to make clinical treatment recommendations relying on the provided data. Recently, results of the largest multicenter RCT of 2308 patients called "Acetylcysteine for Contrast-Induced Nephropathy Trial" (ACT) have been published [36]. It randomized patients in 46 centers in Brazil, to take 1200 mg of oral NAC or placebo twice daily for 2 doses before and after the procedure. Intravenous hydration with normal saline, 1 mL/kg/h, from 6–12 h before to 6–12 h after angiography, was strongly recommended. NAC was not able to significantly reduce the incidence of CIN (12.7% in the NAC group and 12.7% in the control group, $p = 0.97$) [117].

### *6.1.6 Ascorbic acid*

Ascorbic acid serves as an antioxidant [118]. It does this via reacting with most biologically relevant free radicals and oxidants such as superoxide ions and hydroxyl ion [119]. It donates an electron to devastating oxidizing radicals [120]; this one-electron oxidation leads to the formation of $AH^-$ the ascorbyl radical also called semidehydroascorbic acid [121]. Consequently, the reactive free radical is reduced [122]. Ascorbic acid has been reported to result in vasodilatation in coronary [123] and brachial arteries [124]. Thus, vitamin C can have favorable effects on vascular dilatation, through its antioxidant actions on nitric oxide, but these findings are not consistent [125]. Through which pathway vitamin C may offer nephron protection against CIN is still currently uninvestigated. The first clinical use of ascorbic acid for CIN prevention was reported by Spargias and his colleagues [116]. Two hundred and thirty-one patients were summoned and randomized to obtain either 3 g of ascorbic acid supplied in chewable tablets or placebo at least 2 h prior to the beginning of the required procedure. This was followed by 2 g of ascorbic acid or placebo the night and the morning post-procedure. Intravenous hydration with normal saline at a rate of 50–125 mL/h was started in every patient till at least 6 h post-procedure. Incidence of CIN was less in ascorbic acid group (9%) and 20% in control group ($p = 0.02$). A considerable change in the antioxidant state was noticed in the group treated with ascorbic acid. Since then various RCTs have been performed [126, 127]. Pooled analysis of these trials assumed that patients who receive ascorbic acid have 33% less risk of CIN in comparison with patients receiving placebo or alternative pharmacological therapy (RR: 0.67 (95% CI: 0.46–0.96), $p = 0.03$) [100]. This indicates that ascorbic acid provides effective nephron protection in the face of CIN and may form a part of efficient prophylactic pharmacological regimens. However, the utilization of ascorbic acid has not yet been recommended by the contrast media safety committee.

### 6.2 Statins

Statins maintain nitric oxide formation, lower oxidative stress, and beneficially affect the endothelial function [101]. In one retrospective study of more than 1,000 patients with renal impairment undergoing coronary angiography, the risk of CIN was markedly decreased in patients who are receiving a statin before the procedure [128]. Another study of more than 29,000 patient recorded in a percutaneous cardiac intervention registry demonstrated that patients who received statins before the procedure had both a lower CIN incidence ($p < 0.0001$) and nephropathy that required dialysis ($p < 0.03$) [181]. Further studies looking into the benefit from statins are warranted [129].

#### *6.2.1 High-dose versus low-dose statins*

High-dose statin therapy may be theoretically more efficacious regarding CIN prevention as a result of acute suppression of inflammatory chemokines [130]. Xie and his colleagues investigated the potency of high-dose statins (simvastatin 80mg, atorvastatin 40 and 80 mg) compared with low-dose statins (simvastatin 20 mg, atorvastatin 10 and 20mg) and revealed that high-dose statins lowered the incidence of CIN [131]. These results were backed up by a recent meta-analysis which showed that high-dose statins (atorvastatin 80 mg, simvastatin 80 mg) in comparison with low-dose statins (atorvastatin 10 and 20 mg, simvastatin 20 mg) in patients having acute coronary syndromes resulted in a relative risk ratio for CIN of 0.46 (4.5 vs 10.2%, $p = 0.004$); however, it was not of considerable significance among patients performing elective procedures [132]. However, high-dose statins are guideline recommended medications to lower the risk of CIN.

#### *6.2.2 Theophylline*

Adenosine has been implicated to be a responsible factor for mediating CM-enhanced renal vasoconstriction [133–135]: hence the use of adenosine antagonists appears logical [136]. Theophylline and aminophylline have been often used to measure their efficacy as adenosine receptor antagonists in guarding against contrast-induced acute kidney injury (CI-AKI). Various randomized trials have used theophylline [20, 137, 138]. A meta-analysis of those studies guided to the fact that theophylline considerably lowers the risk of CIN (RR: 0.48; 95% CI: 0.26–0.89;

p = 0.02). There was moderate heterogeneity that suggests cautious interpretation of these results. Furthermore, patients with baseline renal insufficiency did not show any benefit from theophylline.

*6.2.3 Allopurinol*

This drug is a xanthine oxidase inhibitor which may hamper the fall in the GFR following CM exposure by limiting oxygen free radical production, inhibiting adenine nucleotide degradation, and limiting the vasodilator reaction to intrarenal adenosine. A trial that included 159 patients randomized patients performing coronary angiography procedures to allopurinol (300 mg orally) with hydration or hydration alone, showed that allopurinol can guard against CIN in high-risk patients receiving CM [139]. However, these effects of allopurinol in the prevention of CIN need further larger studies.

*6.2.4 Dopamine*

Dopamine (in a renal dose 0.5–2.5 μg/kg/min) has a vasodilator action on the renal vasculature and has an ability to increase renal blood flow and GFR with a potential benefit in the prevention of CIN. Trials with positive results were small, not randomized and with questionable endpoints [140]. On the contrary, negative trials were large, randomized, controlled, and with adequate statistical power [141]. Thus, the usage of dopamine in guarding against CIN is no longer recommended.

*6.2.5 Targeted renal therapy*

A suggested theory for failure of various drugs used for kidney protection is that systemically administered drugs may not achieve adequate drug level in the renal vasculature in order to be successful regarding the prevention of CIN. This has led to the technique of direct infusion of a drug in a selective manner into the kidneys via the renal arteries, which is known as targeted renal therapy (TRT). This should have the ability of decreasing the systemic side effects of that drug. Fenoldopam is a dopamine-1 agonist that acts as a vasodilator and thus has a potential to attenuate the vasoconstriction induced by CM in the renal vessels. Although it was not possible to demonstrate its benefit in reducing the incidence of CIN [142], it was observed that a large number of patients could not tolerate low doses of fenoldopam as a result of drug-induced hypotension, which is itself a risk predictor of CIN. Employing TRT, selective bilateral renal artery catheterization may be performed for localized drug delivery. In a pilot study on patients undergoing endovascular aneurysm repair, Benephit PV Infusion System (Flow Medica, Inc., Fremont, CA, USA) was used for selective catheterization of both renal arteries through brachial artery puncture. There was no episode of hypotension, thus every patient received fenoldopam at a rate of 0.4 μg/kg/min for the duration of the aneurysm repair [143]. If the pigtail catheter is inserted in the aorta just over the level of the renal artery avoiding selective catheterization, this appears to be a simple way but would lead to considerable systemic drug effects as a result of infusion of the drug into the systemic circulation [143]. The safety and performance of TRT were also assessed by retrospective analysis of 285 patients who received fenoldopam via TRT, as a part of "The Benephit System Renal Infusion Therapy (Be-RITe)" registry [144]. Benephit Infusion System (Flow Medica, Inc., Fremont, CA, USA) was used. Bilateral renal artery cannulation achieved success in 94.2%, with a mean cannulation time of 2 min. Incidence of CIN was 71% less than predicted, with the greatest benefit in patients with highest risk of CIN. Prospective studies and RCTs are therefore required in order to assess real ability of this technique.

### 6.2.6 *Ischemic preconditioning*

Ischemic preconditioning includes exposure to short episodes of ischemia followed by reperfusion to make the target organ prepared against the main ischemic insult. If the site of generation of these short episodes of ischemic reperfusion is remote from the site of target organ, it is called remote ischemic preconditioning. This technique has been used with only variable success in offering myocardial and renal protection in cardiovascular medicine [145–151]. Results of an RCT propose usefulness from remote ischemic preconditioning in preventing CIN [152]. The likely usefulness may arise from its capability to attenuate the CM-induced ischemia reperfusion injury. Recently, ischemic preconditioning has lost its credibility as it was unable to translate successful results in laboratories into clinical practice [153].

## 7. Sequelae

Patients who develop CIN have greater complications, a worse prognosis, more serious long-term outcomes, and longer duration of hospital stay, which result in elevated medical costs [154, 155]. Less than 0.5–2% of patients who develop CIN require dialysis [156]. Those requiring dialysis are more likely to exhibit serious short- and long-term outcomes. Nearly 30% of those patients experience chronic renal impairment [154]. CIN may also be linked to an increased mortality which is independent of other risk factors [157]. Hospital death rates in such patients have been reported as 36% and the 2-year survival rate as only 19% [158, 159]. Levy et al. compared 181 inpatients that developed CIN with matched control patients who did not develop it; both groups underwent contrast-related procedures [156]. The mortality rate in the control group was 7%, compared to 34% in the CIN group. In another study of 7230 patients who underwent percutaneous coronary interventions, patients who developed CIN had more common myocardial infarctions, more hospital stays, and higher 1-year mortality rates compared to those without CIN. CIN patients are more likely to have target vessel revascularization after 1 year, bypass surgery, bleeding which mandates transfusion, and various vascular complications [160]. Patients who undergo a primary percutaneous intervention for acute myocardial infarction and the procedure complicates by CIN were reported to be significantly more likely to have major complications within hospital admission such as acute pulmonary edema, the need for pacemaker insertion, cardiogenic shock, and respiratory failure [160]. Patients with renal insufficiency are at more significant risk of developing atherosclerosis [19]. Actually, following a contrast procedure, a rise in serum creatinine is a more significant indicator of late mortality compared to an elevated creatine kinase-MB isoenzyme [160].

## 8. Conclusion

Contrast-induced nephropathy is a not an uncommon sequela of coronary angioplasty. It can lead to increased morbidity and mortality. One should be aware of the risk factors that increase its incidence and thus limit the amount of contrast so as to avoid such a deleterious complication. Prevention is better than treatment in this case.

## Author details

Ahmed Shawky Elserafy* and Tarek Abdelsalam
Cardiology Department, Ain Shams University, Cairo, Egypt

*Address all correspondence to: ahmedshawkyelserafy@med.asu.edu.eg

## References

[1] McCullough PA, Wolyn R, Rocher LL, Levin RN, O'Neill WW. Acute renal failure after coronary intervention: Incidence, risk factors, and relationship to mortality. The American Journal of Medicine. 1997;**103**:368-375

[2] Perrin T, Descombes E, Cook S. Contrast-induced nephropathy in invasive cardiology. Swiss Medical Weekly. 2012;**142**:w13608

[3] McCullough PA, Adam A, Becker CR, Avidson C, Lameire N, Stacul F, et al. Epidemiology and prognostic implications of contrast-induced nephropathy. The American Journal of Cardiology. 2006;**98**:5-13

[4] Costa N. Understanding contrast media. Journal of Infusion Nursing. 2004;**27**(5):302-312

[5] Bettmann MA. Contrast medium-induced nephropathy: Critical review of the existing clinical evidence. Nephrology, Dialysis, Transplantation. 2005;**20**(Suppl1):2-17

[6] Maddox TG. Adverse reactions to contrast material: Recognition, prevention, and treatment. American Family Physician. 2002;**66**(7):1229-1234

[7] McCullough PA, Stacul F, Davidson C, et al. Overview. Contrast-induced nephropathy: Clinical insights and practical guidance. A report from the CIN consensus working panel. The American Journal of Cardiology. 2006;**98**(6A):2-4

[8] Cruz DN, Goh CY, Marenzi G, Corradi V, Ronco C, Perazella MA. Renal replacement therapies for prevention of radiocontrast-induced nephropathy: A systematic review. The American Journal of Medicine. 2012;**125**:66-78.11

[9] Hou SH, Bushinsky DA, Wish JB, Cohen JJ, Harrington JT. Hospital acquired renal insufficiency: A prospective study. The American Journal of Medicine. 1983;**74**:243-248

[10] Bolognese L, Falsini G, Schwenke C, Grotti S, Limbruno U, Liistro F, et al. Impact of iso-osmolar versus low-osmolar contrast agents on contrast-induced nephropathy and tissue reperfusion in unselected patients with ST-segment elevation myocardial infarction undergoing primary percutaneous coronary intervention (from the Contrast Media and Nephrotoxicity Following Primary Angioplasty for Acute Myocardial Infarction [CONTRAST-AMI] Trial). American Journal of Cardiology. 2012;**109**:67-74

[11] Chen SL, Zhang J, Yei F, Zhu Z, Liu Z, Lin S, et al. Clinical outcomes of contrast-induced nephropathy in patients undergoing percutaneous coronary intervention: A prospective, multicenter, randomized study to analyze the effect of hydration and acetylcysteine. International Journal of Cardiology. 2008;**126**:407-413

[12] Kooiman J, Pasha SM, Zondag W, Sijpkens YW, van der Molen AJ, Huisman MV, et al. Meta-analysis: Serum creatinine changes following contrast enhanced CT imaging. European Journal of Radiology. 2012;**81**:2554-2561

[13] Karlsberg RP, Dohad SY, Sheng R. Contrast-induced acute kidney injury (CI-AKI) following intra-arterial administration of iodinated contrast media. Journal of Nephrology. 2010;**23**:658-666

[14] Chuang FR, Chen TC, Wang IK, Chuang CH, Chang HW, Ting-Yu Chiou T, et al. Comparison of iodixanol and iohexol in patients undergoing intravenous pyelography: A prospective controlled study. Renal Failure. 2009;**31**:181-188

[15] Morcos SK, Thomsen HS, Webb JA. Contrast media induced nephrotoxicity: A consensus report. Contrast Media Safety Committee of the European Society of Urogenital Radiology (ESUR). European Radiology. 1999;**9**:1602-1613

[16] Rudnick MR, Goldfarb S, Wexler L, Ludbrook PA, Murphy MJ, Halpern EF, et al. Nephrotoxicity of ionic and nonionic contrast media in 1196 patients: A randomized trial. The Iohexol Cooperative Study. Kidney International. 1995;**47**:254-261

[17] Dangas G, Iakovou I, Nikolsky E, Aymong ED, Mintz GS, Kipshidze NN, et al. Contrast-induced nephropathy after percutaneous coronary interventions in relation to chronic kidney disease and hemodynamic variables. The American Journal of Cardiology. 2005;**95**:13-19

[18] Lindsay J, Canos DA, Apple S, Pinnow E, Aggrey GK, Pichard AD. Causes of acute renal dysfunction after percutaneous coronary intervention and comparison of late mortality rates with postprocedure rise of creatine kinase-MB versus rise of serum creatinine. The American Journal of Cardiology. 2004;**94**:786-789

[19] Poukkanen M, Wilkman E, Vaara ST, et al. Hemodynamic variables and progression of acute kidney injury in critically ill patients with severe sepsis in Finnish intensive care units. Critical Care. 2013;**57**(7):863-872

[20] Katholi RE, Taylor GJ. Nephrotoxicity from contrast media: Attenuation with theophylline. Radiology. 1995;**195**:17-22

[21] Bakris GL, Lass N, Gaber AO, et al. Radiocontrast medium-induced declines in renal function: A role for oxygen free radicals. The American Journal of Physiology. 1990;**258**:115-120

[22] Gruberg L, Mehran R, Dangas G, et al. Acute renal failure requiring dialysis after percutaneous coronary interventions. Catheterization and Cardiovascular Interventions. 2001;**52**:409-416

[23] Hall KA, Wong RW, Hunter GC, et al. Contrast-induced nephrotoxicity: The effects of vasodilator therapy. The Journal of Surgical Research. 1992;**53**:317-320

[24] Yang DW, Jia RH, Yang DP, Ding GH, Huang CX. Dietary hypercholesterolemia aggravates contrast media-induced nephropathy. Chinese Medical Journal. 2004;**117**(4):542-546

[25] Levey AS, Bosch JP, Lewis JB, et al. A more accurate method to estimate glomerular filtration rate from serum creatinine: A new prediction equation. Modification of diet in renal disease study group. Annals of Internal Medicine. 1999;**130**:461-470

[26] Nikolsky E, Mehran R, Turcot D, et al. Impact of chronic kidney disease on prognosis of patients with diabetes mellitus treated with percutaneous coronary intervention. The American Journal of Cardiology. 2004;**94**:300-305

[27] Lasser EC, Lyon SG, Berry CC. Reports on contrast media reactions: Analysis of data from reports to the US Food and Drug Administration. Radiology. 1997;**203**:605-610

[28] Berns AS. Nephrotoxicity of contrast media. Kidney International. 1989;**36**:730-740

[29] Iakovou I, Dangas G, Mehran R, Lansky AJ, Ashby DT, Fahy M, et al. Impact of gender on the incidence and outcome of contrast-induced nephropathy after percutaneous coronary intervention. The Journal of Invasive Cardiology. 2003;**15**(1):18-22

[30] Rihal CS, Textor SC, Grill DE, Berger PB, Ting HH, Best PJ, et al. Incidence and prognostic importance of acute renal failure after percutaneous coronary intervention. Circulation. 2002;**105**(105):2259-2264

[31] Nikolsky E, Mehran R, Lasic Z, Mintz GS, Lansky AJ, Na Y, et al. Low hematocrit predicts contrast-induced nephropathy after percutaneous coronary interventions. Kidney International. 2005;**67**(2):706-713

[32] Toprak O, Cirit M, Esi E, Postaci N, Yesil M, Bayata S. Hyperuricemia as a risk factor for contrast-induced nephropathy in patients with chronic kidney disease. Catheterization and Cardiovascular Interventions. 2007;**67**(2):227-235

[33] Toprak O, Cirit M. Investigating the volume status before contrast nephropathy studies. Nephrology, Dialysis, Transplantation. 2005;**20**(2):464

[34] Bartholomew BA, Harjai KJ, Dukkipati S, Boura JA, Yerkey MW, Glazier S, et al. Impact of nephropathy after percutaneous coronary intervention and a method for risk stratification. The American Journal of Cardiology. 2004;**93**(12):1515-1519

[35] Gupta RK, Kapoor A, Tewari S, Sinha N, Sharma RK. Captopril for preventing of contrast-induced nephropathy in diabetic patients: A randomized study. Indian Heart Journal. 1999;**51**(5):521-526

[36] Berwanger O. Acetylcysteine for prevention of renal outcomes in patients undergoing coronary and peripheral vascular angiography: Main results from the randomized acetylcysteine for contrast-induced nephropathy trial (ACT). Circulation. 2011;**124**(11):1250-1259

[37] Toprak O, Cirit M, Bayata S, Aslan SL, Sarioglu F, Cetinkaya GS. Is there any relationship between left ventricul ejection fraction and contrast induced nephropathy? Türkiye Klinikleri Journal of Medical Sciences. 2003;**23**(2):104-107

[38] Sadeghi HM, Stone GW, Grines CL, Mehran R, Dixon SR, Lansky AJ, et al. Impact of renal insufficiency in patients undergoing primary angioplasty for acute myocardial infarction. Circulation. 2003;**108**(22):2769-2775

[39] Rich MW, Crecelius CA. Incidence, risk factors, and clinical course of acute renal insufficiency after cardiac catheterization in patients 70 years of age or older. A prospective study. Archives of Internal Medicine. 1990;**150**(6):1237-1242

[40] Brezis M, Rosen S. Hypoxia of the renal medulla—Its implications for disease. The New England Journal of Medicine. 1995;**332**:647-655

[41] Brezis M, Rosen S, Silva P, Epstein FH. Selective vulnerability of the medullary thick ascending limb to anoxia in the isolated perfused rat kidney. The Journal of Clinical Investigation. 1984;**73**:182-190

[42] Heyman SN, Brezis M, Reubinoff CA, et al. Acute renal failure with selective medullary injury in the rat. The Journal of Clinical Investigation. 1988;**82**:401-412

[43] Arakawa K, Suzuki H, Naitoh M, et al. Role of adenosine in the renal responses to contrast medium. Kidney International. 1996;**49**:1199-1206

[44] Heyman SN, Goldfarb M, Carmeli F, et al. Effect of radiocontrast agents on intrarenal nitric oxide (NO) and NO synthase activity. Experimental Nephrology. 1998;**6**:557-562

[45] Dawson P. Cardiovascular effects of contrast agents. The American Journal of Cardiology. 1989;**64**:2-9

[46] Neagley SR, Vought MB, Weidner WA, Zwillich CW. Transient oxygen desaturation following radiographic contrast medium administration. Archives of Internal Medicine. 1986;**146**:1094-1097

[47] Kim SJ, Salem MR, Joseph NJ, et al. Contrast media adversely affect oxyhemoglobin dissociation. Anesthesia and Analgesia. 1990;**71**:73-76

[48] Liss P, Nygren A, Ulfendahl HR, Erikson U. Effect of furosemide or mannitol before injection of a non-ionic contrast medium on intrarenal oxygen tension. Advances in Experimental Medicine and Biology. 1999;**471**:353-359

[49] Heyman SN, Brezis M, Greenfeld Z, Rosen S. Protective role of furosemide and saline in radiocontrast-induced acute renal failure in the rat. American Journal of Kidney Diseases. 1989;**14**:377-385

[50] Solomon R, Werner C, Mann D, et al. Effects of saline, mannitol, and furosemide to prevent acute decreases in renal function induced by radiocontrast agents. The New England Journal of Medicine. 1994;**331**:1416-1420

[51] Heyman SN, Rosen S, Rosenberger C. Renal parenchymal hypoxia, hypoxia adaptation, and the pathogenesis of radiocontrast nephropathy. Clinical Journal of the American Society of Nephrology. 2008;**3**(1):288-296

[52] Workmann RJ, Shaff MI, Jackson RV, et al. Relationship of renal hemodynamic and functional changes following intravascular contrast to the renin-angiotensin system and renal prostacyclin in the dog. Investigative Radiology. 1983;**18**:160-166

[53] Hackstein N, Schneider C, Eichner G, et al. Effect of IV injection of radiographic contrast media on human renal blood flow. American Journal of Radiology. 2007;**188**:1367-1372

[54] Tumlin JA, Wang A, Murray PT, et al. Fenoldopam mesylate blocks reductions in renal plasma flow after radiocontrast dye infusion; a pilot trial in the prevention of contrast nephropathy. American Heart Journal. 2002;**143**:894-903

[55] Hardiek K, Katholi RE, Ramkumar V, Deitrick C. Proximal tubule cell response to radiographic contrast media. American Journal of Physiology. Renal Physiology. 2001;**280**:61-70

[56] Hizoh J, Strater CS, Schick S, et al. Radiocontrast-induced DNA fragmentation of renal tubular cells in vitro: Role of hypertonicity. Nephrology, Dialysis, Transplantation. 1998;**13**:911-918

[57] Beeri R, Symon Z, Brezis M, et al. Rapid DNA fragmentation from hypoxia along the thick ascending limb of rat kidneys. Kidney International. 1995;**47**:1806-1810

[58] Haller CS, Schick M, Zorn W. Cytotoxicity of radiocontrast agents on polarized renal epithelial cell monolayers. Cardiovascular Research. 1997;**33**:655-665

[59] Schnackenberg CG. Physiological and pathophysiological roles of oxygen radicals in the renal microvasculature. American Journal of Physiology, Regulatory, Integrative and Comparative Physiology. 2002;**282**:335-342

[60] Taliercio CP, Vlietstra RE, Fisher LD, Burnett JC. Risks for renal dysfunction with cardiac angiography. Annals of Internal Medicine. 1986;**104**(4):501-504

[61] Rudnick MR, Goldfarb S, Wexler L, Ludbrook PA, Murphy MJ, Halpern EF, et al. Nephrotoxicity of ionic and nonionic contrast media in 1196 patients: A randomized trial. The Iohexol Cooperative Study. Kidney International. 1995;**47**(1):254-261

[62] Aspelin P, Aubry P, Fransson SG, Strasser R, Willenbrock R, Berg KJ. Nephrotoxic effects in high-risk patients undergoing angiography. The New England Journal of Medicine. 2003;**348**(6):491-499

[63] Chalmers N, Jackson RW. Comparison of Iodixanol and Iohexol in renal impairment. The British Journal of Radiology. 1999;**72**(859):701-703

[64] Grainger RG. Renal toxicity of radiological contrast media. British Medical Bulletin. 1972;**28**(3):191-195

[65] Anto HR, Chou S-Y, Porush JG, Shapiro WB. Infusion intravenous pyelography and renal function. Effects of hypertonic mannitol in patients with chronic renal insufficiency. Archives of Internal Medicine. 1981;**141**(12):1652-1656

[66] Eisenberg RL, Bank WO, Hedgock MW. Renal failure after major angiography can be avoided with hydration. American Journal of Roentgenology. 1981;**136**(5):859-861

[67] Solomon R, Werner C, Mann D, D'Elia J, Silva P. Effects of saline, mannitol, and furosemide on acute decreases in renal function induced by radiocontrast agents. New England Journal of Medicine. 1994;**331**(21):1416-1420

[68] Trivedi HS, Moore H, Nasr S, et al. A randomized prospective trial to assess the role of saline hydration on the development of contrast nephrotoxicity. Nephron Clinical Practice. 2003;**93**(1):C29-C34

[69] Taylor AJ, Hotchkiss D, Morse RW, McCabe J. PREPARED: Preparation for angiography in renal dysfunction: A randomized trial of inpatient vs outpatient hydration protocols for cardiac catheterization in mild-to-moderate renal dysfunction. Chest. 1998;**114**(6):1570-1574

[70] Dussol B, Morange S, Loundoun A, Auquier P, Berland Y. A randomized trial of saline hydration to prevent contrast nephropathy in chronic renal failure patients. Nephrology, Dialysis, Transplantation. 2006;**21**(8):2120-2126

[71] Wróbel W, Sinkiewicz W, Gordon M, Woźniak-Wiśniewska A. Oral versus intravenous hydration and renal function in diabetic patients undergoing percutaneous coronary interventions. Kardiologia Polska. 2010;**68**(9):1015-1020

[72] Alpern RJ. Renal Acidification Mechanisms. 6th ed. Philadelphia, PA, USA: WB Saunders; 2000

[73] Halliwell B, Gutteridge JMC. Role of free radicals and catalytic metal ions in human disease: An overview. Methods in Enzymology. 1990;**186**:1-85

[74] Cohen G. The Fenton Reaction. Boca Raton, Fla, USA: CRC Press; 1985

[75] Lindinger MI, Franklin TW, Lands LC, Pedersen PK, Welsh DG, Heigenhauser GJF. $NaHCO_3$ and $KHCO_3$ ingestion rapidly increases renal electrolyte excretion in humans. Journal of Applied Physiology. 2000;**88**(2):540-550

[76] O'Sullivan S, Healy DA, Moloney MC, Grace PA, Walsh SR. The role of N-acetylcysteine in the prevention of contrast-induced nephropathy in patients undergoing peripheral angiography: A structured review and meta-analysis. Angiology. 2012

[77] Teruel JL, Marcen R, Herrero JA, Felipe C, Ortuño J. An easy and effective procedure to prevent radiocontrast agent nephrotoxicity in high-risk patients. Nephron. 1989;**51**(2):282

[78] Merten GJ, Burgess WP, Gray LV, et al. Prevention of contrast-induced nephropathy with sodium bicarbonate: A randomized controlled trial. Journal of the American Medical Association. 2004;**291**(19):2328-2334

[79] Hogan SE, L'Allier P, Chetcuti S, et al. Current role of sodium bicarbonate-based preprocedural hydration for the prevention of contrast-induced acute kidney injury: A meta-analysis. American Heart Journal. 2008;**156**(3):414-421

[80] Navaneethan SD, Singh S, Appasamy S, Wing RE, Sehgal AR. Sodium bicarbonate therapy for prevention of contrast-induced nephropathy: A systematic review and meta-analysis. American Journal of Kidney Diseases. 2009;**53**(4):617-627

[81] Zoungas S, Ninomiya T, Huxley R, et al. Systematic review: Sodium bicarbonate treatment regimens for the prevention of contrast-induced nephropathy. Annals of Internal Medicine. 2009;**151**(9):631-638

[82] Brar SS, Hiremath S, Dangas G, Mehran R, Brar SK, Leon MB. Sodium bicarbonate for the prevention of contrast induced-acute kidney injury: A systematic review and meta-analysis. Clinical Journal of the American Society of Nephrology. 2009;**4**(10):1584-1592

[83] Tepel M, Van Der Giet M, Schwarzfeld C, Laufer U, Liermann D, Zidek W. Prevention of radiographic-contrast-agent-induced reductions in renal function by acetylcysteine. New England Journal of Medicine. 2000;**343**(3):180-184

[84] Li Y, Liu Y, Fu L, Mei C, Dai B. Efficacy of short-term high-dose statin in preventing contrast-induced nephropathy: A meta-analysis of seven randomized controlled trials. PLoS ONE. 2013;**7**(4):e34450

[85] Sadat U. Contrast-induced nephropathy: Do statins offer protection? Current Opinion in Cardiology. 2011;**26**(4):334-337

[86] Trivedi H, Daram S, Szabo A, Bartorelli AL, Marenzi G. High-dose N-acetylcysteine for the prevention of contrast-induced nephropathy. American Journal of Medicine. 2009;**122**(9):874-8e9

[87] Sun Z, Fu Q, Cao L, Jin W, Cheng L, Li Z. Intravenous N-acetylcysteine for prevention of contrast-induced nephropathy: A meta-analysis of randomized, controlled trials. PLoS ONE. 2013;**8**(1):e55124

[88] Zafarullah M, Li WQ, Sylvester J, Ahmad M. Molecular mechanisms of N-acetylcysteine actions. Cellular and Molecular Life Sciences. 2003;**60**(1):6-20

[89] Aruoma OI, Halliwell B, Hoey BM, Butler J. The antioxidant action of N-acetylcysteine: Its reaction with hydrogen peroxide, hydroxyl radical, superoxide, and hypochlorous acid. Free Radical Biology and Medicine. 1989;**6**(6):593-597

[90] Skrzydlewska E, Farbiszewski R. Protective effect of N-acetylcysteine on reduced glutathione, reduced glutathione-related enzymes and lipid peroxidation in methanol intoxication. Drug and Alcohol Dependence. 1999;**57**(1):61-67

[91] Nakano H, Boudjema K, Alexandre E, et al. Protective effects of N-acetylcysteine on hypothermic ischemia-reperfusion injury of rat liver. Hepatology. 1995;**22**(2):539-545

[92] Nitescu N, Ricksten S, Marcussen N, et al. N-acetylcysteine attenuates kidney

injury in rats subjected to renal ischaemia-reperfusion. Nephrology, Dialysis, Transplantation. 2006;**21**(5):1240-1247

[93] Dobashi K, Singh I, Orak JK, Asayama K, Singh AK. Combination therapy of N-acetylcysteine, sodium nitroprusside and phosphoramidon attenuates ischemia-reperfusion injury in rat kidney. Molecular and Cellular Biochemistry. 2002;**240**(1-2):9-17

[94] Ahmad A, Mondello S, Di Paola R, et al. Protective effect of apocynin, a NADPH-oxidase inhibitor, against contrast-induced nephropathy in the diabetic rats: A comparison with n-acetylcysteine. European Journal of Pharmacology. 2012;**674**(2-3):397-406

[95] Saitoh T, Satoh H, Nobuhara M, et al. Intravenous glutathione prevents renal oxidative stress after coronary angiography more effectively than oral N-acetylcysteine. Heart and Vessels. 2011;**26**(5):465-472

[96] Conesa EL, Valero F, Nadal JC, et al. N-acetyl-L-cysteine improves renal medullary hypoperfusion in acute renal failure. American Journal of Physiology. 2001;**281**(3):R730-R737

[97] Loscalzo J. N-acetylcysteine potentiates inhibition of platelet aggregation by nitroglycerin. Journal of Clinical Investigation. 1985;**76**(2):703-708

[98] Salom MG, Ramírez P, Carbonell LF, et al. Protective effect of N-acetyl-L-cysteine on the renal failure induced by inferior vena cava occlusion. Transplantation. 1998;**65**(10):1315-1321

[99] Girouard H, Chulak C, Wu L, Lejossec M, De Champlain J. N-acetylcysteine improves nitric oxide and α-adrenergic pathways in mesenteric beds of spontaneously hypertensive rats. American Journal of Hypertension. 2003;**16**(7):577-584

[100] Boscheri A, Weinbrenner C, Botzek B, Reynen K, Kuhlisch E, Strasser RH. Failure of ascorbic acid to prevent contrast-media induced nephropathy in patients with renal dysfunction. Clinical Nephrology. 2007;**68**(5):279-286

[101] Wolfrum S, Jensen KS, Liao JK. Endothelium-dependent effects of statins. Arteriosclerosis, Thrombosis, and Vascular Biology. 2003;**23**(5):729-736

[102] Efrati S, Berman S, Ilgiyeav I, Siman-Tov Y, Averbukh Z, Weissgarten J. Differential effects of N-acetylcysteine, theophylline or bicarbonate on contrast-induced rat renal vasoconstriction. American Journal of Nephrology. 2009;**29**(3):181-191

[103] Kelly AM, Dwamena B, Cronin P, Bernstein SJ, Carlos RC. Meta-analysis: Effectiveness of drugs for preventing contrast-induced nephropathy. Annals of Internal Medicine. 2008;**148**(4):284-294

[104] Birck R, Krzossok S, Markowetz F, Schnülle P, Van Der Woude FJ, Braun C. Acetylcysteine for prevention of contrast nephropathy: Meta-analysis. The Lancet. 2003;**362**(9384):598-603

[105] Isenbarger DW, Kent SM, O'Malley PG. Meta-analysis of randomized clinical trials on the usefulness of acetylcysteine for prevention of contrast nephropathy. American Journal of Cardiology. 2003;**92**(12):1454-1458

[106] Alonso A, Lau J, Jaber BL, Weintraub A, Sarnak MJ. Prevention of radiocontrast nephropathy with N-acetylcysteine in patients with chronic kidney disease: A meta-analysis of randomized, controlled trials. American Journal of Kidney Diseases. 2004;**43**(1):1-9

[107] Pannu N, Manns B, Lee H, Tonelli M. Systematic review of the impact of N-acetylcysteine on contrast nephropathy. Kidney International. 2004;**65**(4):1366-1374

[108] Guru V, Fremes SE. The role of N-acetylcysteine in preventing radiographic contrast-induced nephropathy. Clinical Nephrology. 2004;**62**(2):77-83

[109] Bagshaw SM, Ghali WA. Acetylcysteine for prevention of contrast-induced nephropathy after intravascular angiography: A systematic review and meta-analysis. BMC Medicine. 2004;**2**:38

[110] Nallamothu BK, Shojania KG, Saint S, et al. Is acetylcysteine effective in preventing contrast-related nephropathy? A meta-analysis. American Journal of Medicine. 2004;**117**(12):938-947

[111] Duong MH, MacKenzie TA, Malenka DJ. N-acetylcysteine prophylaxis significantly reduces the risk of radiocontrast-induced nephropathy: Comprehensive meta-analysis. Catheterization and Cardiovascular Interventions. 2005;**64**(4):471-479

[112] Goldenberg I, Shechter M, Matetzky S, et al. Oral acetylcysteine as an adjunct to saline hydration for the prevention of contrast-induced nephropathy following coronary angiography: A randomized controlled trial and review of the current literature. European Heart Journal. 2004;**25**(3):212-218

[113] Misra D, Leibowtiz K, Gowda RM, Shapiro M, Khan IA. Role of N-acetylcysteine in prevention of contrast-induced nephropathy after cardiovascular procedures: A meta-analysis. Clinical Cardiology. 2004;**27**(11):607-610

[114] Liu R, Nair D, Ix J, Moore DH, Bent S. N-acetylcysteine for the prevention of contrast-induced nephropathy: A systematic review and meta-analysis. Journal of General Internal Medicine. 2005;**20**(2):193-200

[115] Zagler A, Azadpour M, Mercado C, Hennekens CH. N-acetylcysteine and contrast-induced nephropathy: A meta-analysis of 13 randomized trials. American Heart Journal. 2006;**151**(1):140-145

[116] Gonzales DA, Norsworthy KJ, Kern SJ, et al. A meta-analysis of N-acetylcysteine in contrast-induced nephrotoxicity: Unsupervised clustering to resolve heterogeneity. BMC Medicine. 2007;**5**:32

[117] Efrati S, Berman S, Siman-Tov Y, et al. N-acetylcysteine attenuates NSAID-induced rat renal failure by restoring intrarenal prostaglandin synthesis. Nephrology, Dialysis, Transplantation. 2007;**22**(7):1873-1881

[118] Podmore ID, Griffiths HR, Herbert KE, Mistry N, Mistry P, Lunec J. Vitamin C exhibits pro-oxidant properties. Nature. 1998;**392**(6676):559

[119] Buettner GR, Jurkiewicz BA. Catalytic metals, ascorbate and free radicals: Combinations to avoid. Radiation Research. 1996;**145**(5):532-541

[120] Du J, Cullen JJ, Buettner GR. Ascorbic acid: Chemistry, biology and the treatment of cancer. Biochimica et Biophysica Acta. 2012;**1826**(2):443-457

[121] Padayatty SJ, Sun H, Wang Y, et al. Vitamin C pharmacokinetics: Implications for oral and intravenous use. Annals of Internal Medicine. 2004;**140**(7):533-I61

[122] Bielski BHJ, Richter HW, Chan PC. Some properties of the ascorbate free radical. Annals of the New York Academy of Sciences. 1975;**258**:231-237

[123] Levine GN, Frei B, Koulouris SN, Gerhard MD, Keaney JF, Vita JA. Ascorbic acid reverses endothelial vasomotor dysfunction in patients with coronary artery disease. Circulation. 1996;**93**(6):1107-1113

[124] Motoyama T, Kawano H, Kugiyama K, et al. Endothelium-dependent vasodilation in the brachial artery is impaired in smokers: Effect of vitamin C. American Journal of Physiology. 1997;**273**(4):1644-1650

[125] Duffy SJ, Gokce N, Holbrook M, et al. Effect of ascorbic acid treatment on conduit vessel endothelial dysfunction in patients with hypertension. American Journal of Physiology. 2001;**280**(2):528-534

[126] Sadat U, Usman A, Gillard JH, Boyle JR. Does ascorbic acid protect against contrast induced-acute kidney injury in patients undergoing coronary angiography—A systematic review with meta-analysis of randomized controlled trials. Journal of the American College of Cardiology. 2013

[127] Brueck M, Cengiz H, Boening A. N-acetylcysteine or ascorbic acid versus placebo to prevent contrast-induced nephropathy in patients with renal insufficiency undergoing elective cardiac catheterization: A single center, prospective, double-blind, placebo-controlled, randomized trial. Journal of the American College of Cardiology. 2011;**57**(14, supplement s1):E595

[128] Attallah N, Yassine L, Musial J, et al. The potential role of statins in contrast nephropathy. Clinical Nephrology. 2004;**62**(4):273-278

[129] Khanal S, Attallah N, Smith DE, et al. Statin therapy reduces contrast-induced nephropathy: An analysis of contemporary percutaneous interventions. The American Journal of Medicine. 2005;**118**(8):843-849

[130] Stocul F, Adam A, Becker CR, et al. Strategies to reduce the risk of contrast-induced nephropathy. The American Journal of Cardiology. 2006;**98**(6a):59-77

[131] Piorkowski M, Fischer S, Stellbaum C, Jaster M, Martus P, Morguet AJ, et al. Treatment with ezetimibe plus low-dose atorvastatin compared with higher-dose atorvastatin alone: Is sufficient cholesterol-lowering enough to inhibit platelets? Journal of the American College of Cardiology. 2007;**49**:1035-1042

[132] Xinwei J, Xianghua F, Jing Z, Xinshun G, Ling X, Weize F, et al. Comparison of usefulness of simvastatin 20 mg versus 80 mg in preventing contrast-induced nephropathy in patients with acute coronary syndrome under-going percutaneous coronary intervention. The American Journal of Cardiology. 2009;**104**:519-524

[133] Osswald H. Renal effects of adenosine and their inhibition by theophylline in dogs. Naunyn-Schmiedebergs Archiv für Pharmakologie. 1975;**288**(1):79-86

[134] Arend LJ, Thompson CI, Spielman WS. Dipyridamole decreases glomerular filtration in the sodium-depleted dog. Evidence for mediation by intrarenal adenosine. Circulation Research. 1985;**56**(2):242-251

[135] Arend LJ, Bakris GL, Burnett JC, Megerian C, Spielman WS. Role for intrarenal adenosine in the renal hemodynamic response to contrast media. Journal of Laboratory and Clinical Medicine. 1987;**110**(4):406-411

[136] Erley CM, Duda SH, Schlepckow S, et al. Adenosine antagonist theophylline prevents the reduction of glomerular filtration rate after contrast media application. Kidney International. 1994;**45**(5):1425-1431

[137] Gandhi MR, Brown P, Romanowski CA, et al. The use of theophylline, an adenosine antagonist in the prevention of contrast media induced nephrotoxicity. British Journal of Radiology. 1992;**65**(777):838

[138] Kolonko A, Wiecek A, Kokot F. The nonselective adenosine antagonist theophylline does prevent renal dysfunction induced by radiographic contrast agents. Journal of Nephrology. 1998;**11**(3):151-156

[139] Erol T, Tekin A, Katırcıbaşı MT, Sezgin N, Bilgi M, Tekin G, et al. Efficacy of allopurinol pretreatment for prevention of contrast-induced nephropathy: A randomized controlled trial. International Journal of Cardiology. 2013;**167**(4):1396-1399

[140] Kapoor A, Sinha N, Sharma RK, Shrivastava S, Radhakrishnan S, Goel PK, et al. Use of dopamine in prevention of contrast induced acute renal failure—A randomised study. International Journal of Cardiology. 1996;**53**(3):233-236

[141] Abizaid AS, Clark CE, Mintz GS, et al. Effects of dopamine and aminophylline on contrast-induced acute renal failure after coronary angioplasty in patients with preexisting renal insufficiency. American Journal of Cardiology. 1999;**83**(2):260-263

[142] Stone GW, McCullough PA, Tumlin JA, et al. Fenoldopam mesylate for the prevention of contrast-induced nephropathy: A randomized controlled trial. Journal of the American Medical Association. 2003;**290**(17):2284-2291

[143] Allie DE, Lirtzman MD, Wyatt CH, et al. Targeted renal therapy and contrast-induced nephropathy during endovascular abdominal aortic aneurysm repair: Results of a feasibility pilot trial. Journal of Endovascular Therapy. 2007;**14**(4):520-527

[144] Weisz G, Filby SJ, Cohen MG, et al. Safety and performance of targeted renal therapy: The Be-RITe! Registry. Journal of Endovascular Therapy. 2009;**16**(1):1-12

[145] Rahman IA, Mascaro JG, Steeds RP, et al. Remote ischemic preconditioning in human coronary artery bypass surgery: From promise to disappointment? Circulation. 2010;**122**(11):S53-S59

[146] Ali ZA, Callaghan CJ, Lim E, et al. Remote ischemic preconditioning reduces myocardial and renal injury after elective abdominal aortic aneurysm repair: A randomized controlled trial. Circulation. 2007;**116**(11):I98-I105

[147] Walsh SR, Sadat U, Boyle JR, et al. Remote ischemic preconditioning for renal protection during elective open infrarenal abdominal aortic aneurysm repair: Randomized controlled trial. Vascular and Endovascular Surgery. 2010;**44**(5):334-340

[148] Xie J, Liao X, Chen W, et al. Remote ischaemic preconditioning reduces myocardial injury in patients undergoing heart valve surgery: Randomised controlled trial. Heart. 2012;**98**(5):384-388

[149] Venugopal V, Hausenloy DJ, Ludman A, et al. Remote ischaemic preconditioning reduces myocardial injury in patients undergoing cardiac surgery with cold-blood cardioplegia: A randomised controlled trial. Heart. 2009;**95**(19):1567-1571

[150] Hausenloy DJ, Mwamure PK, Venugopal V, et al. Effect of remote ischaemic preconditioning on myocardial injury in patients undergoing coronary artery bypass graft surgery: A randomised controlled trial. The Lancet. 2007;**370**(9587):575-579

[151] Pedersen KR, Ravn HB, Povlsen JV, Schmidt MR, Erlandsen EJ, Hjortdal VE. Failure of remote ischemic preconditioning to reduce the risk of postoperative acute kidney injury in children undergoing operation for complex congenital heart disease: A randomized single-center study. Journal of Thoracic and Cardiovascular Surgery. 2012;**143**(3):576-583

[152] Er F, Nia AM, Dopp H, et al. Ischemic preconditioning for prevention of contrast medium-induced nephropathy: Randomized pilot RenPro Trial (Renal Protection Trial). Circulation. 2012;**126**(3):296-303

[153] Ludman AJ, Yellon DM, Hausenloy DJ. Cardiac preconditioning for ischaemia: Lost in translation. DMM Disease Models and Mechanisms. 2010;**3**(1-2):35-38

[154] McCullough PA, Adam A, Becker CR, et al. Epidemiology and pragmatic implications of contrast-induced nephropathy. The American Journal of Cardiology. 2006;**98**(6A):5-13

[155] Maeder M, Klein M, Fehr T, et al. Contrast nephropathy: Review focusing on prevention. Journal of the American College of Cardiology. 2004;**44**(9):1763-1771

[156] Levy EM, Viscoli CM, Horwitz RI. The effect of acute renal failure on mortality: A cohort analysis. JAMA. 1996;**257**(19):1489-1494

[157] Foley RN, Parfrey PS, Sarnak MJ. Clinical epidemiology of cardiovascular disease in chronic renal failure. American Journal of Kidney Diseases. 1998;**32**(5 Suppl 3):S112-S119

[158] McCullough PA, Adam A, Becker CR, Davidson C, Lameire N, Stacul F, et al. Risk prediction of contrast-induced nephropathy. The American Journal of Cardiology. 2006;**98**(6A):27-36

[159] Persson PB, Hansell P, Liss P. Pathophysiology of contrast medium-induced nephropathy. Kidney International. 2005;**68**(1):14-22

[160] Benko A, Fraser-Hill M, Magner P, et al. Canadian Association of Radiologists Canadian Association of Radiologists: Consensus guidelines for the prevention of contrast-induced nephropathy. Canadian Association of Radiologists Journal. 2007;**58**(2):79-87

Section 5

# Management

Chapter 10

# Preventing Rupture: Clipping of Unruptured Intracranial Aneurysms

*Ioan Alexandru Florian, Teodora Larisa Timis, Cristina Caterina Aldea and Ioan Stefan Florian*

## Abstract

Unruptured intracranial aneurysms (UIAs) represent a major public health issue due to their unpredictable natural history. Whether to actively treat them or to maintain them under observation remains a hotly disputed topic. In this chapter, we present a review of the literature regarding the history of clipping and its use in UIAs, as well as the experience of our senior author in this field. We performed an extensive Medline and Google Academic search of the relevant literature. We have also made a retrospective analysis on patients harboring UIAs and multiple intracranial aneurysms (MIAs) clipped by the senior author between 1997 and 2017. About 89 patients had solitary UIAs, alongside 101 with MIAs possessing 257 individual aneurysms in total. All UIA patients were discharged with a favorable neurological outcome and no mortality. Concerning MIAs, the majority of cases had 2 aneurysms, the highest number being 6. And, 61 patients from this group had a favorable outcome. In the hands of experienced vascular neurosurgeons, clipping remains a safe option for both UIAs and MIAs. This procedure offers a long-lasting protection from aneurysmal rupture. In the future, new clip technologies and intraprocedural methods of verifying vessel patency and aneurysmal occlusion may further enhance postoperative results.

**Keywords:** intracranial aneurysm, multiple aneurysms, unruptured, surgery, clipping

## 1. Introduction

Once considered as the definitive curative option for intracranial aneurysms (IAs), clipping has steadily lost its footing in the face of the less invasive and lower-risk-laden endovascular procedures. Successful clipping implies completely occluding the aneurysmal sack at its origin on the parent artery, significantly diminishing the risk of rupture and ensuing morbidity. The procedure is especially indicated for ruptured aneurysms. However, there is ongoing debate regarding the necessity for surgery in the case of unruptured intracranial aneurysms (UIAs). Since many of these patients also harbor more than one aneurysm, another controversial aspect in neurosurgery is whether to treat all aneurysms in the same session or to leave the unruptured lesions for a delayed intervention or even for an endovascular procedure. In this chapter, we present our considerable experience and attitude in the surgical management of unruptured and multiple aneurysms.

Preventing rupture from IAs represents a major concern for neurosurgeons, neuroradiologists, and neurointerventionists, as this represents a catastrophic and potentially life-threatening occurrence in the natural history of this pathology. UIAs are defined as not possessing a known history or signs of rupture or that have been diagnosed incidentally for symptoms unrelated to intracranial hemorrhage. They are a veritable "ticking time bomb" that, under certain conditions, can "detonate" and cause a devastating hemorrhagic stroke with severe and often irreversible consequences. Therefore, preventive surgical treatment of UIAs, especially clipping of the aneurysmal sack, is a valuable and possibly life-saving option.

A successful clipping means that the vascular clip completely isolates the aneurysmal lumen from blood flow at its origin on the parent artery. This point of origin is generally located at either a bifurcation or a sharp turn of an artery. Surgical clipping may prevent rupture of that particular aneurysm, although an incomplete occlusion can result in recurrence. Since the development of less invasive endovascular techniques, clipping has lost most of its standing in the treatment of UIAs, being reserved for hemorrhagic lesions or those otherwise unsuitable for endovascular procedures. Certain highly experienced centers still favor the intracranial approach for UIAs due to the longevity of procedure and excellent postoperative neurological outcome.

Additionally, some patients may harbor more than one aneurysm, occurring either concomitantly or sequentially. These may be diagnosed incidentally, during the rupture of at least one of the aneurysms or at a variable point in time during postprocedural control. The treatment of multiple intracranial aneurysms (MIAs) to this day remains a highly debated topic, lacking a general consensus regarding indications, timing, and modality. Our experience supports the single-stage single-opening surgical treatment of multiple UIAs.

## 2. Short history and evolution of aneurysm surgery

Although the pathology of intracranial aneurysms had been scrupulously studied by the beginning of the twentieth century, treatment options were scarce and most often fruitless [1]. Harvey Cushing (1869–1939) himself doubted whether these lesions could be approached surgically due to the technical limitations, reduced accessibility and visibility of the lesions, as well as a general lack of experience in the surgical community [1–3]. Up until that point, the treatment of intracranial aneurysms relied on the proximal ligation technique, as described by John Hunter (1728–1793). This resulted in thrombosis and occlusion inside the aneurysm. In 1885, Sir Victor Horsley (1857–1916) was reportedly the first to successfully perform such an intervention for an intracranial aneurysm by ligating the right common carotid artery [1, 2, 4]. Cushing is credited with developing the wrapping technique for the treatment of intracranial aneurysms; however, in 1931 his pupil, Dott Norman McComish (1897–1973), performed the first elective frontal craniotomy in order to wrap and reinforce a ruptured aneurysm with autologous muscle from the patient's thigh [3–5]. Axel Herbert Olivecrona (1891–1980) was the first to perform a successful surgical trapping and removal of an intracranial aneurysm in 1932, a technique then further elaborated by Walter Dandy (1886–1946) [5]. In 1937, Dandy used a modified version of the Cushing clip to occlude a posterior communicating artery (PCoA) aneurysm via a "hypophyseal approach," being the first ever documented intervention of its kind [1, 2–5].

Since then, aneurysm clipping has undergone extensive improvements in both technique and instrumentation. The Cushing clip was malleable; however, according to Kenneth George McKenzie (1892–1964), the two sides of the clips were frequently of unequal length, had rough ends, and had a habit of turning in the holder [6]. Furthermore, it could not be reopened or repositioned; thus, an improper placement could compromise the entire intervention [5]. In 1927, McKenzie conceived a more versatile alternative to the instruments used [6–9]. In 1949, Duane William Jr. changed the McKenzie-modified clip holder to punch out more effective U-shaped clips [5]. Olivecrona made a considerable redesign of the clips in 1953 that allowed reopening and repositioning of the clips [4, 5, 9]. However, the drawback to these clips were crushing the aneurysmal neck and producing shearing and tearing of the fragilized vascular walls. Thus, Henry Schwartz introduced the cross-action alpha clip, basically a miniaturized spring forceps that could close by itself [3, 5, 9]. Despite this concept being brilliant, its utilization in aneurysm surgery was problematic due to its large size and the bulkiness of its applicator. In 1952, Frank Mayfield and George Kees Jr. made delicate yet crucial enhancements to clip technology, significantly reducing the size of the shank, while also constructing clips of diverse lengths and angles, as well as having wider blade openings [3–5, 9–11]. They were also responsible for the bayoneted design of the clip that would permit better visualization during manipulation. Joseph McFadden suggested a modification of Kees' design, with rounded blades and blunted tips [3, 11].

Charles Drake (1920–1998) was credited with developing the fenestrated clip in 1969, which could allow placement of the clips on more inaccessible aneurysms without compromising the parent vessel [1, 3, 4]. This was especially useful for treating posterior fossa aneurysms, for which Drake also pioneered innovative techniques and surgical approaches (such as the subtemporal approach for aneurysms of the basilar apex) [4]. George Smith (1916–1964) also made an essential innovation with a vessel-encompassing clip that could occlude aneurysms on the opposite side of the affected artery [3, 12]. Elaborating on this concept, Thoralf Sundt (1930–1992) devised a Teflon-lined clip-graft that could also mend small tears or irregularities in the artery [1, 3–5, 12, 13]. At present, adjustments are still made regarding configuration, instrumentation, and clip composition.

The next most important bound in aneurysm surgery came in the form of the operating microscope, allowing better visualization and illumination of the aneurysm neck and surrounding vessels [1, 4, 5, 14]. Gazi Yasargil, the father of microneurosurgery, had probably the greatest contribution in this field by not only standardizing the use of the operating microscope in aneurysm surgery but also by developing and refining procedures and instruments now commonly used in vascular neurosurgery [1, 3, 4]. The clips he created were specifically designed for use alongside microscopic magnification. Moreover, he also underscored the necessity of understanding cisternal and microvascular anatomy in neurosurgery. Drake's seemingly most remarkable addition to vascular neurosurgery was comprehending the intricate anatomy of posterior circulation aneurysms, as well as improving outcomes following their surgical treatment [4, 5]. Magnetic resonance imaging (MRI) became crucial in the diagnosis of cerebrovascular pathologies. Although, since the first clips introduced in neurosurgery were made of stainless steel, they were not compatible with MRI. After rigorous compatibility testing, Robert Spetzler introduced the pure titanium clips as a nonferromagnetic alternative with the same mechanical properties as other clips available at that time [4, 5, 15, 16].

Yasargil also described the end-to-side anastomosis between the superficial temporal artery and middle cerebral artery (MCA), which bypassed the blood flow from the extracranial circulation to the intracranial compartment [5]. The bypass techniques are currently used in the management of more complex giant aneurysms, however with less satisfactory outcomes than the standard surgical approaches for smaller aneurysms [5, 17]. A more recent advancement has been the introduction of intraoperative videoangiography by means of fluorescent dyes such as fluorescein sodium or indocyanine green [18]. Charles Wrobel first described this method in 1994 for real-time testing of aneurysmal obliteration and the patency of adjacent arteries [5, 19]. This tool renders intraoperative catheter-based angiography or Doppler ultrasonography obsolete in certain cases and allows repositioning of inconveniently placed clips before the onset of permanent damage [5, 18–20]. Other contemporary innovations include the endoscopic endonasal approaches in order to clip skull base aneurysms; however, this technique awaits further validation [5, 21–23].

Evidently, not all aneurysms were amenable to clipping. Before the dawn of endovascular procedures, surgeons attempted various methods of introducing foreign materials into the aneurysm sack to achieve thrombosis, with variable results. The materials ranged from heated silver enameled wire [24], copper wire [25], and silk sutures [26], to magnetically guided iron suspensions [27] to even animal hair from horse or dog [28]. Despite these techniques being mostly obsolescent, they indisputably paved the way to endovascular treatment of intracranial vasculopathies. The most important step in this direction belonged to the invention of the angiography as a superior instrument for diagnosing intracranial pathologies. The first cerebral angiography was performed by Egas Moniz (1874–1955) in 1927, a technique which remained the only dependable diagnostic method for identifying intracranial lesions until the introduction of computed tomography (CT) nearly 50 years later [1, 4, 29–31]. Fascinatingly enough, an editorial published in The Lancet in 1931 predicted the probability of not only diagnosing intracranial aneurysms through this tool but also as an opportunity for therapy in later years [1, 29]. The endovascular coils presently used were preceded by detachable balloons that could be deployed inside vascular lesions and would harden to result in a controlled localized thrombosis [1, 4, 32]. However, this technique resulted in significant complications and was soon replaced. The first successful treatment of an intracranial aneurysm via coiling belonged to Ira Braun in 1985 [1, 4]. Guido Guglielmi undoubtedly had the most significant role in developing modern coils that were electrolytically detachable [33–35].

Ever since, the role of microneurosurgery in the treatment of aneurysms has diminished in the face of a safer, easier, less invasive, and satisfyingly durable procedure with a shorter hospital stay and faster recovery time [36–38]. Many other endovascular techniques and tools have been elaborated in the wake of this innovation the technology experiencing an exponential growth. A thorough description of such instruments is beyond the scope of this chapter. In what follows, we detail the microsurgical treatment options for unruptured solitary and multiple aneurysms, with a special emphasis on clipping, its effects, outcome, and consequences while also sharing our operative experience.

## 3. Natural history of unruptured aneurysms

To quote physicist Niels Bohr (1885–1962), "Prediction is very difficult, especially about the future." This also applies to UIAs regarding what can cause them to bleed and when. There is a high variability between populations in the prevalence of UIAs, being cited between 1% and as much as 7% of the general population [39–42]. They are more commonly found in the anterior circulation, at more advanced ages, and more often in women. The natural history seems to differ according to the shape, location, and size of the lesion, with a significant incongruity between the number of incidentally discovered aneurysms each year (2000–4000 per 100,000 persons/year) and the annual incidence of aneurysmal subarachnoid hemorrhage (aSAH) (approximately 10 per 100,000 persons/year) [43]. In other words, out of 200 to 400 patients diagnosed yearly with an intracranial aneurysm, chances are that only one of these may rupture. The annual and cumulative risk of rupture has been appraised at approximately 1%/year and at 9% at 9 years for the Japanese and Korean populations [44], similar to that of Western countries (0.2–1.6%/year and 10% at 10 years) [45–48]. Factors attributed to impact the natural history of UIAs may be related to the aneurysm itself, the patient, or even external influences.

Concerning patient-related factors, it seems that women have a higher prevalence of UIAs than men, and the peak incidence was found between the fifth and sixth decades of age. Patients with polycystic kidney disease, type IV Ehlers-Danlos syndrome, and Marfan syndrome are more likely to develop UIAs during their lifetime. Hypertension is the comorbidity most likely associated with this finding, while a positive family history is also an important risk factor among siblings. Up to 15–30% of these patients harbor at least two UIAs, either concomitantly or sequentially. The most common modifiable risk factors attributed to UIAs are smoking, alcohol and drug abuse, as well as using oral contraceptives [49].

According to the results of the PHASE 2 of the International Study of Unruptured Intracranial Aneurysms (ISUIA) trial, patients that had no previous aSAH and harbored aneurysms under 7 mm in diameter possessed no risk of rupture for UIAs in the anterior circulation [50]. However, the risk of bleeding was 2.5%/year for aneurysms located at the PCoA and the posterior cerebral circulation. Concerning patients with a history of aSAH, the risk of rupture for aneurysms smaller than 7 mm in the anterior cerebral circulation reached 1.5%/year, whereas for the posterior circulation, it rose to 3.4%/year. Similarly, the Unruptured Cerebral Aneurysm Study (UCAS) performed in Japan proved that size influenced the risk of rupture, starting from 0.36% for microaneurysms (between 3 and 4 mm), climbing at 4.37% for lesions between 10 to 24 mm to reaching as much as 33.4% for giant aneurysms (≥25 mm) [42]. Analogous results were also reported for the South Korean population [44]. Apparently, as an aneurysm swells, the risk of subsequent rupture rises [51]. However, according to Serrone et al., the single predictor of aneurysm enlargement was the initial size of the lesion, with the annual risk of growth being evaluated at a mean of 3.5%, though higher for larger aneurysms [52]. The morphology of the aneurysm was also incriminated in influencing the risk of rupture, especially the formation of a daughter sac, the shape of the sac, and regions possessing a thinned arterial wall [53]. Pertaining to UIAs selected for conservative treatment, Ramachandran stated that "None of the metrics—including aneurysm size, nonsphericity index, peak wall tension, and low shear stress area—differentiated the stable from unstable groups with statistical significance," suggesting that there might not actually be such a thing as a "stable" intracranial aneurysm [54].

Aneurysmal rupture can also occur during stressful or strenuous activities such as sexual intercourse, labor, defecation, physical exertion, or sports [55]. However, these external factors may in fact conceal the climate impact, as numerous studies indicate a higher incidence of aneurysm rupture during the winter season, as well as during daytime [56–59]. Our experience of operated aneurysms also supports this statement, as illustrated in **Figure 1**.

In summary, the natural history of aneurysms is complicated and shrouded in uncertainty, except for one surety: UIAs do not spontaneously heal.

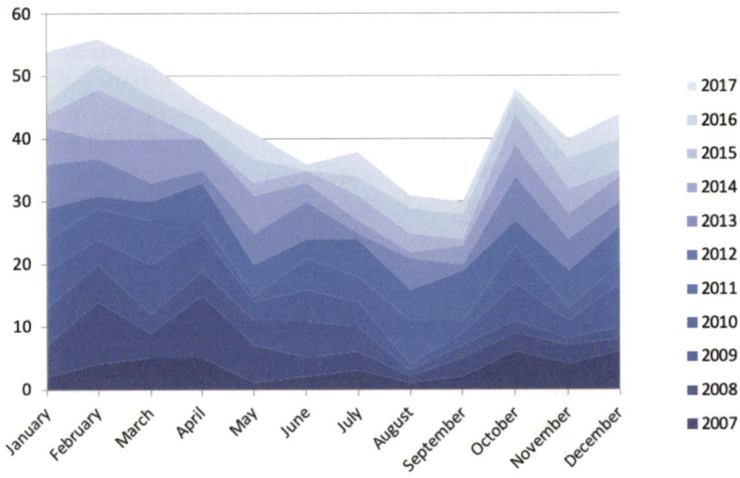


**Figure 1.**
*Multiannual incidence of aneurysmal rupture, as hospitalized and surgically treated in our institution between January and December 2017.*

## 4. Treatment strategies

The purpose of active treatment for UIAs is to permanently and safely occlude the aneurysmal lumen while preserving the normal cerebral vasculature. In order to achieve this, two types of approaches have been conceived: surgical (via craniotomy), which includes clipping and bypass procedures, or endovascular. As certain lesions cannot be safely and efficiently removed from arterial circulation either by clipping or by endovascular procedures, bypass surgery has been elaborated to remove the aneurysm and its parent vessel, without sacrificing arterial supply to the involved tissues.

Currently, there are no controlled randomized studies that single out the superior form of treatment for UIAs. Optimal treatment should focus on the following aspects:

- Age and clinical features of the patient
- Anatomy, size, and location of the aneurysm
- Institutional and personal experience in a certain field
- Technical capabilities of the facility

Since the majority of studies in the reported literature are retrospective in nature, they may suffer from bias. As of yet, the best sources of information regarding the outcome of UIA treatment originate from comparative studies between natural history and complication rates of certain therapies [60]. As our surgical experience exceeds that of endovascular procedures, as well as our standing concerning its importance in the prevention of rupture, we will exclusively present the technical breakdown of aneurysm clipping, according to our practice.

## 5. Aneurysm clipping: technical breakdown

Although seemingly easy in theory, placing a clip at the neck of the aneurysm (i.e., its point of origin) represents a genuine surgical challenge because of the need to preserve the anatomical and functional integrity of the normal vasculature, brain parenchyma, and cranial nerves. This not only implies a good proximal control of the arteries but also adequate exposure of the aneurysm and the vessels, beginning with the craniotomy. In the following paragraphs, we describe the key points of aneurysmal clipping.

### 5.1 Positioning

This is a crucial stage that can either facilitate or hinder the surgical intervention. The patient is placed in a dorsal decubitus. The patient's head should be positioned so that the planned craniotomy is easy to perform, while ensuring that there is no substantial jugular compression (i.e., if the head is rotated excessively to one side) or that proper ventilation is not impeded (i.e., much too little distance between the tip of the mandible and the sternum). The head can be immobilized by a headholder, if this does not hamper venous drainage. We recommend shaving the head, or at the very least the area around the incision, to minimize the risk of infection. Using cutaneous antiseptics such as iodine solution or chlorhexidine, the skin must be thoroughly cleansed, with special attention toward the auricle and the external ear canal.

### 5.2 Surgical exposure

The skin incision should always be larger than the bone opening, considering the possible need to enlarge the craniotomy. A wide enough craniotomy must be performed for an ideal surgical exposure. Brain relaxation increases visibility and motility, while also diminishing the risk of damaging the brain and vessels. This is vital for certain aneurysms, especially of the skull base (internal carotid artery (ICA), anterior communicating artery (AcoA), basilar apex, etc.) or when attempting to clip mirror aneurysms during the same opening. There are a few methods to achieve brain relaxation, such as hyperventilation, cerebrospinal fluid (CSF) drainage (realized via lumbar drainage or ventriculostomy), intracisternal drainage (the most effective form of intraoperative brain relaxation in our experience, performed by opening the basal cisternae and the Sylvian valley), or with intravenous diuretics (mannitol or furosemide).

### 5.3 Craniotomy

The bone opening should be entirely adapted to the location, size, and morphology of the aneurysm. It must be able to reveal the Circle of Willis and be spacious enough to allow the exploration of the main blood vessels. The most commonly used craniotomy for aneurysms of the anterior circulation and of the basilar apex is the frontolateral approach as described by Samii, the classical pterional opening being used in MCA aneurysms and for contralateral clipping in the case of multiple aneurysms. A burr hole is placed at the orbitofrontal angle (keyhole), being careful not to open the orbit or the frontal sinus (if it is large enough to reach this point). The craniotome can then be used to complete the flap. Additional burr holes may be needed. In the classical pterional approach, the sphenoid wing should be drilled as close as possible to the anterior cranial fossa. In the event of a tensioned dura, slight elevation of the head and opening the lumbar drainage will result in proper brain relaxation.

### 5.4 Dura mater incision

The dura can be opened in a cross-shape or a C shape. We favor the latter, leaving the tip of the convexity upward and at least 2 cm above the sphenoid bone. By suspending the dural flap, we ensure a wide enough opening. The rest of the dura is left in place to protect the brain.

### 5.5 Arachnoidal dissection

Although sometimes difficult due to extensive adhesions, this step is mandatory for exploring the optochiasmatic region. The opening in the Sylvian valley is made just above the ipsilateral optic nerve, the most constant landmark and the place where the arachnoid is the furthest from the cortex. Next, the opening is extended both laterally and medially using a thin aspirator and microsurgical scissors. Evacuation of the CSF will further relax the brain and offer a large operating field. Dissection resumes medially for ACoA aneurysms and laterally for PCoA aneurysms, whereas it continues along the artery itself for internal carotid artery lesions. Once the valley has been opened, the bifurcation of the ICA is visible, and the neck of the aneurysm can be distinguished. The neck is then dissected and isolated from the surrounding normal vasculature. For middle cerebral artery aneurysms, the ICA should be dissected laterally, as well as the proximal portion of the MCA. This type of opening has some drawbacks, as it first brings the surgeon to the tip of the aneurysmal sac and the proximal control is lacking at this moment. But a delicate dissection proximal to the aneurysm will shortly offer the visibility over the M1 segment, where a temporary clip could be safely placed. The interoptic triangle allows access toward basilar apex aneurysms; however, accessing the neck of the aneurysm itself is much more challenging, especially since the first element that "greets" the surgeon in this approach is the aneurysmal fundus.

The parent vessel has to be exposed proximally to the aneurysm to ensure blood flow control in the case of intraoperative rupture. The main vessel should be adequately exposed before the neck of the aneurysm, which, in turn, should be dissected before the fundus. The perforators adjacent to the lesion must be separated from the neck before placing the permanent clip. If the aneurysm sac is too wide and complex to be clipped, prudent use of the bipolar coagulator can adjust its diameter. Immediately after the clip is placed, the permeability of surrounding vessels and perforators must be demonstrated. If intraoperative rupture occurs, lowering arterial pressure, tamponing, temporary clipping of parent vessel, and aspirating the aneurysmal sac will favor neck definition and placement of definitive clip.

### 5.6 Clipping

Once the aneurysm has been successfully dissected from the surrounding vessels, a permanent clip is placed at the aneurysmal neck. It has to be parallel to the parent artery in order to avoid stretching or occluding it. The length and shape of the clip should be adapted to the morphology of the aneurysm and must trap the neck entirely, without also trapping perforators or adjacent structures. Sometimes, it is necessary to reduce the volume of the aneurysm by applying a temporary clip proximal to the aneurysm. Timing in this step is crucial, as more than 10 min of temporary occlusion of a major vessel such as the MCA or ICA can lead to severe consequences. Once the aneurysm has shrunk enough, the permanent clip can be carefully applied (**Figure 2**).

### 5.7 Intraoperative aneurysmal rupture (IAR)

This is a dreadful but preventable incident, more hazardous if it occurs early, such as during induction of anesthesia or while opening of the dura. Arguably

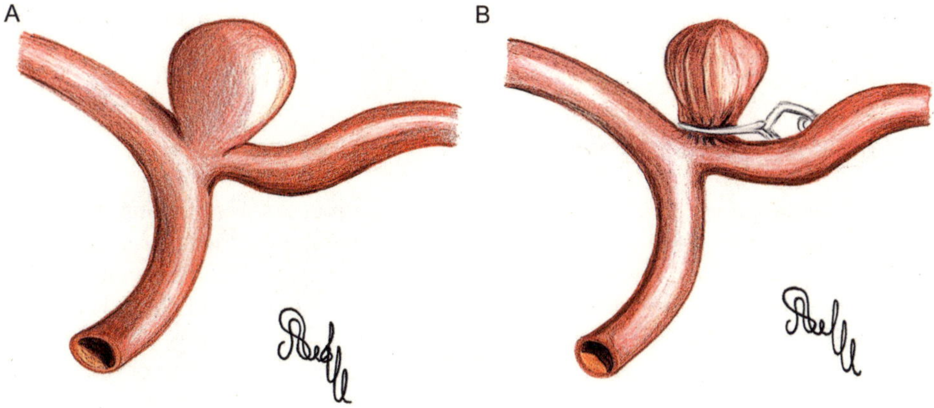


**Figure 2.**
*Representation of an unruptured aneurysm before (A) and after clipping (B) (drawings provided by the first author of this chapter).*

the most challenging of IARs may be those of basilar apex aneurysms. The aims in this scenario are hemostasis, avoiding further aneurysmal damage, preventing accidental injury to main vessels and perforators, and, finally, clipping the aneurysm. Certain steps should be followed to avoid IAR: careful positioning of the head to minimize brain traction; vigilant induction of anesthesia and ensuring that hypertension bouts do not occur; a sufficiently wide craniotomy that guarantees appropriate access, as well as adequate brain relaxation (using diuretics or a preoperative lumbar drainage); and last but not least, sharp instruments are safer for dissection than blunt instruments. Ensuring proximal control before aneurysmal neck dissection can diminish the risk of IAR. Also, using the anatomical paths through the arachnoidal planes will also lower the chance of IAR. In our practice, we apply temporary clips if we anticipate a difficult dissection, for example, giant aneurysms, polylobulated aneurysms, or those that have recently bled. Even so, the occlusion via temporary clip should not exceed a cumulative 20–25 min with repeated placements. However, temporary clips are the most useful in IAR if placed as early as possible.

### 5.8 Closure

Without exception, this is performed after thorough hemostasis. For this, we employ hemostatic materials (Surgicel® or Gelfoam®) and the judicious use of the bipolar coagulator. Patience is essential, as rushing this step can compromise the entire operation. In nearly all our surgeries, we use autologous periosteum to perform dural plasty. In our opinion, near-watertight closure of the dura with a 5/0 thread (either with continuous or separate sutures) is sufficient. The bone is inserted back into place and fixed either with titanium mesh and screws or sutures with thick threads passing through small burr holes. Placing an external drainage under the aponeurosis for a period of 24 h is mandatory. The skin closure is performed either continuously or with separate sutures or staples.

### 5.9 Postoperative control

We usually perform a CTA after closure, with the patient still sedated and intubated. It is much safer to make sure that the vessels are angiographically permeable, or to correct any abnormality under the same anesthesia, than to wait for the patient to awake and develop ischemic complications. We have also used intraoperative fluorescence angiography to not only verify the occlusion of the aneurysmal sack but also the patency of the surrounding normal vessels.

## 6. Hemodynamic consequences of aneurysm clipping

The hemodynamic characteristics of intracranial aneurysms are thought to play a pivotal role in their development, evolution, and eventual rupture, interfering and modifying the local biology of the vascular wall [61–63]. The theory suggests that the wall is exposed to a higher degree of sheer stress than it can physiologically withstand. This leads to a local weakening and abnormal remodeling, which in time will form an aneurysm. Its growth can be a result of local proliferation of mural cells, a distention of the cellular and intercellular structures, or possibly a mixture of the two. A meticulous in vitro study affirmed that growth cannot be entirely the result of simple fluid physics [64], a non-Newtonian model being more precise in ascertaining the altered hemodynamics in intracranial aneurysms [65]. However, as it is impossible to perform direct measurements on hemodynamic stress in patients or living experimental models, methods implying computational fluid dynamics are used to estimate these phenomena [65–67].

Aneurysmal rupture results from the mechanical weakening of the arterial wall that is subsequently unable to contain the force of the flowing blood [68]. The wall sheer stress is defined as the tangential frictional force that the blood exerts upon the endothelium, being the highest at the neck and the apex of the aneurysm [65]. The innerworkings of endovascular procedures are closely linked to these hemodynamic conditions, as the presence of a coil determines alterations in wall shear stress and blood flow that conclude with the intraluminal thrombosis of the aneurysm [69]. In MIA, wall sheer stress is apparently increased in UIAs distal to a ruptured aneurysm after treatment, whether surgical or endovascular, leading to a theoretical rise in the risk of rupture [66]. Moreover, also in MIA, ruptured aneurysms may possess a more irregular shape, larger size, and dome-to-neck ratio, as well as a lower minimum wall shear stress than with their unruptured counterparts [70].

After clipping, a series of local and distal changes in hemodynamics may occur. Nevertheless, these are not as intensely analyzed as for untreated aneurysms. Successful surgical obliteration of the aneurysm results in the complete cessation of blood flow inside the lumen. However, it is not clear what impact the presence of the aneurysmal clip itself has on the wall shear stress or its effects on the vascular wall. A residual neck (i.e., a portion of the neck that was not occluded by the blades of the clip) may in time lead to aneurysmal regrowth, depending on the size of the remnant as well as its location [71]. Apparently, a distal remnant is at a higher risk for aneurysmal regrowth than a proximal residue. Therefore, it is crucial to ensure an adequate placement of the clip during surgery and to adjust its position if required. The alterations in dynamic flow can also be observed systemically after clipping or coiling, especially in the period after vasospasm caused by aneurysmal rupture [72]. In the study conducted by Inoue et al., patients treated by coiling presented a significantly lower cardiac index, as well as a significantly higher systemic vascular resistance index than the group managed via clipping, although this might have been the result of systemic therapy for managing vasospasm and aggressive volume loading rather than of the procedure itself, especially as the patients in the coiling group arrived in a worse neurological state than those of the clipping group. Needless to say, more studies are required to discern the actual impact that clipping has on the cerebral vasculature, especially concerning aneurysmal regrowth, reoccurrence, and rerupture.

## 7. Clipping of solitary unruptured aneurysms

The cerebrovascular diseases causing such controversy in regard to treatment are few in number [73]. The reasoning behind this continuous debate is that the prophylactic management of UIAs must be justified by a suitable procedure-related outcome when compared to the anticipated natural history [74]. Despite clipping once being the management centerpiece, the swift refinement of endovascular procedures and innovation of flow diversion devices have steadily replaced surgery as the first line of therapy for UIAs. However, certain countries still favor clipping due to its longevity, effectiveness, and the lower risk of recanalization than endovascular techniques, as well as lower procedure-related costs [75–77]. Consequently, whereas older patients who are unsuitable for surgery may benefit the most from endovascular procedures, clipping is considered preferable for younger patients with lower-grade aneurysms and that may be able to tolerate this intervention [76, 78]. The unruptured intracranial aneurysm treatment score (UIATS) provides a fast and easy method of triaging between the two treatment options; however, it has not yet been prospectively tested on patients harboring UIAs [79].

Studies such as ISAT, ISUIA, and UCAS are among the most cited concerning aneurysm treatment and natural history. The first of these revealed superior 1-year clinical outcomes for ruptured aneurysms by coiling in comparison to clipping, yet these results cannot be accurately extrapolated to clipping of UIAs [80]. The conditions in the unruptured setting are more advantageous, as the purpose of therapy is to ensure lifelong protection against aneurysm rupture, whereas the treatment of ruptured lesions is to allow survival of the patient during the acute phase of SAH without rebleeding or postoperative morbidity. Likewise, MCA aneurysms, which are generally considered more easily approached by surgery, were grossly underrepresented in this study. Several authors obtained much higher rates of complete obliteration via clipping than through endovascular procedures for aneurysms in this location [77, 81, 82]. This is more likely a consequence of the particular configurations of MCA aneurysms, rendering it more difficult to completely occlude the neck via endovascular procedures (wide-necked, possessing a small dome-to-neck ratio, the neck encompassing one of the arterial branches, etc.) [77]. Moreover, these aneurysms are generally adjacent to or surrounded by small perforators that may prohibit the use of stents. This technique also has the fundamental drawback of postprocedural thromboembolic events that may ensue at a higher frequency [83, 84]. In the largest multicenter study of very small UIAs treated via surgery, Bruneau et al. showed that the lesions found distal to the M1 segment were the safest to treat [85]. Despite additional enquires being required to reach a definitive conclusion, it is still worth regarding surgical clipping as the principal treatment modality for UIAs of the MCA.

Aneurysms of the anterior communicating artery are the most frequently reported in a large number of studies, possessing a higher risk of rupture than other locations while also being amenable to both endovascular and microsurgical techniques [36, 74, 86–89]. The term may actually be overly broad, also including aneurysms of the A1 and A2 junctions of the anterior cerebral artery or belonging entirely to these two segments, but being indistinguishable from true ACoA aneurysms on angiographic studies [88]. This location represents a genuine challenge for either approach. On the one hand, microvascular clipping is made difficult by depth, presence of perforators, and placement along the midline, implying increased cerebral traction in the absence of adequate relaxation [87, 89]. On the other hand, certain intrinsically unfavorable characteristics of aneurysms found in this location, such as a small dome, wide neck, multiple adjacent perforators, acute vessel angles, complex morphology, or posterior projection, can hinder endovascular procedures as well [74, 90]. In their systematic analysis, O'Neill et al. discovered that coiling delivers the most favorable clinical results, while stent-assisted coiling produced the highest incidence of treatment-related morbidity, without improving the rates of angiographically detectable recurrences or retreatment [74]. However, microsurgical clipping offered the most definitive aneurysm repair of the three methods and significantly lower rates of recurrence or reintervention. The best course of action for UIAs of this location remains to be decided.

UIAs of the internal carotid artery, including its smaller branches such as the anterior choroidal artery, ophthalmic artery, hypophyseal artery, and artery PCoA, are also fairly common, some sources citing them as the second most frequent after aneurysms of the ACoA [36, 91, 92]. Because the parent artery is located in proximity to the skull base, the surgical access of these aneurysms is often difficult. In order to address this issue, and many others, the first flow diverter device sanctioned for use was in 2011, being designated for wide-necked intracranial aneurysms of the ICA in adults [37]. Fortunately, small aneurysms of the cavernous segment generally present a low risk of rupture [73]. Therefore, taking into consideration the hemorrhage rates described by ISUIA for aneurysms of this location, it is generally not advisable to treat asymptomatic lesions smaller than 5 mm in any way [39, 73]. Aneurysms larger than 7 mm or those that are symptomatic can be safely treated by either method with satisfactory postoperative results. Once again, endovascular procedures are less invasive, but microsurgical clipping yields a higher rate of complete occlusion [93]. Despite this, due to the hemodynamic charge of the ICA, it is possible that pulsations, differences in wall thickness, and tension may cause clip rotation [94]. Additionally, after retractors are removed, the ensuing brain shift may determine additional kinking and subsequent stenosis of the anterior choroidal artery. ICA bifurcation aneurysms are generally scarce and, as a result, underrepresented in large prospective observational studies, leading to an enigmatic natural history [93]. For aneurysms of the paraclinoid ICA or of the ophthalmic artery, it is advisable to remove the anterior clinoid process to ensure better access and proximal control. This also alleviates the risk of causing postoperative visual disturbances, which represent a common complication of ICA aneurysm management, especially for this segment [95]. Using a bone microrongeur or an ultrasonic aspirator to perform piecemeal removal of the anterior clinoid instead of a high-speed drill leads to fewer such complications [95, 96]. Small UIAs of the paraclinoid ICA that are medially pointing can also be safely approached from the contralateral side, thus diminishing the need of mobilizing the optic nerves as well as of performing anterior clinoidectomy [97]. As a remark, appropriate selection of therapeutic method for unruptured aneurysms of the ICA and its branches should factor in the individualities of the lesions themselves. Ideally, a hybrid unit would allow either approach and the possibility of converting an endovascular procedure into an open surgical intervention in the case of intraprocedural complications (**Figure 3**).

Aneurysms of the posterior circulation, including the basilar artery apex or the posteroinferior cerebellar artery (PICA), have a much higher propensity to rupture [36, 73, 98]. Therefore, a conservative approach would be inadvisable for UIAs of this location. However, there is little data comparing the endovascular and surgical treatment of posterior circulation UIAs. After ISAT and the ensuing paradigm shift, there has been a scarcity of microsurgical reports on basilar apex aneurysms. Tjahjadi et al. reported a significantly higher rate of good and fair outcome (71 and 16%, respectively) after surgery of UIAs of the basilar apex than after clipping of ruptured lesions of the same site (49 and 19%, respectively) [99]. Nanda et al. also reported good outcomes following microsurgical clipping (71.9%) and asserted that a non-dominant PCoA (especially if hypoplastic) can be safely divided in the perforator-free area as to allow additional retraction of the ICA [100]. ISUIA revealed similar clinical outcomes for the patients recruited; however, the

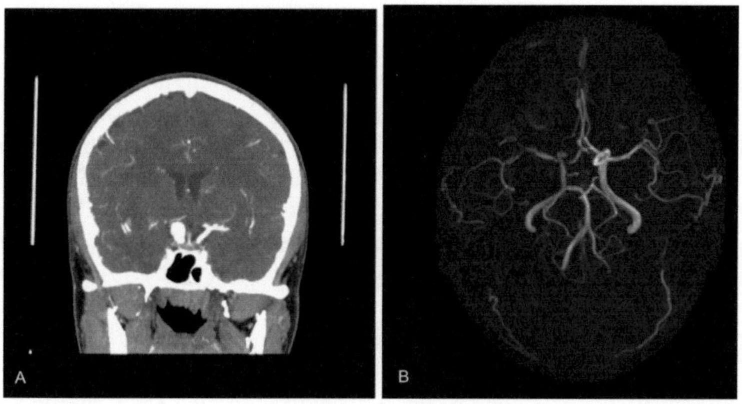


**Figure 3.**
*Illustrative case 1. (A) Preoperative CTA of a 21-year-old male with an incidentally discovered aneurysm of the right internal carotid artery (paraclinoidal segment). Video 1 is available at: https://bit.ly/2Z8W6rm. We used a right frontolateral craniotomy and approached the aneurysm via the Sylvian fissure. We drilled the anterior clinoid process, but the aneurysm ruptured during initial attempt at clipping. Because of its sheer size, we used three fenestrated clips to occlude the aneurysmal sac. The patient was discharged with no neurological deficit. (B) MRI scan, TOF sequence, at 1-year follow-up, showing the presence of the clip and no intraluminal flow.*

endovascular procedures only achieved complete occlusion in approximately half of the cases treated [50, 101]. In contrast, aneurysms of the PICA (and to a certain extent the vertebral artery—VA) are still primarily treated via clipping due to their wide necks, generally multilobulated and nonsacular characteristic, thrombosed lumens, emerging arteries, or distal locations that render coiling substandard [102]. The lower cranial nerves encountered in the surgical field can easily and securely be avoided, especially via the transcondylar approach [103]. Moreover, cases in which microsurgery should be more fervidly supported number those with unfavorable endovascular access, very small aneurysm domes, or contraindications for stent usage (intolerance to dual antiplatelet therapy, nickel allergy, etc.) [85, 101].

The previously mentioned UCAS and ISUIA are regarded as the most prudently devised large studies vis-à-vis the natural history of UIA, with numerous guidelines having been published in their wake in order to improve management decision-making [78]. However, imaging control was not compulsory in ISUIA; therefore, it could not tackle the possibility of aneurysms eventually changing their morphology or size. Moreover, there is the question of the UCAS not being relevant for populations outside Japan. There are still centers that recommend treatment for all small aneurysms possessing risk of developing SAH, the presence of a daughter sack or multiple aneurysms [78, 104]. After the ISAT was published, endovascular techniques gained a boost in popularity in the USA for both ruptured and unruptured aneurysms, overtaking surgical treatment in number of procedures performed [105]. Previous analyses show that coiling was associated with fewer complications, lower mortality, faster hospital discharge, and significantly lower costs than clipping [105, 106]. However, in centers outside the USA, where hospitalization, procedure, and nursing costs are lower, the differences concerning patient expenses are smaller. In South Korea, it seems that coiling is more expensive than clipping for UIAs, and this may also be available for developing countries [106]. The principal reason for this is the cost of endovascular implantable devices themselves (stents, coils and flow diverters, etc.), constituting more than 50% of procedure-related costs [107, 108]. Even so, a previous meta-analysis concluded that coiling generated a higher independent outcome and lower mortality rate, being the more cost-effective method of the two [108].

In aspects to randomized studies comparing endovascular therapy to surgery, the literature is extremely limited. The Collaborative Unruptured Endovascular Versus surgery (CURES) trial, which randomized 104 patients harboring unruptured between 3 and 25 millimeters to either coiling ($n$ = 56) or clipping ($n$ = 48), showed that there were no significant differences regarding in aneurysm occlusion rate, mortality, and morbidity after 1 year [80, 109]. Nevertheless, there were more patients with perioperative neurological deficit after clipping and with hospitalizations beyond 5 days. Mortality and morbidity rates for CURES were lower than reported in the ISUIA regarding both clipping and coiling [109]. Another prospective study, the trial on endovascular management of unruptured intracranial aneurysms (TEAM), which compared coiling to observational management, was halted less than 3 years after initiation as a result of poor recruitment [110].

Another controversial subject is the management of aneurysm remnant or repermeabilization after clipping or coiling. It has been repeatedly demonstrated that microsurgery leads to fewer such instances [75–82]. Although the issue of hemorrhage after initial treatment and its consequences have been extensively covered for ruptured aneurysms, there is currently no such data for UIAs [39]. Patients should therefore be regularly monitored (we recommend yearly CTA investigations), regardless of the form of treatment and any increase in size or change in morphology be contended judiciously.

Currently, the ideal strategy for solitary unruptured aneurysms is elusive. Although of great consequence, an issue seldom considered in these studies is the experience and proficiency of the neurosurgeon [73]. This is expressly observed in high-volume centers with a large number of operated cases, where outcomes are unquestionably much more favorable. Regardless, surgical prophylaxis of rupture via clipping remains a safe, effective, and possibly curative option. It remains to be seen whether the trends will continue to favor endovascular procedures or if an unexpected shift in balance might rejuvenate the popularity of surgical intervention.

## 8. Clipping of multiple aneurysms

In the Western population, it is estimated that 10–13% of patients with IAs possess MIAs, and it is sometimes difficult to find the source of SAH, but even more so to treat each lesion [70, 111–114]. A number of cases have been correlated with either congenital or chronic disorders such as Gaucher's disease, Fahr's disease, or Behcet's disease, although whether there is an etiologic correlation or merely a diagnostic coincidence is unknown [115–118]. Mirror aneurysms denote a rare condition in which the multiple aneurysms are placed symmetrically in the cerebral hemispheres. The most common sites are the non-cavernous segments of the ICAs [119, 120]. Mirror aneurysms also display a decreased propensity to rupture and improved outcomes than non-mirror aneurysms. Certain risk factors such as female gender (which also strongly influences the number of IAs), advanced age, smoking, uncontrolled hypertension, and increased body mass have been linked to a heightened chance of developing MIA [121, 122]. However, due to contradictory and inconclusive results, it is currently unknown whether the presence of MIAs implies a greater risk of rupture than that of single IAs [122]. Aneurysm morphology and size are thought to play the most important roles in the risk of rupture [91, 70]. Apparently, endovascular procedures lead to fewer neurologic complications than surgical clipping; however clipping yields higher occlusion rates, fewer total complications, and angiographic recurrence [69]. In theory, hemodynamic alterations occurring in an untreated distal UIA after the treatment of a proximal IA might increase the risk of bleeding, underlying the necessity of treating all aneurysms simultaneously and by any means [66]. It is sometimes feasible to treat all aneurysms at the same time during the same sitting and using the same craniotomy, thus lowering hospital stay, surgical exposure, and risk of complications [119, 123–125].

We support the classical pterional approach for tackling multiple aneurysms of the anterior circulation in the same opening. It offers a wide enough opening to approach even the aneurysms of the M1 segment on the opposite side. This is mostly useful for selected patients with simple contralateral UIA with narrow necks and which project inferiorly or anteriorly [119, 123]. The craniotomy should be performed on the side of the most complex aneurysm, or the one which has ruptured. On one hand, this methodology provides the highest visibility of the aneurysm and shortest distance to the dome and hematoma in case of bleeding. On the other hand, because of the hemodynamic changes that might occur during the clipping of the other IAs, it is easier to control bleeding on this side.

Clipping the contralateral aneurysms first may prevent a complicated and hard to manage bleeding on this side. After that, clipping the aneurysms more proximal to the surgeon can be performed. There are, however, some drawbacks to this technique [123, 126]. Firstly, it implies a heightened brain retraction compared to that of the same-side craniotomy, yet this can be managed by adequate brain relaxation. The maneuverability is lower, and the vision is reduced on the opposite side. However, a larger craniotomy, wider arachnoid dissection, and brain relaxation can aid in this situation. Contralateral MCA bifurcation and PCoA aneurysms are more difficult to find and clip, requiring maneuvering around thin perforators and fragile veins. Hemostasis is not as easy on the distal side in the case of rupture, which is why these IAs should be clipped first. Lastly, this technique requires an experienced vascular neurosurgical team; however, surgical simulation with 3D reconstructions may alleviate results [127]. However, this surgery should only be performed in selected cases, as the risks associated with a single challenging surgery do not compensate for the expenses of two easier interventions (**Figure 4**).

From our operative experience, we contraindicate performing two surgeries on two separate days, as the risk of rupture of the remaining untreated UIAs during this interval is not negligible. If a single opening is not indicated, we recommend approaching the more complex aneurysms first through one craniotomy, and afterward, during the same anesthesia, performing another craniotomy and clipping the residual UIAs. However, there is no consensus regarding this treatment method [119, 120, 126]. Alternatively, a combined surgical-endovascular approach can be performed, with surgery reserved for the ruptured and more difficult aneurysms [128, 129]. To summarize, deciding the management of multiple aneurysms should take into account the individual characteristics of the patient and of each the aneurysms, as well as the experience of the neurosurgical team involved.

## 9. Aneurysm clipping in elderly

At present, there are no corroborated management guidelines for UIAs in elderly patients, yet the retrospective reports reveal excellent results for both treatment strategies [130–132]. It has been shown that elderly patients with UIAs are less likely to die following aneurysmal rupture SAH than younger and/or female patients [37, 40, 78, 133, 134]. Therefore, a conservative approach may also be considered especially for small UIAs. Even so, the advanced age in itself supposedly increases the risk of periprocedural complications. Surgical interventions are correlated with larger amounts of blood loss, higher treatment-related costs, and longer hospitalizations than endovascular techniques, though provide a complete and maintainable aneurysmal occlusion

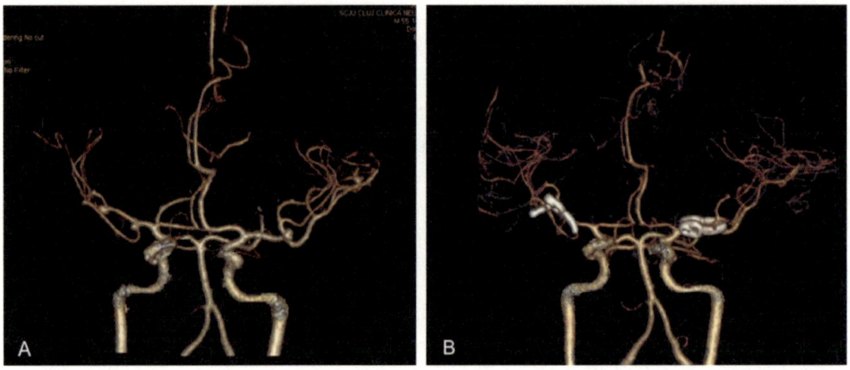


**Figure 4.**
*Illustrative case 2. (A) CTA 3D reconstruction of a 55-year-old male with multiple cerebral aneurysms—two on the right middle cerebral artery and one the left middle cerebral artery bifurcation. He presented to emergency department with right-sided weakness with gradual onset 3 days prior to surgery. Video 2 is available at: https://bit.ly/2Z8W6rm. He underwent microsurgical clipping via a right frontolateral craniotomy. All the clips were placed in the same procedure. (B) Postoperative CTA 3D reconstruction showing proper clip placement. He was discharged without any additional deficit.*

[130, 135, 136]. Despite the differences in regard to mortality being relatively small, they are nonetheless significant and favor endovascular coiling as the safest of the two [136]. Aside from preventing rupture, interventional therapy has demonstrated cognitive improvement without causing further intellectual deficits, in addition to a decrease in anxiety levels [137, 138]. Older patients harboring MIAs without a history of SAH can be managed conservatively, whereas those at risk or with a previous SAH should be treated in a one- or two-staged intervention [119]. Moreover, coiling might prove more appropriate for those with serious comorbidities and in an altered clinical state, while clipping is more suitable in the presence of intracranial vasospasm or hematomas [69]. The same as for younger patients with MIAs, the ruptured lesion should always be managed first and foremost, yet for unruptured MIAs treatment may only be indicated if the risk related to observation outweighs those of therapy.

## 10. Neurological and clinical outcome after clipping

There are conflicting reports regarding the postprocedural outcomes for these interventions. Short-term outcomes generally favor endovascular procedures, with a higher incidence of postinterventional adverse events after surgery [74, 139]. According to Kim et al., there is no significant difference regarding all-cause mortality at 7 years after the elective treatment of UIAs via either clipping or coiling [140]. The meta-analysis performed by Ruan et al. showed similar outcomes for the two procedures [141]. On the other hand, in their meta-analysis, Falk Delgado et al. reported a higher independent outcome and lower mortality after coiling of UIAs [108]. The outcomes may be improved with the intraoperative use of electrophysiological monitoring, fluorescence angiography, or Doppler ultrasonography [142]. Surgical clipping of UIAs does not negatively impact quality of life nor does it affect cognitive functions in such a way that patients are unable to work or drive at 6 weeks or 1 year after the intervention [143, 144]. The risk of poor outcome for patients below the age of 65 stands at around 2–4% and rises with aneurysm size, which when compared to the 0.3–0.9% risk of annual rupture might outclass the natural history in a few years after treatment [89, 103, 145]. Nonetheless, mortality is extremely low, if not inexistent in these series. Therefore, a more aggressive treatment may be acceptable for UIAs in younger patients. Although some series have demonstrated clipping of UIAs is effective and has no mortality even in elderly [131], the risk of a poorer outcome increases in this age group, with higher instances of disability and death than endovascular procedures specifically in the presence of comorbidities [132, 136]. Retreatment of intracranial aneurysms is also associated with a higher mortality rate [146]. However, in our experience, clipping of solitary UIAs yields excellent results, with no mortality and a high degree of functional independence, as will be shown in a later subchapter.

## 11. Complications of surgical clipping

Since clipping is a surgical intervention, there are chances of developing complications related to the procedure, medical and infectious complications as well as those attributable to anesthesia. The following paragraphs will focus on the complications of clipping itself. These can be divided according to timing of onset after the intervention into immediate and delayed complications.

IAR is one of the most frequent and most dreaded periprocedural complications [147]. This is especially the case for inexperienced (and oftentimes reckless) surgeons; however, preoperative GCS has also been shown to play a role in predicting this event [148]. It occurs especially around the time of neck dissection and clip placement or adjustment and is capable of hampering the microsurgical procedure, sometimes being life-threatening [149]. Nevertheless, it is significantly less frequent for UIAs than for the ruptured lesions [147]. A steady technique, proper discovery of the parent artery, temporary clipping proximal to the aneurysm, and aspiration can regain control of the situation and ensure proper clip placement.

Ischemic complications may also arise from improper clip placement or due to thromboembolism from the aneurysm. The type and severity of neurological consequences depend mostly on the location of the aneurysm [150–153]. The most frequent type of postoperative events and possibly even underestimated, ischemia leads to poorer outcomes at discharge and often entails a reintervention [153, 154]. After clipping of UIAs, transcranial Doppler studies show a decrease in transient reduction in cerebrovascular reactivity on the side of the aneurysm, leading to a proneness toward cerebral ischemia [155]. Endovascular procedures apparently bear a higher risk for thromboembolic events and ischemia [156], yet a recent meta-analysis showed that there was no statistical difference between coiling and clipping in respect to this event [141]. Incidence of perforator territory ischemia is higher for aneurysms of the A1 segment, whereas olfactory disturbances are more common for lesions of the ACoA [157]. Silent ischemic lesions are fairly frequent (up to 10% of procedures) and mostly irreversible, though rarely disabling [153, 157]. It has been argued that induced hypertension may reduce the effects of delayed cerebral ischemia [158]. Regardless, there is still no conclusive data to sustain the benefits of induced hypertension, whereas serious adverse events are sometimes unavoidable.

Another undesirable complication is the occlusion of the surrounding arteries, especially deep and subtle perforators. Again, dissection, proper magnification and illumination of the surgical field, and adequate brain relaxation can improve the visibility of the aneurysmal neck and surrounding structures. It is also important to utilize clips adjusted to aneurysm size and morphology. Electrophysiological monitoring, micro-Doppler ultrasonography, or intraoperative angiography can rapidly detect an arterial occlusion and facilitate repositioning of the clip [152, 159].

Clip slippage can happen when advanced atherosclerosis thickens the aneurysmal wall, making it impossible for the clip to close properly [151, 160]. Clip rotation and kinking of the parent vessel can also be the result of uneven arterial walls due to atheromatous degeneration [94]. Using a double-clip technique can often prevent this from occurring, yet certain aneurysms may require more complex techniques [151, 125, 160].

Aneurysmal residue or incomplete occlusion signifies an aneurysm sac or neck that is still permeable and has a significant chance of rupture [37, 80, 86, 161, 162]. Aneurysmal rest (or dog ear) occurs when a small triangular portion of the neck is not occluded by the aneurysmal blades. In time, and under certain hemodynamic conditions, this residual neck can lead to aneurysm regrowth, and eventual rupture, requiring further imaging studies and possibly another intervention [104]. In the microsurgical series described by Nanda, the majority of recurrences were found at the ACoA, followed by ICA, VA, and PICA [163]. Adequate neck dissection and using suitable clips may avoid this complication [164]. Also using intraoperative angiographic procedures can confirm proper clip placement.

Clipping UIAs of the ophthalmic artery can lead to visual disturbances [162]. Apparently, if visual deficit was present before treatment, clipping may offer a higher degree of improvement than coiling [162, 165]. From our own experience, we can add that the clipping of aneurysms of the paraclinoid segment of the ICA or the superior hypophyseal artery may in some cases result in acute pituitary deficiency. Some of these patients will require lifelong hormone substitution therapy.

Cerebral vasospasm is predominantly a complication of ruptured aneurysms, but it has rarely been described as occurring after clipping of UIA [166]. The exact etiological mechanism is unknown, although it might be multifactorial, especially after aggressive manipulation of the vessels.

Cognitive dysfunction after UIA therapy may occur, regardless of treatment method [137]. Nevertheless, the exact effect clipping has on cognitive functions remains uncertain.

Some patients with surgically treated UIAs may develop a chronic subdural hematoma in time, being at a higher risk for this than patients with ruptured lesions [167]. Risk factors include brain atrophy, male sex, chronic antiplatelet use, and advanced age.

As long as the risk of complications remains, the incentive of perfecting microsurgical techniques will persist. The purpose of gaining surgical experience is to ensure a long-term survival of the patient with the best possible neurological outcome, while also striving to lower or eliminate the chance of adverse events.

## 12. Our experience

During many years of practice, we learned that trying to make an asymptomatic patient feel better is ridiculously challenging. As for the patients themselves, the notion of living with an "undetonated bomb" might be daunting. As we have already shown, the issue of UIAs in a patient harboring multiple aneurysms out of which one has bled is equally controversial in the contemporary scientific literature.

We reviewed the experience of a single neurosurgeon (Professor Ioan Ştefan Florian MD, PhD—Iuliu Hatieganu University of Medicine and Pharmacy, Cluj-Napoca, Romania) in microsurgical clipping over 21 years (1997–2017). This amounted to a consecutive series of 872 patients with intracranial aneurysms (1004 separate lesions in total), both ruptured and unruptured.

From this patient pool, 89 (10.2%) presented with solitary UIA, the ages at the two extremes being 11 and 86 years, respectively. Among these, 46 (51.69%) were admitted with Hunt and Hess grade 0, while the remaining 43 (48.31%) were admitted with grade 1a. Regarding clinical outcome, our most important conclusion was that we encountered no mortality in this particular group. Eighty-seven patients (97.8%) were discharged with a Glasgow Outcome Score (GOS) of 5 (**Figure 5**).

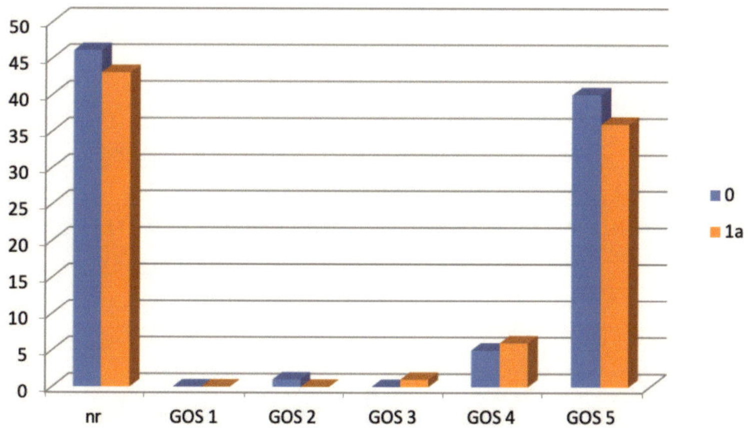


**Figure 5.**
*Outcome of patients with solitary unruptured aneurysms at time of discharge—author's case series (0, Hunt and Hess grade 0; 1a, Hunt and Hess grade 1a; GOS, Glasgow Outcome Score).*

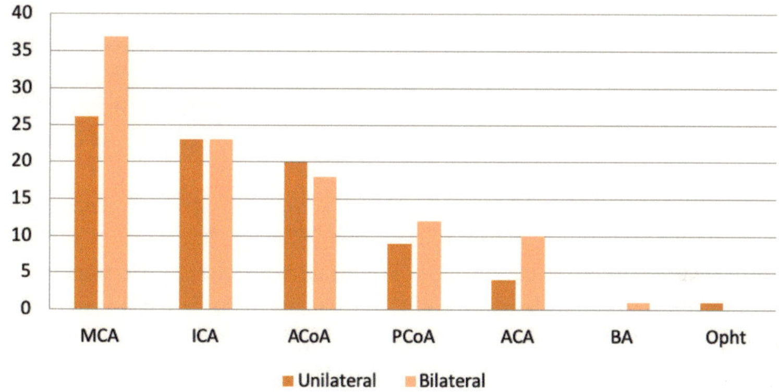


**Figure 6.**
*Location of lesions in the multiple cerebral aneurysms group. MCA, middle cerebral artery; ICA, internal carotid artery; ACoA, anterior communicating artery; PCoA, posterior communicating artery; ACA, anterior cerebral artery; BA, basilar artery; Opht, ophthalmic artery.*

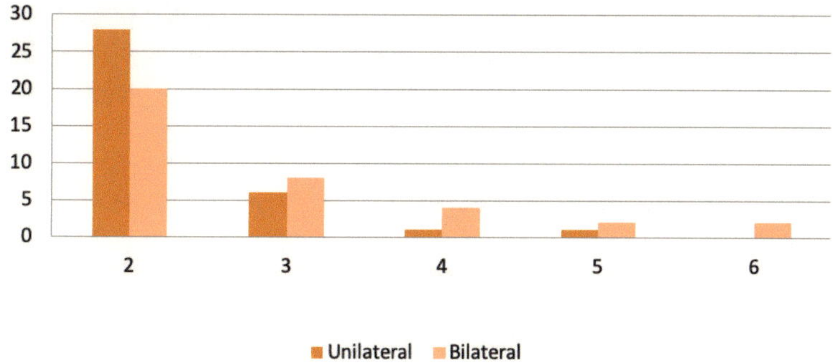


**Figure 7.**
*Number of lesions per patient with multiple intracranial aneurysms. The majority of patients with two aneurysms had both lesions on the same side, whereas for three or more lesions, these were bilateral. The highest number of aneurysms in a single patient was six.*

| Parameter | Statistical test | Odds ratio | Confidence interval 95% | P |
|---|---|---|---|---|
| Hunt and Hess scale | Mann-Whitney U | — | — | 0.588 |
| Associated complications | Chi square | 1.35 | 0.25–7.75 | 0.73 |
| Age | *t* | — | — | 0.25 |
| Preoperative days | *t* | — | — | 0.37 |
| Glasgow Outcome Scale | Chi square | 1.5 | 0.9–11.53 | 0.69 |
| Complications | Chi square | 2.6 | 0.53–13.11 | 0.22 |
| Mortality | Chi square | 0.4 | 0.03–5.24 | 0.47 |

**Table 1.**
*Comparison between the two groups on admission (Hunt and Hess scale, associated complications, and age) and on discharge (preoperative days, Glasgow Outcome Scale, complications, and mortality).*

In our series, we identified 101 patients (11.58%) with multiple aneurysms, harboring a total of 257 lesions. The most common location was the middle cerebral artery, followed by the internal carotid and anterior communicating artery (**Figure 6**). Initially, our approach in treating them was to clip the ruptured aneurysms or the ones with the higher risk, leaving the others for a later procedure. However, after we lost two patients with MIA on the night before the second planned intervention due to the rupture of the single unclipped lesion, we overhauled our methodology. The current goal in all cases is single-stage surgery (unilateral frontopterional approach) with all aneurysms clipped during the same procedure. If this is unfeasible, we perform a second craniotomy during the same anesthesia, as we believe the process of patient waking elevates the risk of rupture of any unclipped UIA.

Most patients presented with two aneurysms (57.6%). The highest number of aneurysms was six (one patient, female). The male-to-female ratio was 1:3, with the higher number of aneurysms leading to an increase of female predominance. Our series too suggests that MIA is primarily a pathology of the female gender (**Figure 7**).

We analyzed the complication rate, mortality, and state at discharge between groups with unilateral and bilateral aneurysms of the anterior circulation. There were no statistically significant differences between the two groups regarding the rate of complications or the outcome ($P > 0.05$, **Table 1**). When we compared patients with mirror middle cerebral aneurysms to the rest of the lot, no statistically significant difference could be observed either ($P > 0.05$). 60.39% of patients (61) were discharged with a favorable neurological outcome (GOS of 4 or 5).

Our data demonstrates that, with an appropriate selection of cases, surgery yields definitive and favorable results in solitary UIAs if handled by an experienced team. "Single-stage, single-opening surgery" is a viable option for treating the unruptured lesions in the context of multiple intracranial aneurysms.

## 13. Final remarks and future directions

Clipping of UIAs remains a valuable treatment option in preventing rupture and subsequent hemorrhagic stroke. In the hands of experienced vascular neurosurgeons, it is still a secure and long-lasting procedure, despite the relative ease and comparable safety and durability of endovascular procedures. Since aneurysmal rupture cannot be accurately predicted, clipping stands as a virtually curative procedure. Nevertheless, being an invasive procedure, it still harbors inherent risks. While our experience shows that clipping of solitary UIAs is not associated with mortality and only minimal morbidity, clipping of MIAs can pose a challenge.

Because any unclipped lesion bears a significant risk of rupture, we strongly advocate for the treatment of all aneurysms in patients with MIAs in the same procedure, and if feasible, through the same opening. The techniques and instruments themselves require constant updates in order to minimize postoperative morbidity and mortality while also ensuring ease and comfort in use. In the future, new clip technologies and intraprocedural methods of confirming the patency of parent or perforating vessels (such as fluorescein angiography) may further alleviate postoperative results. Additionally, new ways of training budding neurosurgeons in vascular pathology via interactive virtual simulations and augmented or virtual reality surgeries may rekindle the interest in surgical clipping for future generations.

## Conflict of interest

The authors declare that there is no conflict of interest.

## Other declarations

All authors contributed equally to the writing of this manuscript.

## Author details

Ioan Alexandru Florian[1,2]*, Teodora Larisa Timis[3], Cristina Caterina Aldea[1,2] and Ioan Stefan Florian[1,2]

1 Clinic of Neurosurgery, Cluj County Emergency Clinical Hospital, Cluj-Napoca, Romania

2 Department of Neurosurgery, Iuliu Hatieganu University of Medicine and Pharmacy, Cluj-Napoca, Romania

3 Department of Physiology, Iuliu Hatieganu University of Medicine and Pharmacy, Cluj-Napoca, Romania

*Address all correspondence to: florian.ioan.alexandru@gmail.com

## References

[1] Prestigiacomo CJ. Historical perspectives: The microsurgical and endovascular treatment of aneurysms. Neurosurgery. 2006;**59:**S3-39-S3-47

[2] Cushing H. Contributions to study of intracranial aneurysms. Guy's Hospital Reports. 1923;**73**:159-163

[3] Louw DF, Asfora WT, Sutherland GR. A brief history of aneurysm clips. Neurosurgical Focus. 2001;**11**(2):E4

[4] Peschillo S, Caporlingua A, Caporlingua F, Guglielmi G, Delfini R. Historical landmarks in the management of aneurysms and arteriovenous malformations of the central nervous system. World Neurosurg. Apr 2016;**88**:661-671. DOI: 10.1016/j.wneu.2015.10.093. PMID: 26555508.

[5] Lai LT, O'Neill AH. History, evolution, and continuing innovations of intracranial aneurysm surgery. World Neurosurgery. 2017;**102**:673-681. DOI: 10.1016/j.wneu.2017.02.006

[6] Duane W Jr. A modification of the McKenzie silver clip. Journal of Neurosurgery. 1950;**7**:92

[7] Botterell EH. Kenneth George McKenzie, M.D., F.R.C.S. 1923-1963. Surgical Neurology. 1982;**17**(2):81-89

[8] Alexander E. Kenneth George McKenzie, Canada's first neurosurgeon. Journal of Neurosurgery. 1974;**41**:1-9

[9] Pertuiset B, Siehez JP, Arthuis F, Bordi L, Haisa T, Siddiqui SA. Haemostatic clips and clamps used in surgical neurology with special reference to nonferromagnetic phynox spring clips by Aesculap. Acta Neurochirurgica (Wien). 1990;**102**:127-132

[10] Dujovny M, Agner C, Ibe O, Perlin A. Self-closing aneurysm clip: A historical review. Neurological Research. 2010;**32**(10):1011-1020

[11] Mayfield FH, Kees G Jr. A brief history of the development of the Mayfield clip. Journal of Neurosurgery. 1971;**35**:97-100

[12] Viers A, Allen MB, Alleyne CH. George W. Smith, M.D. (1916-1964). Journal of Neurosurgery. 2012;**117**(4): 800-803

[13] Sundt TM, Murphey F. Clip-grafts for aneurysm and small vessel surgery. 3. Clinical experience in intracranial internal carotid artery aneurysms. Journal of Neurosurgery. 1969;**31**(1):59-71. DOI: 10.3171/jns.1969.31.1.0059

[14] Pool JL, Colton RP. The dissecting microscope for intracranial vascular surgery. Journal of Neurosurgery. 1966;**25**:315-318

[15] Shellock FG, Shellock VJ. Spetzler titanium aneurysm clips: Compatibility at MR imaging. Radiology. 1998;**206**: 838-841

[16] Lawton MT, Heiserman JE, Prendergast VC, Zabramski JM, Spetzler RF. Titanium aneurysm clips: Part III—Clinical application in 16 patients with subarachnoid hemorrhage. Neurosurgery. 1996;**38**:1170-1175

[17] Yasargil MG. Microneurosurgery, Clinical Considerations, Surgery of the Intracranial Aneurysms and Results. Vol. II. New York: Thieme; 1984. 398 p

[18] Kacucs C, Florian IA, Ungureanu G, Florian IS. Fluorescein angiography in intracranial aneurysm surgery: A helpful method to evaluate the security of clipping and observe blood flow. World Neurosurgery. 2017;**105**:406-411

[19] Wrobel CJ, Meltzer H, Lamond R, Alksne JF. Intraoperative assessment of

aneurysm clip placement by intravenous fluorescein angiography. Neurosurgery. 1994;**35**:970-973

[20] Washington CW, Zipfel GJ, Chicoine MR, Derdeyn CP, Rich KM, Moran CJ, et al. Comparing indocyanine green videoangiography to the gold standard of intraoperative digital subtraction angiography used in aneurysm surgery. Journal of Neurosurgery. 2013;**118**:420-427

[21] Kassam AB, Gardner PA, Mintz A, Snyderman CH, Carrau RL, Horowitz M. Endoscopic endonasal clipping of an unsecured superior hypophyseal artery aneurysm. Technical note. Journal of Neurosurgery. 2007;**107**:1047-1052

[22] Ensenat J, Alobid I, de Notaris M, Sanchez M, Valero R, Prats-Galino A, et al. Endoscopic endonasal clipping of a ruptured vertebral-posterior inferior cerebellar artery aneurysm: Technical case report. Neurosurgery. 2011;**69**(1 suppl operative):onsE121-onsE127 [discussion: onsE127-onsE128]

[23] Germanwala AV, Zanation AM, et al. Neurosurgery. 2011;**68**(1 suppl operative):234-239 [discussion: 240]

[24] Werner SC, Blakemore AH, King BG. Aneurysm of the internal carotid artery within the skull: Wiring and electrothermic coagulation. Journal of the American Medical Association. 1941;**116**:578-582

[25] Mullan S, Reyes C, Dawley J. Stereotactic copper electric thrombosis of intracranial aneurysms. Progress in Neurological Surgery. 1969;**3**:193-211

[26] Dandy WE. Intracranial arterial aneurysms in the carotid canal. Diagnosis and treatment. Archives of Surgery. 1942;**45**:335-350

[27] Alksne JF, Fingerhut AG, Rand RW. Magnetic probe for the stereotactic thrombosis of intracranial aneurysms. Journal of Neurology, Neurosurgery, and Psychiatry. 1967;**30**:159-162

[28] Gallagher JP: Pilojection for intracranial aneurysms: Report of progress. Journal of Neurosurgery. 1964; 21: 129-134

[29] Artico M, Spoletini M, Fumagalli L, Biagioni F, Ryskalin L, Fornai F, et al. Egas Moniz: 90 years (1927-2017) from cerebral angiography. Frontiers in Neuroanatomy. 2017;**11**:81. DOI: 10.3389/fnana.2017.00081

[30] Moniz E. Cerebral angiography: Its application in clinical practice and physiology. Lancet. 1933;**225**:1144-1147

[31] Wolpert SM. On the radiologic diagnosis of cerebral aneurysms with plain films and cerebral angiography: A historical survey. American Journal of Neuroradiology. 1995;**16**:181-184

[32] Serbinenko FA. Balloon catheterization and occlusion of major cerebral vessels. Journal of Neurosurgery. 1974;**41**:125-145

[33] Guglielmi G, Vinuela F. Endovascular treatment of intracranial saccular aneurysms with GDC platinum detachable coils: Small-necked aneurysms. In: Pasqualin A, Da Pian R, editors. New Trends in Management of Cerebro-Vascular Malformations. Springer, Vienna. 1994; pp 269-271

[34] Phillips TJ, Mitchell P. Endovascular treatment of intracranial aneurysms. Imaging in Medicine. 2010;**2**(6):633-657

[35] Byrne JV, Guglielmi G. Treatment by endosaccular packing with the guglielmi detachable coil. In: Endovascular Treatment of Intracranial Aneurysms. Berlin, Heidelberg: Springer; 1998. pp. 133-165

[36] Seibert B, Tummala RP, Chow R, Faridar A, Mousavi SA, Divani AA.

Intracranial aneurysms: Review of current treatment options and outcomes. Frontiers in Neurology. 2011;**2**:45

[37] Pierot L, Gawlitza M, Soize S. Unruptured intracranial aneurysms: Management strategy and current endovascular treatment options. Expert Review of Neurotherapeutics. 2017. DOI: 10.1080/14737175.2017.1371593

[38] Koebbe CJ, Veznedaroglu E, Jabbour P, Rosenwasser RH. Endovascular management of intracranial aneurysms: Current experience and future advances. Neurosurgery. 2006;**59**(5 Suppl 3):S93-S102 [discussion S3-13]

[39] Ambekar S, Khandelwal P, Bhattacharya P, Watanabe M, Yavagal DR. Treatment of unruptured intracranial aneurysms: A review. Expert Review of Neurotherapeutics. 2016;**16**(10):1205-1216

[40] Aishima K, Shimizu T, Aihara M, Yoshimoto Y. Lifetime effects of small unruptured intracranial aneurysms. World Neurosurgery. 2016;**95**:434-440. DOI: 10.1016/j.wneu.2016.08.060

[41] Chen Y, Fan H, He X, et al. China intracranial aneurysm project (CIAP): Protocol for a prospective cohort study of interventional treatment and craniotomy for unruptured aneurysms. BMJ Open. 2018;**8**:e019333. DOI: 10.1136/ bmjopen-2017-019333

[42] Morita A, Kirino T, Hashi K, et al. The natural course of unruptured cerebral aneurysms in a Japanese cohort. The New England Journal of Medicine. 2012;**366**:2474-2482

[43] Poeata I. Intracranial aneurysms. In: Popescu I, Ciuce C, editors. Treaty of Surgery, Neurosurgery. 2nd ed. Vol. VI. Bucharest: Editura Academiei Române; 2014. pp. 384-391. [Text in Romanian]

[44] Byoun HS, Huh W, Oh CW, Bang JS, Hwang G, Kwon OK. Natural history of unruptured intracranial aneurysms: A retrospective single center analysis. Journal of Korean Neurosurgical Association. 2016;**59**(1):11-16

[45] Güresir E, Vatter H, Schuss P, Platz J, Konczalla J, de Rochement RM, et al. Natural history of small unruptured anterior circulation aneurysms: A prospective cohort study. Stroke. 2013;**44**(11):3027-3031

[46] Müller TB, Sandvei MS, Kvistad KA, Rydland J, Håberg A, Vik A, et al. Unruptured intracranial aneurysms in the Norwegian Nord-Trøndelag Health Study (HUNT): risk of rupture calculated from data in a population-based cohort study. Neurosurgery. 2013;**73**(2):256-261 [discussion 260; quiz 261]

[47] Korja M, Lehto H, Juvela S. Lifelong rupture risk of intracranial aneurysms depends on risk factors: A prospective Finnish cohort study. Stroke. 2014;**45**(7):1958-1963

[48] Le Roux PD, Winn RH. Surgical decision making for the treatment of intracranial aneurysms. In: Winn R, editor. Youmans and Winn Neurological Surgery. 7th ed. Philadelphia: Elsevier; 2017. pp. 3232-3256

[49] Thompson BG, Brown RD Jr, Amin-Hanjani S, Broderick JP, Cockroft KM, Connolly ES Jr, et al. Guidelines for the management of patients with unruptured intracranial aneurysms: A guideline for healthcare professionals from the American Heart Association/ American Stroke Association. Stroke. 2015;**46**(8):2368-2400

[50] Wiebers DO, Whisnant JP, Huston J 3rd, Meissner I, Brown RD Jr, Piepgras DG, et al. Unruptured intracranial aneurysms: natural history, clinical outcome, and risks of surgical

and endovascular treatment. Lancet. 2003;**362**:103-110

[51] Inoue T, Shimizu H, Fujimura M, Saito A, Tominaga T. Annual rupture risk of growing unruptured cerebral aneurysms detected by magnetic resonance angiography. Journal of Neurosurgery. 2012;**117**:20-25

[52] Serrone JC, Tackla RD, Gozal YM, Hanseman DJ, Gogela SL, Vuong SM, et al. Aneurysm growth and de novo aneurysms during aneurysm surveillance. Journal of Neurosurgery. 2016;**125**(6):1374-1382

[53] Suzuki T, Takao H, Suzuki T, Kambayashi Y, Watanabe M, Sakamoto H, et al. Determining the presence of thin-walled regions at high-pressure areas in unruptured cerebral aneurysms by using computational fluid dynamics. Neurosurgery. 2016;**79**(4):589-595

[54] Ramachandran M, Retarekar R, Raghavan ML, Berkowitz B, Dickerhoff B, Correa T, et al. Assessment of image-derived risk factors for natural course of unruptured cerebral aneurysms. Journal of Neurosurgery. 2016;**124**:288-295

[55] Kawai K, Nonaka K, Suzuki H, Kirino T, Tamura A. Differential effects of activity and climate on onset of subarachnoid hemorrhage. Neurologia Medico-Chirurgica (Tokyo). 2001;**41**(5):229-236

[56] Nyquist PA, Brown RD Jr, Wiebers DO, Crowson CS, O'Fallon WM. Circadian and seasonal occurrence of subarachnoid and intracerebral hemorrhage. Neurology. 2001;**56**(2):190-193

[57] Beseoglu K, Hanggi D, Stummer W, Steiger HJ. Dependence of subarachnoid hemorrhage on climate conditions: A systematic meteorological analysis from the Dusseldorf metropolitan area. Neurosurgery. 2008;**62**:1033-1038 [discussion 8-9]

[58] Umemura K, Hirashima Y, Kurimoto M, Kuwayama N, Kubo M, Origasa H, et al. Involvement of meteorological factors and sex in the occurrence of subarachnoid hemorrhage in Japan. Neurologia Medico-Chirurgica (Tokyo). 2008;**48**(3):101-107

[59] de Steenhuijsen Piters WA, Algra A, van den Broek MF, Dorhout Mees SM, Rinkel GJ. Seasonal and meteorological determinants of aneurysmal subarachnoid hemorrhage: A systematic review and meta-analysis. Journal of Neurology. 2013;**260**(2):614-619

[60] Mastorakos P, Ding D, Peterson E, Starke RM. General principles for the management of ruptured and unruptured intracranial aneurysms. In: Principles of Neurological Surgery. Elsevier Inc; 2018. pp. 254-263. e2

[61] Frösen J, Tulamo R, Paetau A, et al. Saccular intracranial aneurysm: Pathology and mechanisms. Acta Neuropathologica. 2012;**123**(6):773-786

[62] Mut F, Hamzei-Sichani F, Doddasomayajula R, et al. Hemodynamic characteristics of ruptured and unruptured multiple aneurysms at mirror and ipsilateral locations. American Journal of Neuroradiology. 2017;**38**(12):2301-2307

[63] Cebral JR, Duan X, Chung BJ, Putman C, Aziz K, Robertson AM. Wall mechanical properties and hemodynamics of unruptured intracranial aneurysms. AJNR. American Journal of Neuroradiology. 2015;**36**(9):1695-1703

[64] Tateshima S, Tanishita K, Omura H, Villablanca JP, Vinuela F. Intra-aneurysmal hemodynamics during the growth of an unruptured aneurysm:

In vitro study using longitudinal CT angiogram database. American Journal of Neuroradiology. Apr 2007;**28**(4):622-627

[65] El-Bassiouny OA, Saqr KM, Shehata AI, Hassan T, el Gibaly A, Diaa O. Effects of non-Newtonian viscosity on the hemodynamics of cerebral aneurysms. Applied Mechanics and Materials. 2016;**819**:366-370

[66] Conde Alonso C, Riveiro Rodríguez A, Díaz Molina J, et al. Hemodynamic changes in the treatment of multiple intracranial aneurysms: A computational fluid dynamics study. World Neurosurgery. 2018;**118**:e631-e638

[67] Mohamied Y, Sherwin SJ, Weinberg PD. Understanding the fluid mechanics behind transverse wall shear stress. Journal of Biomechanics. 2017;**50**:102-109

[68] Sforza DM, Putman CM, Cebral JR. Hemodynamics of cerebral aneurysms. Annual Review of Fluid Mechanics. 2009;**41**:91-107

[69] Dong QL, Gao BL, Cheng ZR, et al. Comparison of surgical and endovascular approaches in the management of multiple intracranial aneurysms. International Journal of Surgery. 2016;**32**:129-135

[70] Zhang Y, Yang X, Wang Y, et al. Influence of morphology and hemodynamic factors on rupture of multiple intracranial aneurysms: Matched-pairs of ruptured-unruptured aneurysms located unilaterally on the anterior circulation. BMC Neurology. 2014;**14**(1):253

[71] Byun HS, Rhee K. Intraaneurysmal flow changes affected by clip location and occlusion magnitude in a lateral aneurysm model. Medical Engineering & Physics. 2003;**25**(7):581-589

[72] Inoue T, Iwaasa M, Nagata I, Isotani E, Ishizaka S, Horie N. Impact of clipping versus coiling on postoperative hemodynamics and pulmonary edema after subarachnoid hemorrhage. BioMed Research International. 2014;**2014**(1):1-9

[73] Chen SF, Kato Y, Sinha R, Kumar A, Watabe T, Imizu S, et al. Surgical treatment of patients with unruptured intracranial aneurysms. Journal of Clinical Neuroscience. 2015;**22**(1):69-72

[74] O'Neill AH, Chandra RV, Lai LT. Safety and effectiveness of microsurgical clipping, endovascular coiling, and stent assisted coiling for unruptured anterior communicating artery aneurysms: A systematic analysis of observational studies. Journal of Neurointerventional Surgery. 2017;**9**(8):761-765

[75] Bradac O, Hide S, Mendelow DA, Benes V. Aneurysm treatment in Europe 2010: An internet survey. Acta Neurochirurgica. 2012;**154**(6):971-977. DOI: 10.1007/s00701-012-1340-2

[76] Chua MH, Griessenauer CJ, Stapleton CJ, He L, Thomas AJ, Ogilvy CS. Documentation of improved outcomes for intracranial aneurysm management over a 15-year interval. Stroke. 2016;**47**(3):708-712

[77] Choi JH, Park JE, Kim MJ, Kim BS, Shin YS. Aneurysmal neck clipping as the primary treatment option for both ruptured and Unruptured middle cerebral artery aneurysms. Journal of Korean Neurosurgical Association. 2016;**59**(3):269-275

[78] Tintim C, Machado HS. Clipping versus coiling for intracranial aneurysms: Recent trends. Journal of Anesthesia and Clinical Research. 2017;**08**(06):1-10. DOI: 10.4172/2155-6148.1000732

[79] Etminan N, Brown RD, Beseoglu K, et al. The unruptured intracranial aneurysm treatment score: A multidisciplinary consensus. Neurology. 2015;**85**(10):881-889

[80] Te D, Findlay JM, Magro E, et al. Surgical clipping or endovascular coiling for unruptured intracranial aneurysms: A pragmatic randomised trial. Journal of Neurology, Neurosurgery, and Psychiatry. 2017;**88**:663-668

[81] van Dijk JM, Groen RJ, Ter Laan M, Jeltema JR, Mooij JJ, Metzemaekers JD. Surgical clipping as the preferred treatment for aneurysms of the middle cerebral artery. Acta Neurochirurgica. 2011;**153**(11):2111-2117

[82] Güresir E, Schuss P, Berkefeld J, Vatter H, Seifert V. Treatment results for complex middle cerebral artery aneurysms. A prospective single center series. Acta Neurochirurgica. 2011;**153**:1247-1252

[83] Yahia AM, Latorre J, Gordon V, Whapham J, Malek A, Fessler RD. Tromboembolic events associated with neuroform stent in endovascular treatment of intracranial aneurysms. Journal of Neuroimaging. 2010;**20**:113-117

[84] Yahia AM, Gordon V, Whapham J, Malek A, Steel J, Fessler RD. Complications of neuroform stent in endovascular treatment of intracranial aneurysms. Neurocritical Care. 2008;**8**:19-30

[85] Bruneau M, Amin-Hanjani S, Koroknay-Pal P, Bijlenga P, Jahromi BR, Lehto H, et al. Surgical clipping of very small unruptured intracranial aneurysms: A multicenter international study. Neurosurgery. 2016 Jan;**78**(1):47-52

[86] Proust F, Debono B, Hannequin D, et al. Treatment of anterior communicating artery aneurysms: Complementary aspects of microsurgical and endovascular procedures. Journal of Neurosurgery. 2003;**99**:3-14

[87] Hernesniemi J, Dashti R, Lehecka M, et al. Microneurosurgical management of anterior communicating artery aneurysms. Surgical Neurology. 2008;**70**:8-28 [discussion 29]

[88] Wong H, Banfield J, Hughes N, Shankar JJS. Are anterior communicating aneurysms truly anterior communicating aneurysms? An observational study. World Neurosurgery. 2019. pii: S1878-8750(19)30365-1

[89] Lai LT, Gragnaniello C, Morgan MK. Outcomes for a case series of unruptured anterior communicating artery aneurysm surgery. Journal of Clinical Neuroscience. 2013;**20**:1688-1692

[90] Finitsis S, Anxionnat R, Lebedinsky A, et al. Endovascular treatment of ACom intracranial aneurysms. Report on series of 280 patients. Interventional Neuroradiology. 2010;**16**:7-16

[91] Bhogal P, AlMatter M, Hellstern V, Ganslandt O, Bäzner H, Henkes H, et al. Difference in aneurysm characteristics between ruptured and unruptured aneurysms in patients with multiple intracranial aneurysms. Surgical Neurology International. 2018;**9**:1

[92] Maud A, Rodriguez GJ, Barboza MA. Endovascular treatment of intracranial aneurysms by interventional neurologists: First year single-center experience. Journal of Vascular and Interventional Neurology. 2014;**7**(2):13-16

[93] La Pira B, Brinjikji W, Burrows AM, Cloft HJ, Vine RL, Lanzino G. Unruptured internal carotid artery bifurcation aneurysms: General features and overall results after modern

treatment. Acta Neurochirurgica. 2016;**158**(11):2053-2059

[94] Sakuma J, Suzuki K, Sasaki T, Matsumoto M, Oinuma M, Kawakami M, et al. Monitoring and preventing blood flow insufficiency due to clip rotation after the treatment of internal carotid artery aneurysms. Journal of Neurosurgery. 2004;**100**(5):960-962

[95] Kikuta K, Kitai R, Kodera T, Arishima H, Isozaki M, Hashimoto N, et al. Predictive factors for the occurrence of visual and ischemic complications after open surgery for paraclinoid aneurysms of the internal carotid artery. Acta Neurochirurgica. Supplement. 2016;**123**:41-49

[96] Chang DJ. The "no-drill" technique of anterior clinoidectomy: A cranial base approach to the paraclinoid and parasellar region. Neurosurgery. 2009;**64**(3 Suppl):ons96-ons105 [discussion ons105-6]

[97] Serrano LE, Ayyad A, Archavlis E, Schwandt E, Nimer A, Ringel F, et al. A literature review concerning contralateral approaches to paraclinoid internal carotid artery aneurysms. Neurosurgical Review. 2018. DOI: 10.1007/s10143-018-01063-3 [Epub ahead of print]

[98] Nanda A, Patra DP, Bir SC, Maiti TK, Kalakoti P, Bollam P. Microsurgical clipping of unruptured intracranial aneurysms: A single Surgeon's experience over sixteen years. World Neurosurgery. Apr 2017;**100**: 85-99. DOI: 10.1016/j.wneu.2016.12.099

[99] Tjahjadi M, Kivelev J, Serrone JC, Maekawa H, Kerro O, Jahromi BR, et al. Factors determining surgical approaches to basilar bifurcation aneurysms and its surgical outcomes. Neurosurgery. 2016;**78**(2):181-191

[100] Nanda A, Sonig A, Banerjee AD, Javalkar VK. Microsurgical management of basilar artery apex aneurysms: A single surgeon's experience from Louisiana State University, Shreveport. World Neurosurgery. 2014;**82**(1-2):118-129

[101] Tjahjadi M, Serrone J, Hernesniemi J. Should we still consider clips for basilar apex aneurysms? A critical appraisal of the literature. Surgical Neurology International. 2018;**9**:44. Published Feb 21, 2018. DOI: 10.4103/sni.sni_311_17

[102] Sanai N, Tarapore P, Lee AC, Lawton MT. The current role of microsurgery for posterior circulation aneurysms: A selective approach in the endovascular era. Neurosurgery. 2008;**62**:1236-1249 [discussion 1249-1253]

[103] Palanisamy D, Yasuhiro Y, Kyosuke M, Tsukasa K, Katsumi T, Kato Y. Transcondylar fossa approach to unruptured vertebral artery and vertebral artery–posterior inferior cerebellar artery aneurysms: Surgical outcome. World Neurosurgery. 2018;**119**:e783-e791. DOI: 10.1016/j.wneu.2018.07.268

[104] Dellaretti M, Ronconi D, Batista DM, de Souza RF, de Almeida CER, Fontoura RR, et al. Safety and efficacy of surgical treatment of intracranial aneurysms: The experience of a single Brazilian Center. World Neurosurgery. 2018;**117**:e580-e587

[105] Lin N, Cahill KS, Frerichs KU, Friedlander RM, Claus EB. Treatment of ruptured and unruptured cerebral aneurysms in the USA: A paradigm shift. Journal of Neurointerventional Surgery. 2018;**10**:i69-i76

[106] Zhang X, Tang H, Huang Q, Hong B, Xu Y, Liu J. Total hospital costs and length of stay of endovascular coiling versus neurosurgical clipping for unruptured intracranial aneurysms:

systematic review and meta-analysis. World Neurosurg. 2018;**115**: 393-399. DOI: https://doi.org/10.1016/j.wneu.2018.04.028

[107] Stone DH, Horvath AJ, Goodney PP, Rzucidlo EM, Nolan BW, Walsh DB, et al. The financial implications of endovascular aneurysm repair in the cost containment era. Journal of Vascular Surgery. 2014;**59**(2):283-290. 90.e1

[108] Falk Delgado A, Andersson T, Falk DA. Clinical outcome after surgical clipping or endovascular coiling for cerebral aneurysms: A pragmatic meta-analysis of randomized and non-randomized trials with short- and long-term follow-up. Journal of Neurointerventional Surgery. 2017;**9**(3):264-277

[109] Huang W, Du R. 2016-2017 Clinical trials in cerebrovascular neurosurgery. Journal of Clinical Neuroscience. 2019;**60**:31-35

[110] Raymond J, Darsaut TE, Molyneux AJ, TEAM Collaborative Group. A trial on unruptured intracranial aneurysms (the TEAM trial): Results, lessons from a failure and the necessity for clinical care trials. Trials. 2011;**12**:64. Published Mar 4, 2011. DOI: 10.1186/1745-6215-12-64

[111] Berg P, Beuing O. Multiple intracranial aneurysms: A direct hemodynamic comparison between ruptured and unruptured vessel malformations. International Journal for Computer Assisted Radiology and Surgery. 2018;**13**:83

[112] Murrone D, Romanelli B, Ierardi A. Surgical case series of multiple aneurysms: A single-Centre experience of 16 years. International Journal of Surgery Case Reports. 2018;**42**:191-195

[113] Dammann P, Wrede KH, Sure U, et al. Risk factors for and clinical consequences of multiple intracranial aneurysms. Stroke. 2018;**49**(4):848-855

[114] Orning JL, Shakur SF, Alaraj A, Behbahani M, Charbel FT, Aletich VA, et al. Accuracy in identifying the source of subarachnoid hemorrhage in the setting of multiple intracranial aneurysms. Neurosurgery. 2018;**83**(1):62-68

[115] Reynolds MR, Heiferman DM, Boucher AB, Howard BM, Barrow DL, Dion JE. Multiple intracranial aneurysms in a patient with type I Gaucher disease: A case report and literature review. British Journal of Neurosurgery. 2018;**15**:1-3

[116] Eroglu U, Kahilogullari G, Demirel A, Arat A, Unlu A. Fahr's syndrome associated with multiple intracranial aneurysms: A case report. Turkish Neurosurgery. 2016;**26**(4):643-645

[117] Ha S, Kim J, Kim CG, Jang SJ. Multiple intracranial aneurysms associated with Behçet's disease. Journal of Cerebrovascular and Endovascular Neurosurgery. 2016;**18**(1):32-37

[118] Fkihi A, Argillos K, Belfeki N, Dahmani R, Velmans N. Unruptured multiple intracranial aneurysms associated with Behçet's disease. Journal de Médecine Vasculaire. 2017;**42**(4):234-236

[119] Wu C, Zhang Y-Y, Xue Z, et al. Treatment strategies for intracranial mirror aneurysms. World Neurosurgery. 2017;**100**:450-458

[120] Mehrotra A, Sharma P, Das KK, Bhaisora KS, Sardhara J, Gupta S, et al. Mirror aneurysms among multiple aneurysms: Lesser of the two evils. World Neurosurgery. Aug 2016;**92**:126-132. DOI: 10.1016/j.wneu.2016.04.124

[121] McDowell MM, Sussman E, Claassen J, et al. Demographic and

clinical predictors of multiple intracranial aneurysms in patients with subarachnoid hemorrhage. Journal of Neurosurgery. 2017;**112**:961-968

[122] Pan J-W, Zhu Y, Weng Y-X, Jiang H, Zhan R-Y, Shen J. Patient and aneurysm characteristics associated with rupture risk of multiple intracranial aneurysms in the anterior circulation system. Acta Neurochirurgica. 2016;**158**(7):1367-1375

[123] Rodríguez-Hernández A, Gabarrós A, Lawton MT. Contralateral clipping of middle cerebral artery aneurysms. Operative Neurosurgery. 2012;**71**(September):ons116-ons124

[124] Asiltürk M, Abdallah A. Clinical outcomes of multiple aneurysms microsurgical clipping: Evaluation of 90 patients. Neurologia i Neurochirurgia Polska. 2018;**52**(1):15-24

[125] Fotakopoulos G, Elera-Florez H, Hernesniemi J, Colasanti R, Choque-Velasquez J. Seven cerebral aneurysms: A challenging case from the Andean slopes managed with 1-stage surgery. World Neurosurgery. 2016;**97**:565-570

[126] Guo S, Xing Y. Surgical treatment of multiple intracranial aneurysms. Turkish Neurosurgery. 2014;**24**(2):208-213

[127] Ling C, Wang H, Chen Z, et al. Contralateral approach based on a preoperative 3-dimensional virtual osteotomy technique for anterior circulation aneurysms. Journal of Stroke and Cerebrovascular Diseases. 2019;**28**(4):1099-1106

[128] Kheĭreddin AS, Filatov IM, Belousova OB, Eliava SS, Iakovlev SB, Sazonov IA, et al. Substantiation of differentiated management of patients with multiple cerebral aneurysms [in Russian]. Zhurnal Voprosy Neĭrokhirurgii Imeni N. N. Burdenko. 2012;**76**(3):45-53 [discussion 53]

[129] Ahmed O, Kalakoti P, Hefner M, Cuellar H, Guthikonda B. Seven intracranial aneurysms in one patient: Treatment and review of literature. Journal of Cerebrovascular and Endovascular Neurosurgery. 2015;**17**(2):113-119

[130] Chernyshev OY, Bir SC, Maiti TK, et al. Changing paradigm in the management of elderly patients with intracranial aneurysms: An institutional review. Journal of Clinical Neuroscience. 2017;**43**:94-102

[131] Park JH, Kim YI, Lim YC. Clinical outcomes of treatment for intracranial aneurysm in elderly patients. Journal of Cerebrovascular and Endovascular Neurosurgery. 2014;**16**(3):193

[132] O'Neill AH, Chandra RV, Slater LA, et al. Influence of comorbidities on treatment of unruptured intracranial aneurysms in the elderly. Journal of Clinical Neuroscience. 2019;**62**:38-45

[133] Brown RD, Broderick JP. Unruptured intracranial aneurysms: Epidemiology, natural history, management options, and familial screening. Lancet Neurology. 2014;**13**(4):393-404

[134] Gu Y, Tian Y, Leng B, et al. Treatment strategy for unruptured intracranial aneurysm in elderly patients: Coiling, clipping, or conservative? Cell Transplantation. 2019;**28**(6):767-774

[135] Kim M, Park J, Lee J. Comparative cost analysis for surgical and endovascular treatment of unruptured intracranial aneurysms in South Korea. Journal of Korean Neurosurgical Association. 2015;**57**(6):455-459

[136] Eloy JA, Gandhi CD, Shao B, Silva NA, Sylvester MJ. Unruptured aneurysms in the elderly: Perioperative outcomes and cost analysis of endovascular coiling and

surgical clipping. Neurosurgical Focus. 2018;**44**(May):E4. DOI: 10.3171/2018.1.focus17714

[137] Srinivasan VM, Wagner K, Chen SR, et al. Cognitive sequelae of Unruptured and ruptured intracranial aneurysms and their treatment: Modalities for neuropsychological assessment. World Neurosurgery. 2018;**120**:537-549

[138] Kubo Y, Ogasawara K, Kashimura H, Otawara Y, Kakino S, Sugawara A, et al. Cognitive function and anxiety before and after surgery for asymptomatic unruptured intracranial aneurysms in elderly patients. World Neurosurgery. 2010;**73**:350-353

[139] Song J, Kim BS, Shin YS. Treatment outcomes of unruptured intracranial aneurysm; experience of 1231 consecutive aneurysms. Acta Neurochirurgica. 2015;**157**(8):1303-1311

[140] Kim YD, Bang JS, Lee SU, et al. Long-term outcomes of treatment for unruptured intracranial aneurysms in South Korea: Clipping versus coiling. Journal of Neurointerventional Surgery. 2018;**10**(12):1218-1223

[141] Ruan C, Long H, Sun H, et al. Endovascular coiling vs. surgical clipping for unruptured intracranial aneurysm: A meta-analysis. British Journal of Neurosurgery. 2015;**29**(4):485-492

[142] Jo KI, Kim HR, Yeon JY, Hong SC, Kim JS. Treatment outcomes of surgical clipping for unruptured anterior circulation aneurysm—Single institute experiences in the era of neurophysiologic monitoring and endovascular treatment. Neurosurgical Review. 2015;**38**(4):677-682

[143] O'Donnell JM, Morgan MK, Manuguerra M. Functional outcomes and quality of life after microsurgical clipping of unruptured intracranial aneurysms: A prospective cohort study. Journal of Neurosurgery. 2 Mar 2018;**130**(1):278-285

[144] Koźba-Gosztyła M, Czapiga B, Jarmundowicz W, Tomiałowicz Ł. Unruptured intracranial aneurysms: Surgery still safe as a treatment option. Advances in Clinical and Experimental Medicine. 2016;**25**(5):911-916

[145] SchmalzPGR,Enriquez-MarulandaA, Alturki A, Stapleton CJ, Thomas AJ, Ogilvy CS. Combined outcomes of endovascular or surgical treatment of Unruptured anterior communicating artery aneurysms: Is a more aggressive management strategy warranted? World Neurosurgery. 2018;**115**:e331-e336

[146] Nijeholt GJ LÀ, Moojen WA, MLD B, Hertgers O, Muskens IS. Outcomes of retreatment for intracranial aneurysms—A meta-analysis. Neurosurgery. 2018. DOI: 10.1093/neuros/nyy455 [Epub ahead of print]

[147] Darkwah Oppong M, Pierscianek D, Ahmadipour Y, et al. Intraoperative aneurysm rupture during microsurgical clipping: Risk re-evaluation in the post–international subarachnoid aneurysm trial era. World Neurosurgery. 2018;**119**:e349-e356. DOI: 10.1016/j.wneu.2018.07

[148] Chen XL, Chen Y, Ma L, et al. Translucent appearance of middle cerebral artery bifurcation aneurysms is risk factor for intraoperative aneurysm rupture during clipping. World Neurosurgery. 2017;**101**:149-154

[149] Leipzig TJ, Morgan J, Horner TG, Payner T, Redelman K, Johnson CS. Analysis of intraoperative rupture in the surgical treatment of 1694 saccular aneurysms. Neurosurgery. 2005;**56**(3):455-466

[150] Kurisu K, Matsushige T, Sakamoto S, et al. Asymptomatic ischemic risks in

microsurgical clipping for unruptured intracranial aneurysms in anterior circulation. World Neurosurgery. 2017;**108**:418-426

[151] Park W, Ahn JS, Lee SH, Park JC, Kwun BD. Results of re-exploration because of compromised distal blood flow after clipping unruptured intracranial aneurysms. Acta Neurochirurgica. 2015;**157**(6):1015-1024

[152] Park W, Hong SH, Ahn JS, et al. Intraoperative use of transcranial motor/sensory evoked potential monitoring in the clipping of intracranial aneurysms: Evaluation of false-positive and false-negative cases. Journal of Neurosurgery. 2018;**130**(3):936-948. DOI: 10.3171/2017.8.jns17791

[153] Li M, Wu J, Chen X, et al. Symptomatic and silent cerebral infarction following surgical clipping of unruptured intracranial aneurysms: Incidence, risk factors, and clinical outcome. Neurosurgical Review. 2018;**41**(2):675-682. DOI: 10.1007/s10143-017-0913-1

[154] McCutcheon BA, Kerezoudis P, Shepherd DL, et al. Quantitative analysis of the effect of institutional case volume on complications after surgical clipping of unruptured aneurysms. Journal of Neurosurgery. 2017:1297-1306

[155] Svendsen F, Logallo N, Helland CA, Bøthun ML, Thomassen L, Haaland ØA. Time course of cerebrovascular reactivity in patients treated for unruptured intracranial aneurysms: A one-year transcranial Doppler and acetazolamide follow-up study. BioMed Research International. 2018;**2018**:1-9

[156] Rordorf G, Bellon RJ, Budzik RE Jr, et al. Silent thromboembolic events associated with the treatment of unruptured cerebral aneurysms by use of Guglielmi detachable coils: Prospective study applying diffusion-weighted imaging. American Journal of Neuroradiology. 2001;**22**:5-10

[157] Matsukawa H, Kamiyama H, Miyazaki T, et al. Impacts of a size ratio on outcome in patients with surgically treated unruptured nondissecting anterior cerebral artery aneurysms. World Neurosurgery. 2018;**111**:e250-e260

[158] van der Jagt M, van Rooij WJJ, Müller MC, et al. Induced hypertension for delayed cerebral ischemia after aneurysmal subarachnoid hemorrhage. Stroke. 2017;**49**(1):76-83

[159] Suzuki M, Yoneda H, Ishihara H, et al. Adverse events after unruptured cerebral aneurysm treatment: A single-center experience with clipping/coil embolization combined units. Journal of Stroke and Cerebrovascular Diseases. 2015;**24**(1):223-231

[160] Kwun BD, Ahn JS, Park JC, Park W, Sheen JJ. Microsurgical treatment strategy for large and giant aneurysms of the internal carotid artery. Clinical Neurology and Neurosurgery. 2018;**177**:54-62

[161] Asaid M, O'Neill AH, Bervini D, Chandra RV, Lai LT. Unruptured paraclinoid aneurysm treatment effects on visual function: Systematic review and meta-analysis. World Neurosurgery. 2017;**106**:322-330. DOI: 10.1016/j.wneu.2017.06.135

[162] Tabani H, Safaee MM, Kamide T, Burkhardt J-K, Lawton MT. Microsurgical clipping of ophthalmic artery aneurysms: Surgical results and visual outcomes with 208 aneurysms. Journal of Neurosurgery. 2018:1-11

[163] Nanda A, Patra DP, Bir SC, Maiti TK, Kalakoti P, Bollam P. Microsurgical clipping of unruptured intracranial aneurysms: A single surgeon's experience over 16 years. World Neurosurgery. 2017;**100**:85-99

[164] Jeon HJ, Kim SY, Park KY, Lee JW, Huh SK. Ideal clipping methods for unruptured middle cerebral artery bifurcation aneurysms based on aneurysmal neck classification. Neurosurgical Review. 2016;**39**(2):215-224

[165] Nanda A, Javalkar V. Microneurosurgical management of ophthalmic segment of the internal carotid artery aneurysms: Single-surgeon operative experience from Louisiana State University, Shreveport. Neurosurgery. 2011;**68**(2):355-370 [discussion 370-1]

[166] Tsyben A, Paldor I, Laidlaw J. Cerebral vasospasm and delayed ischaemic deficit following elective aneurysm clipping. Journal of Clinical Neuroscience. 2016;**34**:33-38

[167] Kwon MY, Kim CH, Lee CY. Predicting factors of chronic subdural hematoma following surgical clipping in unruptured and ruptured intracranial aneurysm. Journal of Korean Neurosurgical Association. 2016;**59**(5):458-465

Chapter 11

# Endovascular Treatment of Brain Aneurysms

*David Altschul, Tarini Vats and Santiago Unda*

## Abstract

Topic: Chapter discussing the indications for treatment of brain aneurysms, endovascular techniques, tips and tricks. 1. Pathophysiology of aneurysms: Discuss the formation of aneurysms, current thinking of aneurysm development 2. Prevalence/Incidence of aneurysms: Discussion of current state of aneurysm prevalence and how it differs in different populations 3. Unruptured Aneurysms: Diagnosis, Management and Treatment: Imaging paradigms of brain aneurysms, current thoughts on how to follow aneurysms which are being observed, different treatment options for unruptured aneurysms, including clipping, coiling, stent assisted coiling, flow diverter stent, flow disruptors, including the medical management of stent placement 4. Ruptured Aneurysms: Diagnosis, Management and Treatment: Imaging paradigms of ruptured aneurysms, management options for co-morbidities associated with aneurysm rupture, treatment options including coiling, clipping, flow diverter stents, flow disruptors 5. Complication Avoidance: Tips and tricks to avoid complications in the treatment of brain aneurysms.

**Keywords:** brain aneurysms, subarachnoid hemorrhage, coils, flow diversion, flow disruption

## 1. Pathophysiology of aneurysms

A cerebral aneurysm is defined as a local outpouching of an intracranial artery and can either be saccular or fusiform. The formation of aneurysms is an incompletely understood gradual process [1] involving genetics, epidemiology and pathobiology, in conjugation with the study of biophysics provides a more complete picture on how these factors interact [2]. The natural history of saccular intracranial aneurysms consists of three phases: initiation, growth, and either stabilization or rupture, and the application of scientific principles to biological processes has made it easier to understand the behavior of aneurysm formation and rupture.

### 1.1 Genetic factors

Various genome studies and subsequent replication case control studies suggest genetic components in the formation of intracranial aneurysms (IA), no specific genes strongly associated with formation have yet been identified. A meta-analysis [3], identified three single nucleotide polymorphisms (SNPs) located on chromosome 9 within the *CDKN2B-AS1* gene, on chromosome 8 near the *SOX17* transcription regulator gene, and on chromosome 4 near the endothelin receptor gene associated with the presence of sporadic IAs. A new IA susceptibility locus on 13q was identified [4]. Subsequent genome-wide association studies [5, 6] have found additional loci on chromosome 7 near *HDAC9*, as well as in chromosomal regions 1p34.3–p36.13, 19q13.3, Xp22 and 7q11. The strongest evidence for linkage was with a locus on 7q11 near the perlecan gene that encodes elastin, a protein that is involved in the preservation of vessel wall integrity.

### 1.2 Structural changes and hemodynamics

Cerebral arteries are prone to aneurysm formation due to presence of cerebrospinal fluid, sparse tunica adventitia, lower proportion of elastic fibers and disruption of internal lamina at bifurcation [7–9]. Blood is an active participant in the formation of aneurysms, its flow provides the mechanical triggers for reactions in the vessels at the level of the endothelium, while it is also a biological participant in the inflammatory cascade [10, 11]. This dual function of blood contributes significantly to the degradation of the arterial wall in the formation of aneurysms [2].

Cohort studies on people with a familial preponderance to saccular aneurysm have shown that the geometry of bifurcations around the circle of Willis adds additional stress to the vessel walls, given the significant shifts in flow velocity, dynamic forces, and shear stress. Thus, high flow across a wall that is not "designed" for the exposed pressures results in tissue injury and remodeling. The biological result may be plaque or may be an aneurysm, depending on the presence (or absence) of an intact media [2]. Fluid-dynamic models calculate and visualize wall shear stress or wall shear gradients, intra-aneurysmal flow, impingement zones, and flow patterns or velocities. Wall shear stress constitutes the degree of friction in the intracranial aneurysm wall that results from blood inflow and impingement into the aneurysm. High and low wall shear stress can both be present during aneurysm formation but the relevance of these flow conditions to the pathogenesis, growth and rupture of an aneurysm remain unclear [12]. The role of shear stress is very controversial, responsible for damage at specific phases of aneurysmal development and rupture. Some studies suggest the direct effect of shear stress on the vessel wall resulting in injury and degeneration of the wall's media, leading to aneurysm formation. Others suggest that low shear stress in the aneurysm and the vessel wall may result in small thrombus formation, endothelial reactivity, and inflammation at the site, thus weakening the vessel.

Data generated from fluid-dynamic models could help improve our understanding of aneurysm formation patterns and potential structural deficiencies in aneurysms. The relevance of existing data derived from computational fluid modeling is limited, however, because the majority of studies compared ruptured with unruptured aneurysms. An ideal approach would be to compare the same aneurysm before and after rupture [13–16].

### 1.3 Molecular changes

In response to internal elastic lamina disruption and the subsequent mechanical overload and shift in tensile forces, vascular smooth muscle cells and fibroblasts synthesize collagen types I and V, which are the main molecular constituents of intracranial aneurysms [17].

Once the molecular mechanisms fail to compensate for the mechanical overload of the vessel wall and myo-intimal injury, cellular and humoral inflammatory responses become the main drivers of aneurysm formation [17–20]. These responses are mediated by inflammatory cytokines such as tumor necrosis factor (TNF), IL-1β and matrix metalloproteinases (MMPs), promote influx of macrophages and continuous degradation of collagen and elastin fibers. Wall shear stress might also contribute to cellular inflammatory responses during aneurysm formation.

### 1.4 Can aneurysm rupture be predicted?

Aneurysm rupture has been suggested to occur as aneurysm expansion approaches and exceeds the physical limits of the tissue. It has also been suggested that the vibrations induced by pulsatile flow and the subsequent resonant frequency may promote aneurysmal rupture [21, 22]. Although not directly resulting in aneurysmal rupture, vibrational irregularities secondary to the presence of the aneurysm may accelerate the degeneration of the aneurysmal wall and subsequently lead to rupture. A shift to quantitative and not just qualitative analysis, and a focus on flow and flow dynamics as a force of influence in rupture have changed the landscape of research for cerebral aneurysms [2].

## 2. Prevalence and incidence of aneurysms

Although Unruptured Intracranial Aneurysms (UIA) are common [23, 24]. Their prevalence is subject to changes due to the improvements in invasive and non-invasive imaging techniques, the increasing knowledge about the related factors that determines screening in asymptomatic populations and the increase in the life expectancy. Historically, the methods used to address prevalence were retrospective or prospective autopsy studies in the decades from 1950's to the earliest 2000's [25] but non-invasive imaging studies have demonstrated higher prevalence and prevalence ratios compared to autopsy studies (PR 3•5, 95% CI 2•1–6•1)3. To study UIA, the Magnetic Resonance Angiography (MRA) is the most common method for detection in asymptomatic patients [26] and compared to Intra-Arterial Digital Subtraction Angiography (IA-DSA), systematic reviews have found no significant differences in the prevalence reported between these two imaging techniques (more details will be elucidated in the next section of this chapter). However, it's important to highlight that prevalence reported in non-invasive imaging studies can present limitations due to the interobserver agreement, training, experience, quality of equipment and expert's judgment [27].

The IA characteristics are also a major concern in prevalence studies; technical limitations in regard to location, size and morphology can decrease the sensitivity and specificity of the diagnostic methods. Both, large and relatively small [28] cohort's studies had shown that saccular morphology is the most common form of presentation and that among patients without history of subarachnoid hemorrhage (SAH) the distribution of IA in the internal carotid artery (ICA) and middle cerebral artery (MCA) are 24.8 and 22.7% [29] respectively, however in patients with previous history of SAH, the prevalence is higher in the MCA. In regard to the size, modern imaging techniques can easily detect aneurysms from 2 mm, which is extremely important to determine the risks of possible treatments or natural history, so far, the current evidence is that UIA > 5 mm, location in basilar artery apex and decrease in BMI over the follow-up period are related to speed up the 2.9% of aneurysm growth per year. However, irrespective of aneurysm size, the irregular shape and daughter sac are more likely to rupture [30, 31]. Although we know these are contributing factors, there is still a need to understand better the contribution of aneurysm related factors.

The prevalence of UIA among the general population is 3–5% [32] but there are several differences between populations that increase the risk for having a IA or a SAH. The risk factors commonly associated to IA development and rupture whether there's a previous history of SAH or not, are age > 30, female sex, African-American race, smoking, alcoholism, hypercholesterolemia, high blood pressure, first and second-degree relatives with SAH history, and other comorbidities as polycystic kidney disease, connective tissue disorders and brain tumors [33–36]. However, lifelong follow-up studies of UIA suggested that only female sex and smoking status were significant risk factors for aSAH [37]. Across countries, compared to USA prevalence, China, Japan, European countries including (UK, Netherlands, Finland, Germany and Italy) had no significant differences in the prevalence ratios adjusted to age, sex and comorbidities [38–41]. Other studies in Iranian population [42] have shown a prevalence of 3.2% but more studies in non-Caucasian populations are still required to further understand the impact of genetics and cultural practices.

The incidence of aneurysmal SAH (aSAH) reports are questionable, first, in average 20% of the aSAH deaths occur suddenly, away from hospital or in emergency rooms [43]. Therefore, incidence can vary between countries with different autopsy rates and medical study protocols. In the case of Finland, the PHASES study showed a 3–6 times increased risk of aneurysm rupture in compared to other European nations and USA [44]. However, these findings can be a proof of how epidemiological studies need to improve their parameters more than a proof that Finnish people have more risk of aSAH. Finland has high rates of autopsy studies in sudden deaths [45] and all nonhospital deaths and moreover, longer life expectancy and pyramid shrinking due to the increasing of elderly population [46]. So, there's no currently strong evidence to conclude that aSAH in Finland cohorts is truly higher than the other countries included in the PHASES study.

In spite of this evidence, careful consideration must be taken when we think about the pros and cons to treat a patient based on their personal risk factors. Most of the large cohort's publications and meta-analysis have been done in populations where ethnicity diversity was limited, the impact of social stratus had not been assessed and criteria for collecting data and analysis was not standardized. Therefore, perfect epidemiological studies do not exist so, great efforts will be necessary to determine inclusion and exclusion criteria in future prospective cohorts.

## 3. Unruptured intracranial aneurysms

Diagnosis of unruptured intracranial aneurysms (UIA) in most of the cases is incidentally during evaluations of other conditions [44] because the vast majority are asymptomatic or have subtle manifestations. Only, 10 to 15.5% of patients have symptoms related to UIA [45]. These symptoms generally are associated to mass effect due to the aneurysm size and growth, rarely cranial neuropathy or even more rare with sentinel hemorrhage, due to minimal blood leaking with the consequent meningeal irritation [45]. Symptomatic UIA often present with neurological deficits as visual dysfunction, ocular nerve palsy, bilateral temporal hemianopsia and other neurological symptoms as headaches, embolic cerebral ischemia, poorly defined spells, and seizures [46, 47]. Patients with symptomatic UIA need more attention because this can be a manifestation about riskier distribution and morphological [45] characteristics of the aneurysm, and a warning sign of an impending rupture [48]. The diagnoses modality after incidental discovery of an UIA, is based on which imaging modality is more sensitive depending on aneurysms characteristics, patients related factors, medical history and moreover, methods available in each center. Therefore, there is no specific diagnoses algorithm for UIA. The decision of screening or further imaging after finding an incidental aneurysm is still on the specialist judgment. These considerations are discussed below:

It has been mentioned that most of the UIA are diagnosed incidentally, and some of the non-invasive imaging methods have also been mentioned in the "prevalence" section of this chapter. However, there are still different evidences about the rates of diagnosis and prevalence reported through these non-invasive imaging methods as the MRA or CTA and IA-DSA, the current gold standard [22, 49]. Many authors had suggested that the MRA and CTA to be the best methods for preliminary screening of IA [50, 51], the sensitivity and specificity of both methods are 87 and 95% for MRA and 90 and 86% for CTA [47]. But the effectiveness of the diagnoses can decrease depending on the IA characteristics; in UIA < 3 mm, MRA and CTA sensitivity plummet to 38 and 61%, respectively [52]. Moreover, the high rates of comorbidities in people with UIA product of common pathophysiology (like hypertension with the consequent kidney failure) or to the old age of patients can limit the use of the contrast dye in CTA for screening. Therefore, MRA is the most frequent tool for screening nowadays. Other non-invasive techniques like transcranial Doppler (TCD) have been explored, but whether power Doppler is done with or without contrast enhancement, it's sensitivity and specificity together are not superior to MRA and CTA [51]. Nevertheless, TCD can be a screening tool in countries were the expensive costs of MRA or CTA makes them inaccessible.

Sensitivity and specificity of imaging methods for diagnostic are important, but more considerations should be taken to study UIA characteristics. IADSA, provides the better spatial resolution than other techniques [44], but this method may not provide a good sense of aneurysm volume and can present difficulties when vessels are overlapped, and therefore 3D reconstructions are often needed to fully evaluated for intracranial aneurysms. Moreover, IADSA as an invasive method, can carry risks; 2.3% of patients can present transient neurological complications, 0.4% permanent neurological complications and 14.7% of non-neurological complications [52]. Novel imaging methods as the Optical coherence tomography (OCT) can be useful to assess key factors in aneurysm structure due to the power to increase 10 times image resolution compared to other current techniques [44] and furthermore, OCT has a nearly-biopsy resolution [53] and enhance resolution of birefringent tissues as artery laminas [54] which is major concern in pathophysiology, as mentioned before in this chapter.

Furthermore, considerations need to be taken as to imaging modality if the patient has had previously treated aneurysms. MRA is not sensitive for patients with previously treated clipped aneurysms. For these patients CTA is preferred. MRA is still sensitive for previously coiled aneurysms. For patients treated with flow diverter stents either MRA with contrast or CTA can be used. If the patient had coils with any kind of stent, then MRA with contrast is the preferred modality.

Taken together the results of imaging for UIA, the neuro-interventional team consider the possible treatments for each patient based on the risks and benefits between prevent treatment and natural history, however due to lack of evidence of the natural history in some categories of UIA is not uncommon to balance the pros and cos between prevent treatment and aSAH outcomes. Some of the current available treatments will be discussed below.

### 3.1 Conservative management

First of all, having an aneurysm does not imply always the need to undergo surgical or endovascular treatment. Most of the UIA will never cause symptoms neither rupture or at least the probability of this events will not be over 1% per year. Therefore, many patients decide to take the risk of conservative management over the risks of preventive treatments. However, conservative management is not equal to doing nothing, this management bear intervention from the physician to educate well the patient about the risk factors that will increase the probabilities of rupture and an active participation of the patients to modify their risky habits. There is strong evidence that supports the conservative management when lifetime risk of morbidity and mortality is low [42] as represented in **Figure 1**.

Nevertheless, in patients under conservative management, imaging follow-ups at 1 year intervals have been recommended with CTA or MRA [25] to assess aneurysm

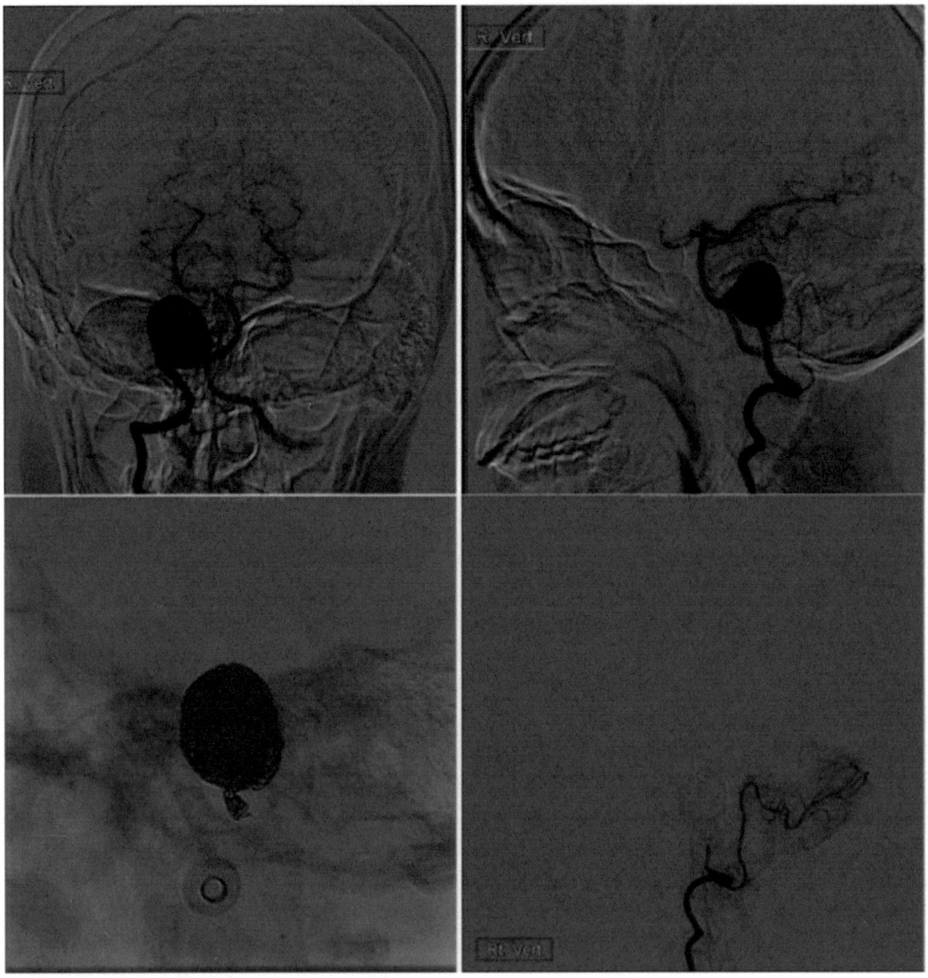

**Figure 1.**
*Giant right vertebral aneurysm before and after coiling.*

growth, although it is unclear whether this frequency of time-interval is truly necessary. However, is not uncommon to have mixed factors in UIA patients, to make it clear, a systematic review showed that if hypertension and history of SAH are present (considering this both as major risk factors) in a patient under 70 years, with an <10 mm UIA in the anterior circulation, we will still be talking about a probability of risk of ~1% per year [24]. So, a standardized timing for imaging follow-ups according to each patients and aneurysm related factors does not exist, in part because aneurysm growing is discontinuous but the ELAPSS score (mentioned in **Figure 1**) can be helpful to determine the need of follow-up at 3 or 5 years based on the risk of aneurysm growth [55]. These patients who choose conservative management live with a small very definite risk of rupture. Recently, a study showed that patients with untreated UIA, may decrease their quality of life (QoL) and moreover, trigger mental disorder as anxiety and depression [56, 57] possibly due to the uncertainty of whether their aneurysm is going to burst and when.

### 3.2 Surgical management

Successful surgery is achieved in most of the cases by excluding aneurysms from circulation but currently, there is a lack of prospective, multicenter and randomized trials that report outcomes in a uniform way. Moreover, most of the studies were done in patients with previous aSAH like the ISAT trial [58], which makes difficult to extrapolate those results to patients with UIA and no history of aSAH. The ISUIA-2 study did evaluate the surgical outcomes of nearly 1500 patients. They reported a mortality rate of 2.7% at 1 year and poor outcome (mRS 3–5) of 1.4% at 1 year. In this study, age > 70, posterior circulation and giant aneurysms were all associated with higher surgical morbidity and mortality. A meta-analysis done in the US with patients without previous history of aSAH that underwent to elective surgical clipping (SC) 14,411 and to endovascular treatment (EVT) 16,659 reported that iatrogenic stroke, intracranial hemorrhage, pulmonary complications, sepsis and status epilepticus were significantly higher after SC [59]. Moreover, the reduced recovery time and shorter stays in hospital [60] play a major role in the final decision of patient to avoid surgery. Nowadays, SC is usually reserved to younger patients that will benefit more from an immediate occlusion of the aneurysm, less need to have follow-up imaging, less probability of retreatment and the ones with large and giant aneurysms or locations in the MCA.

### 3.3 Endovascular treatment (EVT)

Since its conception, endovascular treatment has rapidly taken over as the major treatment for most intracranial aneurysms. While there is supporting data for ruptured intracranial aneurysms from the ISAT trial, there is no randomized controlled trial comparing surgery and endovascular treatment to surgical clipping for unruptured aneurysms. Relative indications for endovascular treatment are poor surgical candidate, favorable aneurysm and vascular anatomy, high risk for anesthesia complications and posterior circulation aneurysms. In 2012, a systematic review and meta-analysis reported different outcomes between endovascular treatments; >52 years, >10 mm and posterior circulation location were main risk factors to poor outcomes [61]. Coiling alone was safer compared to the percent of complications reported with balloon-assisted coiling 7.1% (99% CI 3.9–12.7), 9.3% (99% CI 4.9–16.9) with stent-assisted coiling and 11.5% (99% CI 4.9–24.6) with flow-diverting stents. However, the increase of the complications reported with additional devices can be due to the more-complex aneurysm cases or due to the number and type of devices placed. Furthermore, in the last decade the neuro-interventional procedures have improved their outcomes with increased understanding of the various treatments and technological innovation improving safety and efficacy.

### 3.4 Coiling

EVT emerged in the 1990's with coiling [62]. Since then, technological advances in coil properties made neuro-interventional procedures safer with improved outcomes. Recently, a single center study reported 0% of poor outcomes when coiling was used [25], however >20% of poor outcomes have been reported after coiling in aneurysms >10 mm size, with wide necks, unfavorable dome-to-neck ratio < 2 and fusiform configuration [63]. So, using coiling alone must be used just in aneurysms with specific characteristics, otherwise new devices must be considered.

### 3.5 Stent assisted coiling

This method represents a solution for aneurysms in which coiling alone will not be the best option (mentioned in **Figure 1**), as coiling this endovascular technique has the same concerns about patient selection, recovery and risks. However, when leaving a stent placed in the artery it is important to manage the tolerance and adherence of the patient to dual anti-platelet therapy (DAPT) (**Figure 2**) [64].

### 3.6 Flow diversion

This method was developed in the 2000s. The concept of Flow Diversion is that a high-mesh density stent placed in the parent artery will disrupts blood flow into the aneurysm with the subsequent thrombosis of the aneurysm, this process takes 6 weeks to 6 months in average in radiographic follow-ups. Moreover, the stent in parent artery provides a scaffold for which endothelium can grow [62]. In 2011, the FDA approved the Pipeline Embolization Device (PED) for large or giant (≥10 mm) wide-necked intracranial aneurysms from the petrous to the superior hypophyseal segments of the ICA [65]. Since then, a second flow diverter stent (Surpass) has come to market. Flow diverter stents now have expanded indications, including smaller aneurysms, and aneurysm up to the internal carotid artery bifurcation. Recently, a multicenter group published a retrospective study of follow-ups after PED placement [66], in this report overall complications were 3.4% and in multivariate analysis older age > 70, larger diameter > 15 mm and fusiform were identified as independent variables with higher rates of incomplete occlusion in 6-month follow-up. However, currently there is not a standardized scale to report

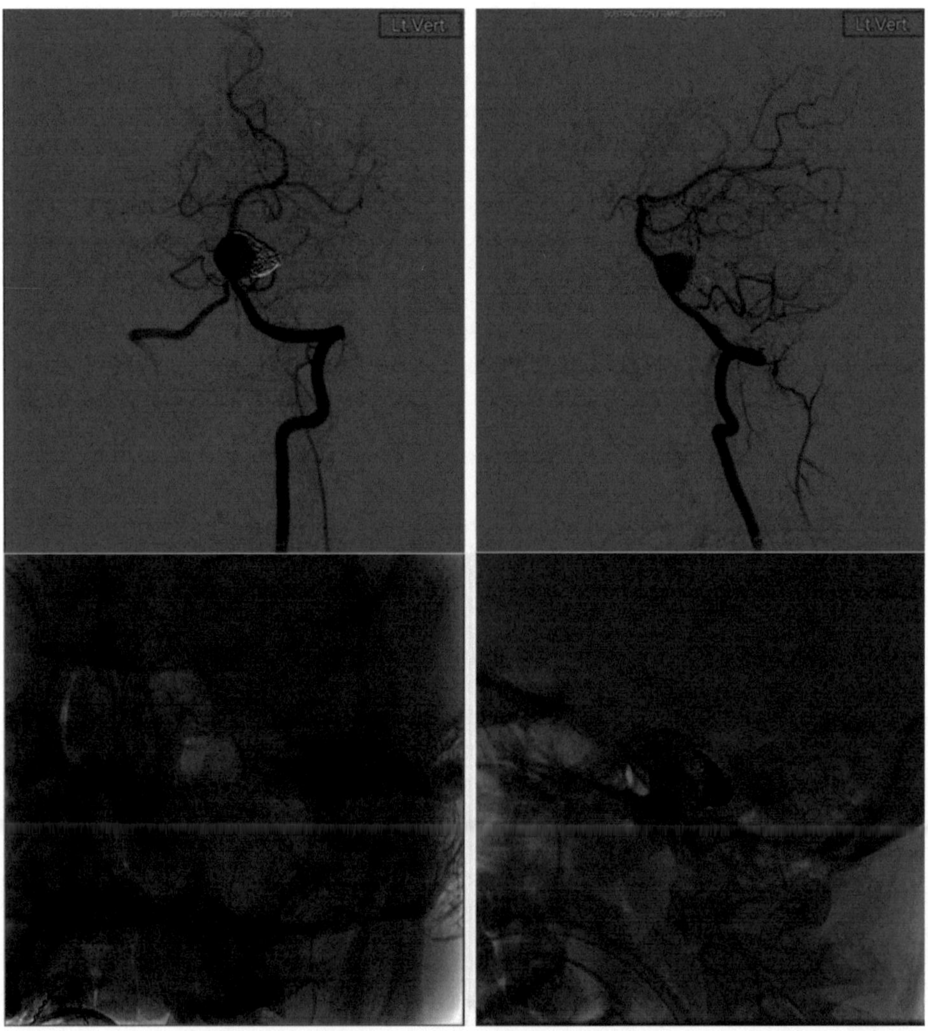

**Figure 2.**
*Pipeline placement in a wide neck aneurysm in the left vertebral artery.*

radiographic outcomes that can be useful to meta-analysis studies or to new prospective randomized cohorts. Flow diverter stents are currently also limited usually to unruptured aneurysms, given the need for DAPT, however their use has found a niche in the treatment of ruptured blister aneurysms. Consequently, the next generation of this technology is looking into the possibility of special coating to mitigate the need for DAPT. Further investigation is still needed before this advancement will come to market.

### 3.7 Flow disruptors and web endoluminal bridge (WEB)

Although flow diversion devices can work out for many types of aneurysms as off-label uses; aneurysms located in bifurcations with wide neck and dome-to-neck ratio > 1 and < 2 remains a challenge for this technology. Therefore, the WEB device was created in regard of these concerns in flow diversion and has proven promising to overcome those limitations. The WEB device is placed intra-aneurysm with a subsequent change in the blood flow at the aneurysm neck [67]. In European multicenter prospective studies, the WEB device placed in basilar, MCA, Acomm and ICA bifurcation showed 2.7% of morbidity and at 1 year of follow-up, 56% of aneurysm complete occlusion [68]. Owing this method does not require to put the patient under DAPT unlike the PED, it can be used also in aSAH cases. Further investigation is needed as to the long-term outcomes for this device (**Figures 3** and **4**).

### 3.8 Medical management after flow diverter placement

All the patients that can be good candidates for PED placement based on their UIA characteristics needs also to be eligible for prolonged DAPT. Acetylsalicylic acid (ASA) plus clopidogrel is the DAPT of reference used for preventing thrombosis in such procedures [69]. The laboratory tests pre and post-procedure are yet to be standardized; due to the risk of clopidogrel resistant (28–68%) [70], is has been considered necessary to assess platelet reactivity. High platelet reactivity (HPR) is related with thromboembolic evens after stenting arteries [71]. Depending on institutional protocols, some neuro-interventional teams use the VerifyNow P2Y12 assay which has been widely studied however, the results of this tests may not be completely reliable [72] due to the fact that P2Y12 response units (PRU) cannot differentiate aspirin-induced platelet inhibition in patients administered clopidogrel. Other studies recommend the use of the Thromboelastography (TEG), which is dynamic and real time tool to measure clot formation. The advantages of VerifyNow assay is that can be done very fast with instant results, however in patients with programed procedures for UIA stenting this concerning may not be transcendental.

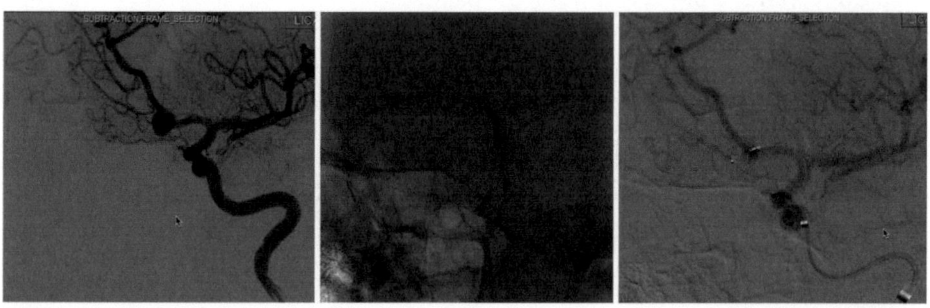

**Figure 3.**
*Web Endoluminal bridge placement in left ICA bifurcation.*

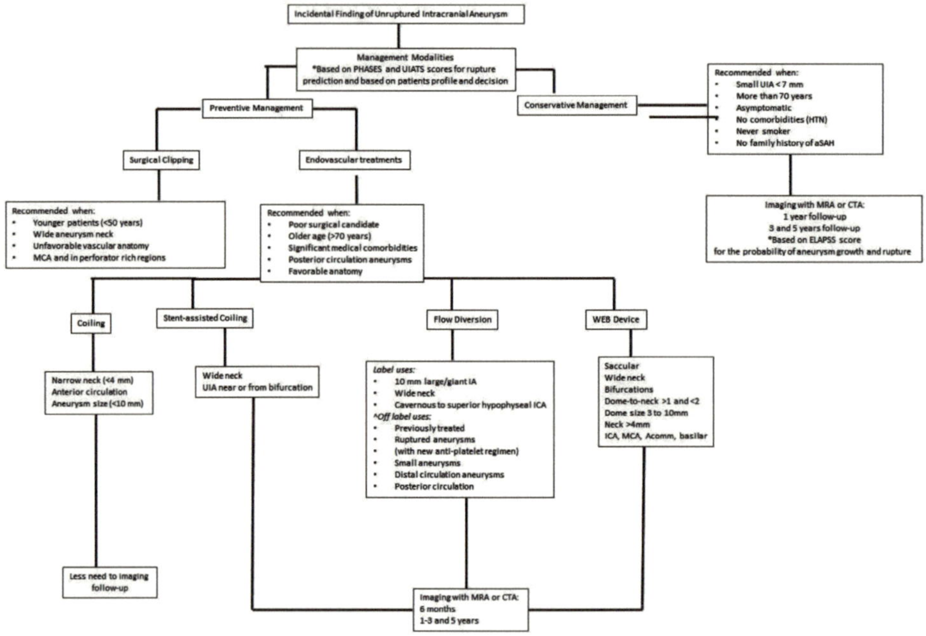


**Figure 4.**
*Flowchart of management after incidental UIA diagnosis.*

VerifyNow can overestimate the rate of clopidogrel resistance when compared to TEG. However, there is currently no randomized trials that have assessed the utility of this tests. Moreover, there's no strong evidence to support that the assessment of platelet reactivity improves clinical and imaging outcomes after stent placement. Nevertheless, the neuro-interventional teams at these days usually starts the DAPT with 325 mg of ASA and 75 mg of clopidogrel 7 days prior and maintain for 3–6 months after PED placement.

## 4. Ruptured intracranial aneurysms

A 50-year-old female was preparing her children for school when she experienced a headache severe enough to make her lie down on the sofa. She managed to get the children off to school, but the headache did not abate. She was used to headaches, as she had migraines periodically that were controlled with over-the-counter medications, but this one was different and much more intense. She took a couple of acetaminophen, and when the pain was not relieved, she brought herself to the emergency department (ED) [73].

Headache is seen in up to 2% of patients, presenting to the emergency department (ED). Most are benign, but it is imperative to understand and discern the life-threatening causes of headache when they present. Headache caused by a subarachnoid hematoma (SAH) from a ruptured aneurysm is one of the deadliest, but fortunately, also rare, comprising only 1% of all headaches presenting to the ED [74].

Rupture is the most serious consequence of intracranial aneurysms. Subarachnoid hemorrhage (SAH) from a leaking aneurysm is a neurological emergency. While SAH is typical of aneurysmal rupture, it is also associated with intraventricular hemorrhage, intracerebral hemorrhage, and subdural hematoma. The force of rupture and location of an aneurysm determine the presence of the other types of hemorrhage. Although the prevalence of aneurysms is high, the global annual incidence of subarachnoid hemorrhage is 10/100,000person years, so the best possible treatment plan would be to determine exactly those aneurysms that will rupture and the ones that never will.

### 4.1 Presentation

The presenting symptom of SAH is acute headache, generally described as "the worst headache of my life."

Some cohort studies mention it as "thunderclap" headache that peaks at headache onset or reaches severity within minutes to an hour of onset [75].

1. Signs of meningeal irritation-meningismus, photophobia

2. Signs of intracranial hypertension-nausea, vomiting, diminished level of consciousness

3. Epileptic seizures

4. Focal neurological deficits

5. Intraocular hemorrhage [76, 77]

    - Terson syndrome: hemorrhage in vitreous humor, associated with high mortality [78]

    - Subhyaloid (pre-retinal) hemorrhage [79].

### 4.2 Scoring system

Several scoring systems have been developed to predict patient outcomes for those with aneurysm related sub-arachnoid hemorrhage (a-SAH). The Hunt and Hess score and World Federation of Neurological Surgeons grading system are both used to predict patient outcome, and the Fisher grade helps to predict vasospasm [80, 81].

The severity of neurologic impairment and the amount of subarachnoid bleeding on admission are the strongest predictors of neurologic complications and outcome [82]. Therefore, it is essential that patients with SAH be scored promptly after arrival and stabilization. The World Federation of Neurological Surgeons Scale (WFNSS) and the modified Fisher Scale are the most reliable and simple to perform [74, 75]. Higher WFNSS and modified Fisher Scale scores are associated with worse clinical outcome and a higher proportion of neurologic complications. The modified Fisher scale is designed to predict the development of delayed cerebral ischemia (DCI) which is the most common cause of disability secondary to rupture next the actual rupture itself (**Tables 1–3**).

### 4.3 Initial imaging

With such a large number of patients presenting to the ED with a chief complaint of headache [79–84], the description of headache can help differentiating those with a benign cause from those with an emergent etiology such as SAH. The diagnosis of SAH should be considered in any patient with a severe and sudden onset or rapidly escalating headache (**Figure 5**).

| Grade | Glasgow coma scale (GCS) | Neurological exam |
|---|---|---|
| 1 | 15 | No motor deficit |
| 2 | 13–14 | No motor deficit |
| 3 | 13–14 | Motor deficit |
| 4 | 7–12 | With/without motor deficit |
| 5 | 5–6 | With/without motor deficit |

**Table 1.**
*World Federation of Neurological Surgeons Grading System for Subarachnoid Hemorrhage - (WFNS) scale.*

| Grade | Criteria | Survival |
|---|---|---|
| I | Asymptomatic, mild headache, slight nuchal rigidity | 70% |
| II | Moderate to severe headache, nuchal rigidity, no neurological deficit other than cranial nerve palsy | 60% |
| III | Drowsiness/confusion and mild focal neurological deficit | 50% |
| IV | Stupor, moderate to severe hemiparesis | 20% |
| V | Coma, decerebrate positioning | 10% |

**Table 2.**
*Hunt and Hess scale.*

| Grade | Appearance of blood on CT | Risk of cerebral hemorrhage |
|---|---|---|
| 0 | No sub arachnoid hemorrhage (SAH) or ventricular hemorrhage (VH) | 0% |
| 1 | Minimal SAH, No VH in 2 lateral ventricles | 6% |
| 2 | Minimal SAH, VH in 2 lateral ventricles | 14% |
| 3 | Large SAH, No VH in 2 lateral ventricles | 12% |
| 4 | Large SAH, VH in 2 lateral ventricles | 28% |

**Table 3.**
*Modified fisher grading system [82].*

### 4.4 Management

Once the patient has been diagnosed with an SAH, treatment should focus on limiting secondary neurologic injuries to improve the patient's functional outcome.

- Resuscitation of a patient with SAH should follow all established protocols with immediate attention to airway and circulatory support.
- After stabilization of the airway and circulation, treatments specific to SAH can begin.

### 4.5 Pharmacologic treatments

#### *4.5.1 Antiepileptic drugs*

In patients with a suspected ruptured aneurysm, seizures can lead to aneurysmal rebleeding and result in intracranial hypertension and herniation, the

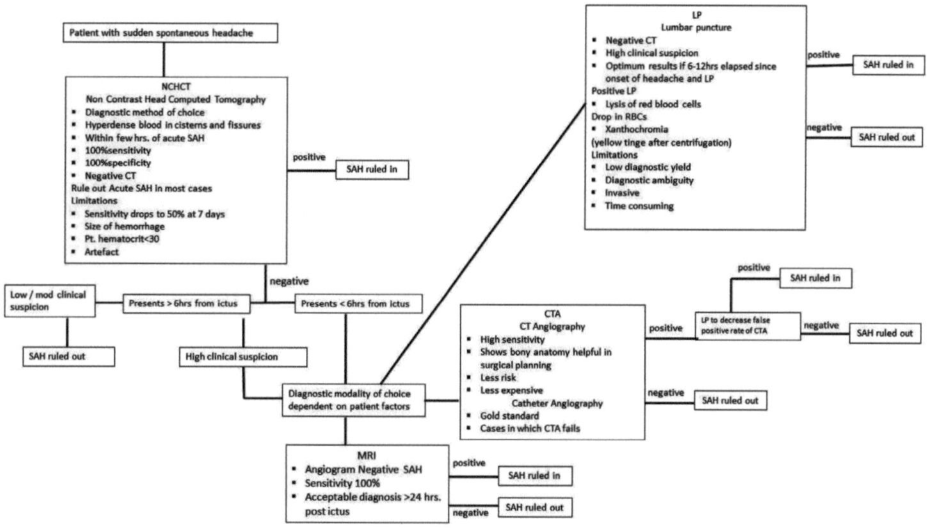


**Figure 5.**
*Flowchart of management aSAH [1, 10–12].*

risk of being highest in patients with poor Hunt and Hess grade and those with thick subarachnoid blood [85]. Routine prophylactic antiepileptic drug use in patients with SAH is a common practice despite limited evidence The American Stroke Association (ASA) guideline recommends consideration of short-term prophylactic antiepileptic drug use in the immediate post hemorrhage period [86]. No randomized controlled trials have investigated the safety and effectiveness of antiepileptic drugs in SAH [87].

### 4.6 Nimodipine

Delayed cerebral ischemia (DCI) is one of the most serious complications associated with SAH, occurring in one-third of patients surviving the initial hemorrhage and results in poor outcome in half of the patients with this complication [86]. Nimodipine is a calcium antagonist that is thought to reduce the rate of cerebral vasospasm by reducing the influx of calcium into the vascular smooth muscle cells. The administration of nimodipine to reduce the risk of poor outcome and DCI is the only level IA evidence recommended by the ASA [86].

### 4.7 Blood pressure management

There is general consensus that hypertension should be controlled after SAH and until the ruptured aneurysm is secured. However, specific parameters for blood pressure have not been defined and data are sparse. Early retrospective studies suggest a higher rate of rebleeding with SBP greater than 160 mm Hg and severity of initial hemorrhage [88]. Therefore, the ASA and Neurocritical Care Society recommend maintaining SBP less than 160 mm Hg and mean arterial pressure less than 110 mm Hg before the ruptured aneurysm is secured to reduce the risk of rebleeding [86, 87, 89, 90]. The ideal antihypertensive to use in SAH would be a parenteral agent that produces a rapid and reproducible dose response while concurrently minimizing adverse cerebral effects. Labetalol, nicardipine, and clevidipine are agents recommended by the ASA [86].

### 4.8 Antifibrinolytics

When early definitive treatment of the ruptured aneurysm is not possible, antifibrinolytic therapies such as amino epsilon caproic acid or tranexamic acid can be considered to reduce the risk of early aneurysmal rebleeding. Early studies showed a reduction in rebleeding but an increase in cerebral ischemia with prolonged use of antifibrinolytics [88]. Neither aminocaproic acid or tranexamic acid is approved by the US Food and Drug Administration for prevention of aneurysmal rebleeding, thus the use of antifibrinolytic therapies should be discussed on a case-by-case basis.

### 4.9 Rebleeding

Rebleeding can occur before the ruptured aneurysm is secured, and is associated with significant mortality and poor prognosis for functional recovery, most common within the first 24 hours, with some studies reporting peak time of rebleeding within 2 hours [88]. Factors associated with rebleeding include longer time to aneurysm treatment, worse neurologic status on presentation, initial loss of consciousness, previous sentinel headaches, larger aneurysm size, and possibly SBP greater than 160 mm Hg [91]. Although early definitive treatment of ruptured aneurysms can reduce the risk of rebleeding, approximately 12–15% of patients die before reaching the hospital [90].

### 4.10 External ventricular drainage

Acute hydrocephalus is common in patients with SAH and is a common cause of early neurologic decline. Treatment of symptomatic hydrocephalus often requires placement of an external ventricular drain, which allows ICP monitoring as well as CSF drainage. Untreated hydrocephalus can lead to intracranial hypertension and cerebral ischemia with potential cerebral herniation. Identification of the presence of hydrocephalus on CT and communication of this finding with neurosurgical consultants are key steps in the management of SAH.

### 4.11 Microsurgical clipping versus endovascular coiling

Definitive treatment of SAH is early microsurgical clipping or endovascular coiling of the ruptured aneurysm to prevent rebleeding and its associated complications. Choice of treatment modality depends on aneurysm size, characteristics, and location, as well as the patient's clinical grade and comorbidities [92]. The International Subarachnoid Aneurysm Trial (ISAT) [93] is a multicenter, randomized clinical trial, which compares a policy of neurosurgical clipping with a policy of endovascular treatment with detachable platinum coils in patients with ruptured intracranial aneurysms considered suitable for either treatment. The results show that endovascular intervention with detachable platinum coils in patients with ruptured intracranial aneurysms can improve the chances of independent survival compared with neurosurgical intervention to clip the neck of the aneurysm.

### 4.12 Pipeline embolization device

The PED has mostly been used to treat unruptured aneurysms, whereas its use for acutely ruptured aneurysms has been limited and is theoretically contraindicated, given the need for dual antiplatelet therapy as it increases the risk of re-hemorrhage [94].

However, in certain cases of complex ruptured aneurysms, the PED may still serve as a good alternative (and sometimes may be the only available option) because these aneurysms are anatomically and technically more difficult to treat using standard techniques [93]. Furthermore, certain anticoagulation protocols can be put into place to prevent the feared consequences associated with PED placement in ruptured aneurysms due to dual antiplatelet therapy. The standard management for the prevention of thromboembolic events when using flow diverters is pretreatment with aspirin and clopidogrel for 7–10 days prior to the procedure. When treating ruptured aneurysms with the PED in conjunction with this dual antiplatelet therapy, there is a concern for hemorrhagic complications. Chalouhi and colleagues [95] described a new regimen for anticoagulation that was recently implemented in the hope of minimizing the risk of thromboembolic and hemorrhagic complications. In summary, the PED may be particularly helpful in acutely ruptured aneurysms that are not amenable to coiling or clipping. It can also be used in a staged fashion 1 or 2 weeks after partial coiling of the aneurysm dome. It is generally preferable to place an external ventricular drain if treatment with the PED is contemplated [96].

## 5. Future directions

The future of neuroendovascular surgery is bright. The technology platforms for access, delivery and treatment continue to improve at exponential rates. As it is there has been a rapid change in the number of brain aneurysm patients treated with endovascular treatment versus open surgical clipping. With this change comes a great void in experience and skill in the open surgical management of brain aneurysms. It remains to be seen whether this skill will be needed in the future [97].

### 5.1 Flow disruptor

Currently there is only one flow disruptor available in the US market; the WEB device. Currently, its limitations lie in the fact that it is only available in sizes to treat aneurysms 3–10 mm in size. The second limitation exists in its delivery system which, at larger sizes requires a 33-microcatheter, and at smallest sizes requires a 21-microcatheter. As newer generations come to market over the next 5 years, we expect there to be improved deliverability, different shapes available, and smaller designs for smaller ruptured aneurysms [98].

### 5.2 Flow diverter

Currently there are two flow diverter stents available in the US Market, the Pipeline Flex (2nd generation), and the Surpass. Currently the bulk of innovation required with this technology is in finding a coating for the stent that might mitigate the need for dual anti-platelet therapy. The second area of innovation is in the deliverability of the stents, currently needing 27-microcatheter for delivery, there is an expectation that these stents can be delivered through a 21-microcatheter in the near future, with also smaller diameter stent sizes available to treat more distal aneurysms. We fully expect the indications on which type of aneurysms can be treated in the near future.

### 5.3 Endosaccular coiling

Coiling has likely reached its technological pinnacle. There has been little advancement in this technology over the last 5 years. One area of interest is in endosaccular flow disruptor type coils such as the Medina system. This is not as of yet FDA approved and remains to be seen whether this is efficacious or safe. Also the adjunctive tools for coiling continue to improve such as the Atlas stent, Pulserider stent and barrel stent which all are improvements for the treatment of bifurcation aneurysms and make difficult to coil aneurysms easier. We expect further improvements in these designs, and with improvements in deliverability. In addition to stents, the balloons available for balloon assisted coiling continue to improve in shape, design and deliverability which are particularly helpful in the setting of a ruptured small or wide necked aneurysm [99].

### 5.4 Imaging and aneurysm rupture prediction

Currently other than aneurysm size, and certain bio-social risk factors, there is no way to accurately predict which aneurysms are at risk for rupture. Over the next 5 years we expect to see, further advancement in the arena of MR vessel wall imaging, and flow-modeling. We hope that this will help improve our predictive models.


## Author details

David Altschul*, Tarini Vats and Santiago Unda
Montefiore Medical Center, Bronx, NY, USA

*Address all correspondence to: david.altschul@gmail.com

## References

[1] Etminan N, Rinkel GJ. Unruptured intracranial aneurysms: Development, rupture and preventive management. Nature Reviews Neurology. 2016;**12**:699-713

[2] Prestigiacomo. Endovascular surgical neuroradiology: Theory and clinical practice; the biophysics of aneurysm formation and rupture. Journal of Vascular and Interventional Radiology. 2015; Thieme Medical Publishers, 2015

[3] Alg VS, Sofat R, Houlden H, Werring DJ. Genetic risk factors for intracranial aneurysms: A meta-analysis in more than 116,000 individuals. Neurology. 2013;**80**:2154-2165

[4] Santiago-Sim T, Depalma SR, Ju KL, McDonough B, Seidman CE, Seidman JG, et al. Genomewide linkage in a large Caucasian family maps a new locus for intracranial aneurysms to chromosome 13q. Stroke. 2009;**40**:57-60

[5] Ruigrok YM, Rinkel GJ. Genetics of intracranial aneurysms. Stroke. 2008;**39**:1049-1055

[6] Foroud T, Lai D, Koller D, Van't Hof F, Kurki MI, Anderson CS, et al. Genome-wide association study of intracranial aneurysm identifies a new association on chromosome 7. Stroke. 2014;**45**:3194-3199

[7] Fang H. in Cerebrovascular Diseases; Wright, I. S. & Millikan, C. H. Grune and Stratton, 1958. 17-22

[8] Lasheras JC. The biomechanics of arterial aneurysms. Annual Review of Fluid Mechanics. 2007;**39**:293-319

[9] Frosen J. Smooth muscle cells and the formation, degeneration, and rupture of saccular intracranial aneurysm wall—A review of current pathophysiological knowledge. Translational Stroke Research. 2014;**5**:347-356

[10] Nixon AM, Gunel M, Sumpio BE. The critical role of hemodynamics in the development of cerebral vascular disease. Journal of Neurosurgery. 2010;**112**:1240-1253

[11] Berk BC. Atheroprotective signaling mechanisms activated by steady laminar flow in endothelial cells. Circulation. 2008;**117**(8):1082-1089

[12] Meng H, Tutino VM, Xiang J, Siddiqui A. High WSS or low WSS? Complex interactions of hemodynamics with intracranial aneurysm initiation, growth, and rupture: Toward a unifying hypothesis. AJNR. American Journal of Neuroradiology. 2014;**35**:1254-1262

[13] Cebral JR et al. Wall mechanical properties and hemodynamics of unruptured intracranial aneurysms. AJNR. American Journal of Neuroradiology. 2015;**36**:1695-1703

[14] Wong GK, Poon WS. Current status of computational fluid dynamics for cerebral aneurysms: The clinician's perspective. Journal of Clinical Neuroscience. 2011;**18**:1285-1288

[15] Alfano JM, Kolega J, Natarajan SK, Xiang J, Paluch RA, Levy EI, et al. Intracranial aneurysms occur more frequently at bifurcation sites that typically experience higher hemodynamic stresses. Neurosurgery. 2013;**73**:497-505

[16] Jing L et al. Morphologic and hemodynamic analysis in the patients with multiple intracranial aneurysms: Ruptured versus unruptured. PLoS One. 2015;**10**

[17] Frösen J, Tulamo R, Paetau A, Laaksamo E, Korja M, Laakso A, et al. Saccular intracranial aneurysm: pathology and mechanisms. Acta Neuropathologica. 2012;**123**:773-786

[18] Kurki MI, Häkkinen SK, Frösen J, Tulamo R, Fraunberg M, Wong G, et al. Upregulated signaling pathways in ruptured human saccular intracranial aneurysm wall: An emerging regulative role of toll-like receptor signaling and nuclear factor-κB, hypoxia-inducible factor-1A, and ETS transcription factors. Neurosurgery. 2011;**68**:1667-1675

[19] Starke RM, Chalouhi N, Ali MS, Jabbour PM, Tjoumakaris SI, Gonzalez LF, et al. The role of oxidative stress in cerebral aneurysm formation and rupture. Current Neurovascular Research. 2013;**10**:247-255

[20] Chalouhi N, Hoh BL, Hasan D. Review of cerebral aneurysm formation, growth, and rupture. Stroke. 2013;**44**:3613-3622

[21] Kleinloog R et al. RNA sequencing analysis of intracranial aneurysm walls reveals involvement of lysosomes and immunoglobulins in rupture. Stroke. 2016;**47**:1286-1293

[22] Aoki T et al. PGE2-EP2 signaling in endothelium is activated by hemodynamic stress and induces cerebral aneurysm through an amplifying loop via NF-κB. British Journal of Pharmacology. 2011;**163**:1237-1249

[23] UCAS Japan Investigators et al. The natural course of unruptured cerebral aneurysms in a Japanese cohort. The New England Journal of Medicine. 2012;**366**:2474-2482

[24] The International Study of Unruptured Intracranial Aneurysms Investigators. Unruptured intracranial aneurysms—Risk of rupture and risks of surgical intervention. International study of Unruptured intracranial aneurysms investigators. The New England Journal of Medicine. 1998;**339**:1725-1733

[25] Vlak M, Algra A, Brandenburg R, Rinkel G. Prevalence of unruptured intracranial aneurysms, with emphasis on sex, age, comorbidity, country, and time period: A systematic review and meta-analysis. Lancet Neurology. 2011;**10**:626-636

[26] Runge, Imaging of Cerebrovascular Disease: A Practical Guide. ISBN 978-1-62623-248-8

[27] Ogilvy C, Jordan N, Ascanio L, Enriquez-Marulanda A, Salem M, Moore M, et al. Surgical and endovascular comprehensive treatment outcomes of unruptured intracranial aneurysms: Reduction of treatment bias. World Neurosurgery. 2019. DOI: 10.1016/j.wneu.2019.03.005

[28] Harrigan M, Deveikis J. Handbook of Cerebrovascular Disease and Neurointerventional Technique. 2nd ed2013. 483p

[29] Lindgren A, Koivisto T, Bjorkman J, von Und Zu M, Heilin K, Jaaskelainen J, et al. Irregular shape of intracranial aneurysm indicates rupture risk irrespective of size in a population-based cohort. Stroke. 2016;**47**:1219-1226

[30] Backes D et al. Difference in aneurysm characteristics between ruptured and unruptured aneurysms in patients with multiple intracranial aneurysms. Stroke. 2014;**45**:1299-1303

[31] Giordan E, Sorenson TJ, Brinjikji W, et al. Risk factors for growth of conservatively managed unruptured intracranial aneurysms. Acta Neurochirurgica. 2018;**160**:2419. https://doi.org/10.1007/s00701-018-3729-z

[32] Bir S, Bollam P, Nanda A. Distribution of ABO blood groups in the patients with intracranial aneurysm and association of different risk factors with particular blood type. Asian Journal of Neurosurgery. 2015;**10**:153-157

[33] Wakabayashi T, Fujita S, Ohbora Y, Suyama T, Tamaki N, Matsumoto S. Polycystic kidney disease and intracranial aneurysms. Early angiographic diagnosis and early operation for the unruptured aneurysm. Journal of Neurosurgery. 1983;**58**:488-491

[34] Raaymakers TW, Rinkel GJ, Ramos LM. Initial and follow-up screening for aneurysms in families with familial subarachnoid hemorrhage. Neurology. 1998;**51**:1125-1130

[35] Bourekas EC, Newton HB, Figg GM, Slone HW. Prevalence and rupture rate of cerebral aneurysms discovered during intra-arterial chemotherapy of brain tumors. AJNR. American Journal of Neuroradiology. 2006;**27**:297-299

[36] Korja M, Lehto H, Juvela S. Lifelong rupture risk of intracranial aneurysms depends on risk factors: A prospective Finnish cohort study. Stroke. 2014;**45**:1958-1963

[37] Ujiie H, Sato K, Onda H, et al. Clinical analysis of incidentally discovered unruptured aneurysms. Stroke. 1993;**24**:1850-1856

[38] Sugai Y, Hamamoto Y, Ookubo T, So K. Angiographical frequency of unruptured incidental intracranial aneurysms. No Shinkei Geka. 1994;**22**:429-432

[39] Heman LM, Jongen LM, van der Worp HB, Rinkel GJ, Hendrikse J. Incidental intracranial aneurysms in patients with internal carotid artery stenosis: A CT angiography study and a metaanalysis. Stroke. 2009;**40**:1341-1346

[40] Ronkainen A, Miettinen H, Karkola K, et al. Risk of harboring an unruptured intracranial aneurysm. Stroke. 1998;**29**:359-362

[41] Mostafazadeh B, Farzaneh SE, Afsharian ST, Seraji FN, Salmasian H. The incidence of berry aneurysm in the Iranian population: An autopsy study. Turkish Neurosurgery. 2008;**18**:228-231

[42] Korja M et al. Cause-specific mortality of 1-year survivors of subarachnoid hemorrhage. Neurology. 2013;**80**:481-486

[43] Greving J et al. Development of the PHASES score for prediction of risk of rupture of intracranial aneurysms: A pooled analysis of six prospective cohort studies. Lancet Neurology. 2014;**13**:59-66

[44] Lunetta P, Lounamaa A, Sihvonen S. Surveillance of injury-related deaths: Medicolegal autopsy rates and trends in Finland. Injury Prevention. 2007;**13**:282-284

[45] Korja M, Kaprio J. Controversies in epidemiology of intracranial aneurysms and SAH. Nature Reviews Neurology. 2015;**12**:50-55

[46] Keedy A. An overview of intracranial aneurysms. McGill Journal of Medicine. 2006;**9**:141-146

[47] Friedman JA, Piepgras DG, Pichelmann MA, et al. Small cerebral aneurysms presenting with symptoms other than rupture. Neurology. 2001;**57**:1212-1216

[48] Date I. Symptomatic unruptured cerebral aneurysms: Features and surgical outcome. Neurologia Medico-Chirurgica (Tokyo). 2010;**50**:788-799

[49] Wagner M, Stenger K. Unruptured intracranial aneurysms: Using evidence and outcomes to guide patient teaching. Critical Care Nursing Quarterly. 2005;**28**:341-354

[50] Polmear A. Sentinel headaches in aneurysmal subarachnoid haemorrhage:

What is the true incidence? A systematic review. Cephalalgia. 2003;**23**:935-941

[51] Liu Y, Zheng Y, An Q, Song Y, Leng B. Optical coherence tomography for intracranial aneurysms: A new method for assessing the aneurysm structure. World Neurosurgery. 2019;**123**:194-201

[52] Raaymakers TW et al. MR angiography as a screening tool for intracranial aneurysms: Feasibility, test characteristics, and interobserver agreement. American Journal of Roentgenology. 1999

[53] Gasparotti R, Liserre R. Intracranial aneurysms. European Radiology. 2005;**15**:441-447

[54] Turner C, Kirkpatrick P. Detection of intracranial aneurysms with unenhanced and echo contrast enhanced transcranial power Doppler. Journal of Neurology, Neurosurgery, and Psychiatry. 2010;**68**:489-495

[55] Leffers AM, Wagner A. Neurologic complications of cerebral angiography. A retrospective study of complication rate and patient risk factors. Acta Radiologica. 2000;**41**(2):4-10

[56] Thorell W, Chow M, Prayson R, et al. Optical coherence tomography: A new method to assess aneurysm healing. Journal of Neurosurgery. 2005;**102**:348-354

[57] Huang D, Swanson E, Lin C, et al. Optical coherence tomography. Science. 1991;**254**:1178-1181

[58] Backes D et al. ELAPSS score for prediction of risk of growth of unruptured intracranial aneurysms. Neurology. 2017;**88**:1600-1606

[59] Yoshimoto Y, Tanaka Y. Risk perception of unruptured intracranial aneurysms. Acta Neurochirurgica. 2013;**155**:2029-2036

[60] Bonares M, de Oliveira Manoel A, Macdonald R, et al. Behavioral profile of unruptured intracranial aneurysms: A systematic review. Annals of Clinical Translational Neurology. 2014;**1**:220-232

[61] Molyneux A, Kerr R, Yu L. For the international subarachnoid aneurysm trial (ISAT) collaborative group international subarachnoid aneurysm trial (ISAT) of neurosurgical clipping versus endovascular coiling in 2143 patients with ruptured intracranial aneurysms: A randomised comparison of effects on survival, dependency, seizures, rebleeding, subgroups, and aneurysm occlusion. Lancet. 2006;**366**:809-817

[62] Salahuddin H et al. Recent trends in electively treated unruptured intracranial aneurysms. Journal of Stroke and Cerebrovascular Diseases. 2019;**28**:2011-2017

[63] Jalbert J, Isaacs A, Kamel H, et al. Clipping and coiling of unruptured intracranial aneurysms among medicare beneficiaries, 2000 to 2010. Stroke. 2015;**46**:2452-2457

[64] Naggara O et al. Endovascular treatment of intracranial unruptured aneurysms: A systematic review of the literature on safety with emphasis on subgroup analyses. Radiology. 2012;**263**:828-835

[65] Iang B, Paff M, Colby GP, et al. Cerebral aneurysm treatment: Modern neurovascular techniques. Stroke and Vascular Neurology. 2016;**1**:93-100

[66] Dengler J, Maldaner N, Glasker S, et al. Outcome of surgical or endovascular treatment of giant intracranial aneurysms, with emphasis on age, aneurysm location, and unruptured aneurysms—A systematic review and meta-analysis. Cerebrovascular Diseases. 2016;**41**:187-198

[67] FDA. Neurovascular Stents Used for Stent-Assisted Coiling of Unruptured Brain Aneurysms: Letter to Health Care Providers. Division of Industry Communication and Education (DICE) at DICE@FDA.HHS.GOV; 2018

[68] Administration. UFaD. Pipeline Embolization Device PMA P100018. Summary of Safety and Effectiveness Data. 2011. Available from: http://www.accessdata.fda.gov/cdrh_docs/pdf10/p100018b.pdf

[69] Pierot L, Wakhloo AK. Endovascular treatment of intracranial aneurysms: Current status. Stroke. 2013;**44**:2046-2054

[70] Fifi JT, Brockington C, Narang J, et al. Clopidogrel resistance is associated with thromboembolic complications in patients undergoing neurovascular stenting. AJNR. American Journal of Neuroradiology. 2013;**34**:716-720

[71] Yi H, Hwang G, Lee B. Variability of platelet reactivity on antiplatelet therapy in Neurointervention procedure. Journal of Korean Neurosurgical Society. 2018;**62**:3-9

[72] Corliss B, Polifka A, Harris N, Hoh B, Fox W. Laboratory assessments of therapeutic platelet inhibition in endovascular neurosurgery: Comparing results of the VerifyNow P2Y12 assay to thromboelastography with platelet mapping. Journal of Neurosurgery. 2017;**129**:1160-1165

[73] Marcolini E, Hine J. Approach to the diagnosis and management of subarachnoid hemorrhage. Western Journal of Emergency Medicine. 2019;**20**:203-211

[74] Edlow JA, Panagos PD, Godwin SA, et al. Clinical policy: Critical issues in the evaluation and management of adult patients presenting to the emergency department with acute headache. Annals of Emergency Medicine. 2008;**52**:407-436

[75] Perry JJ, Stiell IG, Sivilotti ML, et al. High risk clinical characteristics for subarachnoid hemorrhage in patients with acute headache: Prospective cohort study. BMJ. 2010;**341**:5204

[76] Frizzell RT, Kuhn f MR, Quinn C, Fisher WS. Screening for ocular hemorrhages in patients with ruptured cerebral aneurysm: Prospective study of 99 patients. Nerurosurgery. 1997;**41**:529-533

[77] Ness T, Janknecht P, Berghorn C. Frequency of ocular hemorrhages in patients with subarachnoid hemorrhage. Graefe's Archive for Clinical and Experimental Ophthalmology. 2005;**243**:859-862

[78] McCarron MO, Alberts MJ, McCarron P. A systematic review of Terson's syndrome: Frequency and prognosis after subarachnoid hemorrhage. Journal of Neurology, Neurosurgery, and Psychiatry. 2004;**75**:491-493

[79] Tsementzis SA, Williams A. Opthalmological signs and prognosis in patients with subarachnoid hemorrhage. Neurochirurgia (Stuttg). 1984;**27**:133-135

[80] Rosen DS, Macdonald RL. Subarachnoid hemorrhage grading scales: A systematic review. Neurocritical Care. 2005;**2**:110-118

[81] Hunt WE, Hess RM. Surgical risk as related to time of intervention in the repair of intracranial aneurysms. Journal of Neurosurgery. 1968;**28**:14-20

[82] Suarez JI, Tarr RW, Selman WR. Aneurysmal subarachnoid hemorrhage. The New England Journal of Medicine. 2006;**354**:387

[83] Martin SC, Teo MK, Young AM, et al. Defending a traditional practice in the modern era: The use of lumbar puncture in the investigation of subarachnoid hemorrhage. British Journal of Neurosurgery. 2015;**29**:799-803

[84] Abraham M, Chang W. Subarachnoid hemorrhage. Emergency Medicine Clinics of North America. 2016;**34**:901-916

[85] Choi K, Chun H, Yi K, et al. Seizure and epilepsy following aneurysmal subarachnoid hemorrhage: Incidence and risk factors. Journal of Korean Neurosurgical Association. 2009;**46**:93-98

[86] Connolly ES, Rabinstein AA, Carhuapoma JR, et al. Guidelines for the management of aneurysmal subarachnoid hemorrhage: A guideline for healthcare professionals from the American Heart Association/ American Stroke Association. Stroke. 2012;**43**:1711-1737

[87] Lanzino G, D'Urso PI, Suarez J. Participants in the international multi-disciplinary consensus conference on the critical care management of subarachnoid, hemorrhage seizures and anticonvulsants after aneurysmal subarachnoid hemorrhage. Neurocritical Care. 2011;**15**:247-256

[88] Cha KC, Kim JH, Kang HI, et al. Aneurysmal rebleeding-factors associated with clinical outcome in the rebleeding patients. Journal of Korean Neurosurgical Association. 2010;**47**:119-123

[89] Ohkuma H, Tsurutani H, Suzuki S. Incidence and significance of early aneurysmal rebleeding before neurosurgical or neurological management. Stroke. 2001;**32**:1176-1180

[90] Diringer MN, Bleck TP, Claude Hemphill J, et al. Critical care management of patients following aneurysmal subarachnoid hemorrhage: Recommendations from the neurocritical care society's multidisciplinary consensus conference. Neurocritical Care. 2011;**15**:211-240

[91] Starke RM, Connolly ES. Participants in the international multi-disciplinary consensus conference on the critical care management of subarachnoid, hemorrhage rebleeding after aneurysmal subarachnoid hemorrhage. Neurocritical Care. 2011;**15**:241-246

[92] Boogaarts HD, van Amerongen MJ, de Vries J, et al. Caseload as a factor for outcome in aneurysmal subarachnoid hemorrhage: A systematic review and meta-analysis. Journal of Neurosurgery. 2014;**120**:605-611

[93] International Subarachnoid Aneurysm Trial (ISAT). International subarachnoid aneurysm trial (ISAT) of neurosurgical clipping versus endovascular coiling in 2143 patients with ruptured intracranial aneurysms: A randomised comparison of effects on survival, dependency, seizures, rebleeding, subgroups, and aneurysm occlusion. The Lancet. 2002;**366**:809-817

[94] Lin N, Brouillard AM, Keigher KM, Lopes DK, Binning MJ, Liebman KM, et al. Utilization of pipeline embolization device for treatment of ruptured intracranial aneurysms: US multicenter experience. Journal of NeuroInterventional Surgery. 2015;**7**:808-815

[95] Chalouhi N, Jabbour P, Gonzalez LF, et al. Safety and efficacy of endovascular treatment of basilar tip aneurysms by coiling with and without stent assistance: A review of 235 cases. Neurosurgery. 2012;**71**:785-794

[96] Rabinstein AA, Lanzino G, Wijdicks EF. Multidisciplinary management and emerging therapeutic

strategies in aneurysmal subarachnoid haemorrhage. Lancet Neurology. 2010;**9**:504-519

[97] Maragkos G, Ascanio L, Salem M, Gopakumar S, Gomez-Paz S, Enriquez-Marulanda A, et al. Predictive factors of incomplete aneurysm occlusion after endovascular treatment with the pipeline embolization device. Journal of Neurosurgery. 26 Apr 2019:1-8. DOI: 10.3171/2019.1.JNS183226. [Epub ahead of print]

[98] Papagiannaki C, Spelle L, Januel A, Benaissa A, Gauvrit J, Costalat V, et al. WEB intrasaccular flow disruptor—Prospective, multicenter experience in 83 patients with 85 aneurysms. AJNR. American Journal of Neuroradiology. 2014;**35**:2106-2111

[99] Pierot L, Spelle L, Molyneux A, et al. Clinical and anatomical follow-up in patients with aneurysms treated with the WEB device: 1-year follow-up report in the cumulated population of 2 prospective, multicenter series (WEBCAST and French observatory). Neurosurgery. 2016;**78**:133-141

Chapter 12

# Brain Cooling and Cleaning: A New Perspective in Cerebrospinal Fluid (CSF) Dynamics

*Hira Burhan and Iype Cherian*

## Abstract

The function of the cerebrospinal fluid (CSF) has long been considered for mechanical protection and recently attributed to the supply of nutrients to the brain. However, we hypothesize that the brain is a water-cooled and water-cleaned system. Recent studies on the glymphatic pathways and the introduction of cisternostomy as a surgical procedure for traumatic brain injury reveal a vast and in-depth functionality of the CSF, which works in synchrony with the cardiopulmonary rhythms to act as a buffer for optimum cerebral function. The nasal sinuses are located around the suprasellar cistern, and the evaporating wet mucosa within them during the breathing contributes to local cooling, whereas the nocturnal activation of AQP4 channels allows CSF-ISF exchange. The resultant "cooling and cleaning" of the brain not only maintains a physiological equilibrium but also opens doors for understanding and treating pathophysiology underlying common degenerative and neuro-inflammatory diseases. This chapter describes the novel theory of brain cooling and cleaning and the clinical and experimental evidence to support this hypothesis.

**Keywords:** glymphatic pathway, cisternostomy, CSF shift, Virchow Robin spaces, subarachnoid cisterns, hydrocephalus, aquaporin-4

## 1. Introduction

The cerebrospinal fluid (CSF) is an ultrafiltrate of plasma, which resides in two compartments within the central nervous system (**Figure 1**). The ventricular system comprises four interconnected cavities in the brain and contains a network of ependymal cells forming the choroid plexus which has been believed to be the site of production of the CSF. The ventricular system is continuous with the central canal of the spinal cord (from the fourth ventricle) and allows the CSF to continuously bathe the cranium and the spine. The subarachnoid spaces form openings termed as subarachnoid cisterns which separate the arachnoid and the pia mater, thereby creating an anatomic space between the two meninges. These cisterns are filled with cerebrospinal fluid and form the second compartment where the CSF flows within the cranial cavity.

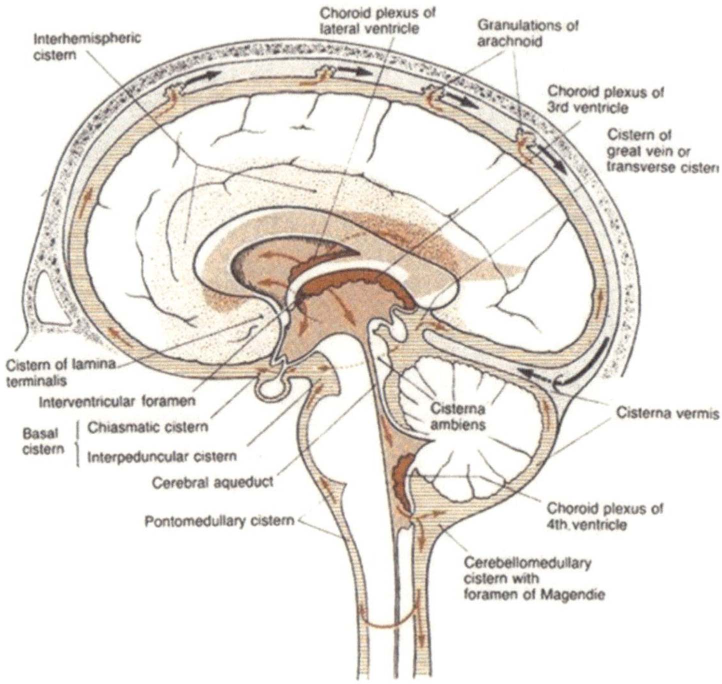


**Figure 1.**
*The anatomy of the fluid compartments of the brain: ventricular and cisternal systems.*

## 2. Cerebrospinal fluid: dynamics and function

Adult CSF volume is estimated to be 150 ml with a distribution of 125 ml within the subarachnoid spaces and 25 ml within the ventricles. This difference in the volume of CSF between the two compartments is important to understand the function of the CSF in a unique perspective.

The CSF secretion varies between individuals, usually ranging between 400 and 600 ml per day in an adult. The constant secretion of CSF contributes to a four to five times turnover per 24-h period. This turnover is of immense importance in exploring the functions of the CSF which have not yet been understood quite well. While the CSF has been considered as a source of nutrition and waste removal and a mechanically buoyant substance, cushioning the brain, the newer insights of the glymphatic pathways have demonstrated a critical role of CSF flow as a physiological buffer for brain functioning.

With a closely regulated composition, the CSF is valuable in analyzing cerebral pathologies. Alterations in the regulation of localized temperatures, malformation of proteins, and impeding clearance of pathologic proteins are the pathophysiological mechanisms for onset and progress of most neurodegenerative disorders as well as secondary brain damage in the setting of trauma. It is, however, interesting to analyze how the impairment of CSF inflow or outflow through the glymphatic system might lead to the cascade of these degenerative and traumatic pathologies.

### 2.1 The glymphatic pathway and the Virchow Robin (paravascular) spaces

The amount of CSF within the CSF compartments is a consequence of the net filtration and absorption of water through the selectively permeable capillary walls traversing through the brain tissue. This net effect is governed by the physiological or pathological conditions prevailing within these compartments. The glymphatic system branches along the course of the arteries, arterioles, capillaries, and venules, forming a paravascular cast. This CSF interacts with the end feet of glia and indirectly with neurons to establish an exchange with the brain ISF (**Figure 2**).

The AQP4 channels mediate the bidirectional transport of water in response to passive osmotic and hydraulic pressure gradients [2, 3], resulting in the CSF-ISF exchange [4]. This makes the glymphatic system extremely pressure dependent. Any increase of pressure in the glymphatic system would produce the passage of fluid toward the interstitial space until the pressure in both compartments is equalized. This exchange drives the removal of exogenous molecules from the interstitial spaces of the brain [5, 6] (**Figure 3**).

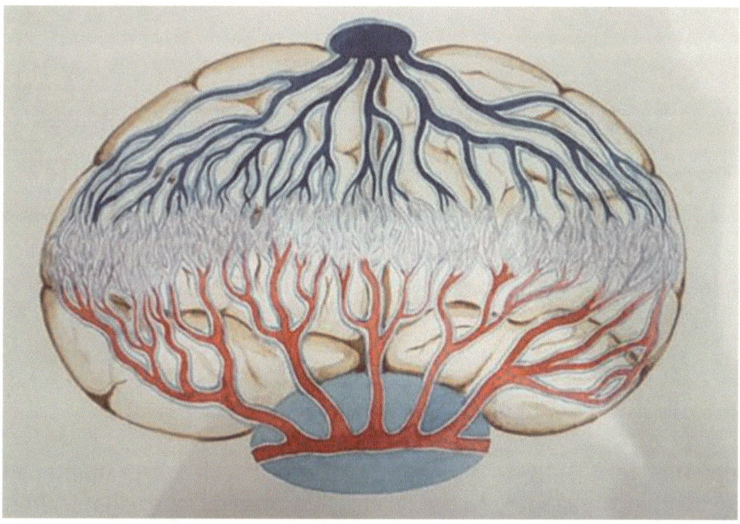

**Figure 2.**
*Artistic representation that depicts the persistence of the paravascular system through the arteries, arterioles, capillaries, venules, and veins. This indicates that just as there is a vascular cast of the brain, there is a paravascular system cast as well. Courtesy: Cherian and Beltran [1].*

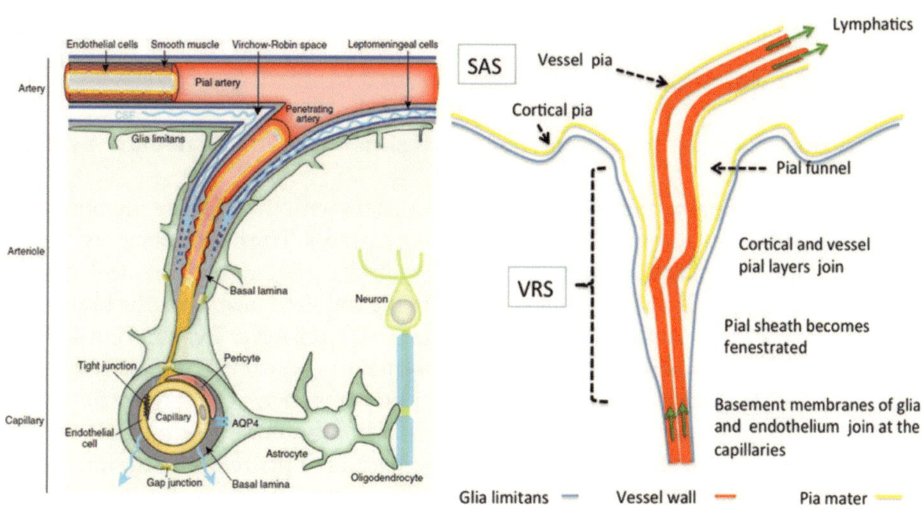


**Figure 3.**
*The anatomy of the Virchow Robin spaces forming an extensive network of communication within the glymphatic pathway. Courtesy: Orešković and Klarica [7].*

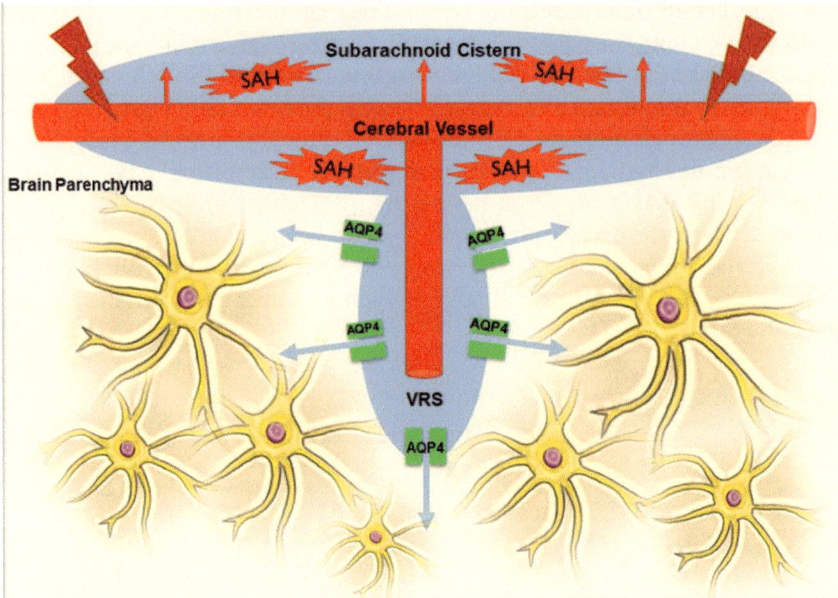


**Figure 4.**
*Schematic representation of the mechanism of CSF-shift edema following traumatic brain injury. The AQP-4 channels on the lining of VRS allow the shift of CSF from the cisterns into the brain parenchyma leading to brain edema.*

### 2.2 Introducing the concept of "CSF-shift" edema

The dependence of AQP4 to pressure gradients in both senses might be the underlying mechanism leading to the recently described "shift edema" following trauma [8] and also would explain the advantages of cisternostomy over craniectomy for the treatment in the short- and long-term follow-up of the patients [9]. Subsequent to subarachnoid hemorrhage, red blood cells are confined to the subarachnoid space and do not enter the VRS as pial membranes between the PVS and the SAS prevent the exchange of large molecules [10] (**Figure 4**).

## 3. Brain as a water-cooled and water-cleaned system

### 3.1 The subarachnoid cisterns and paranasal sinuses: anatomical relationships

The brain can be assumed as a water-cooled system with the CSF as a medium of heat removal and the paranasal sinuses as cooling surfaces. The close contact of the PNS with the suprasellar cisterns helps create a radiation system, and the mechanical process of breathing allows the sinuses to deliver the acquired heat from the brain parenchyma which is dumped by the CSF residing in the cisterns. Evaporation at the sinus surface causes cooling effect that is transmitted to the cisterns, dissipating the heat from the CSF which is acquired from the brain parenchyma [1] (**Figure 5**).

This cooling unit can be hypothesized to be a fundamental thermostat, and any hindrance in CSF flow might explain the cascade of protein misfolding secondary to heat accumulation as seen in neurodegeneration. While brain cooling is a passive process that occurs throughout the day, brain cleaning is more pronounced nocturnally. It is believed that brain cleaning is regulated by AQP4 and exchanges between interstitial fluid and CSF have been demonstrated to be more

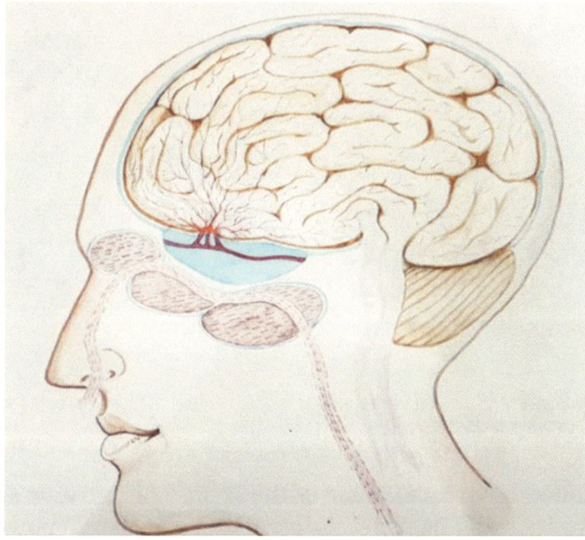

**Figure 5.**
*Close communication of the paranasal sinuses with the cisterns creating a brain cooling unit. Courtesy: Cherian and Beltran [1].*

active during sleep due to an expansion of the extracellular space, being increased by 60% during sleep [11], particularly in the lateral position [12]. The increased glymphatic clearance of the metabolic waste products generated by neural activity in the awake brain occurs during sleep, explaining the need to sleep for restoring alertness and activity.

### 3.2 Hypothesis of the CSF-driven brain cooling and cleaning mechanism

CSF is permanently produced and absorbed in the whole CSF system as a consequence of filtration and reabsorption of water volume through the capillary walls into the surrounding brain tissue. The three- to fourfold turnover rate in CSF production allows for a rigorous cerebral buffering at physiological states which helps maintain brain function. The brain generates tremendous amount of heat throughout the day which needs to be removed essentially to prevent protein misfolding and generation of free radicals. This warrants a system to allow for heat removal in the form of cooling as well as cleaning of metabolic wastes to prevent accumulation of toxic metabolites.

At a physiological state, the difference in arterial and venous hydrostatic and osmotic pressures allows a unidirectional flow of water and other molecules (soluble waste), with water leaving from the arterial end and molecules entering at the venous end. This simultaneous exchange of water and waste at two different ends can thus be regarded as a means of cleaning for the brain [5].

A deeper insight to this simultaneous exchange of water and waste in the blood vessels reveals the orientation of the brain vasculature, which, unlike other organs, runs in an opposite fashion, with the primary arteries lying ventral and more medially, whereas the principal veins run in a dorsal and lateral manner. Additionally, the disposition of white matter tracts creates an anisotropic field that facilitates the direction of fluid and molecules toward the main veins, which is further directed by changes in arteriovenous pressure gradients.

The paravascular system therefore maintains a very intricate and evolved system through extensive branching of vessels in the brain along with its paravascular

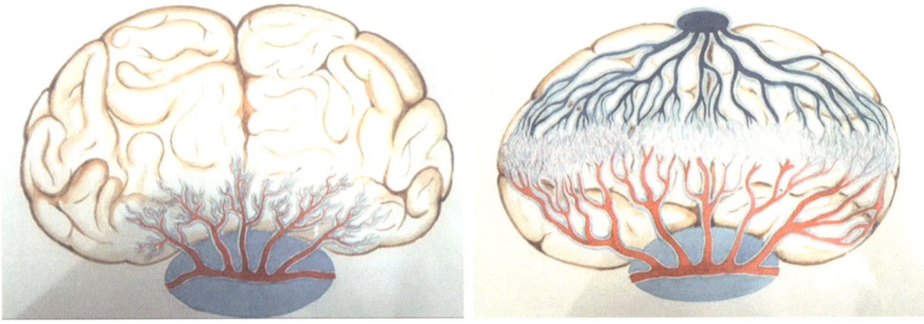

**Figure 6.**
*Schematic representation of the Virchow Robin spaces traveling around the blood vessels from the cisterns into the brain. Courtesy: Cherian and Beltran [1].*

system, thus following the vascular cast of the brain. This intricate system is limited by the selectively permeable capillary walls which is only large enough for a red blood cell to permeate through and may indeed be even more intricate than the vessels, since the limiting dimension of the capillaries is 3 in diameter, which is just large enough for a red blood corpuscle to squeeze through (**Figure 6**).

### 3.3 Role of breathing in brain cooling

The arteriovenous pressure difference described above can lead to the potential role of breathing on the dynamics of CSF flow within the extensive paravascular system. The close relationship of the paranasal sinuses with the basal cisterns provides an excellent radiation chamber that can help in buffering the thermal environment of the brain through continuous evaporation of the mucosa-lined sinus surfaces in contact with the external atmosphere, hence the hypothesis of breathing playing an important role in the cooling of the brain and possibly the clearance of molecules within the paravascular system.

### 3.4 Sleep and aquaporin-4 in brain cleaning

Attributed to the expression and function of the AQP-4 channels, the brain cleaning mechanism is predominant during sleep. Sleep increases the expansion of the extracellular spaces by up to 60% which allows for a maximal exchange of substances to and fro the CSF and the ISF compartments [11]. This phenomenon is particularly observed in the lateral position [12]. Therefore, the restorative properties of sleep may be linked to increased glymphatic clearance of the metabolic waste products that are generated by neural activity in the awake brain. This might underpin the beneficial effects of sleep, in clearance of metabolic byproducts, the phenomenon of jetlag, and the problems with lack of sleep.

## 4. Cardiopulmonary regulation of the CSF flow

The primary CSF delivery mechanism, from the subarachnoid space into the paravascular system and along the paravascular space, appears to be arterial pulsatility [6, 13], coupled with brain compliance [2] (**Figure 7**). Arterial pulsatility, coupled with a perivascular compliance, generates successive physical brain compression and expansion, allowing the brain to act like a sponge by virtue of the cycle-dependent systolic-diastolic circulatory movement of blood through

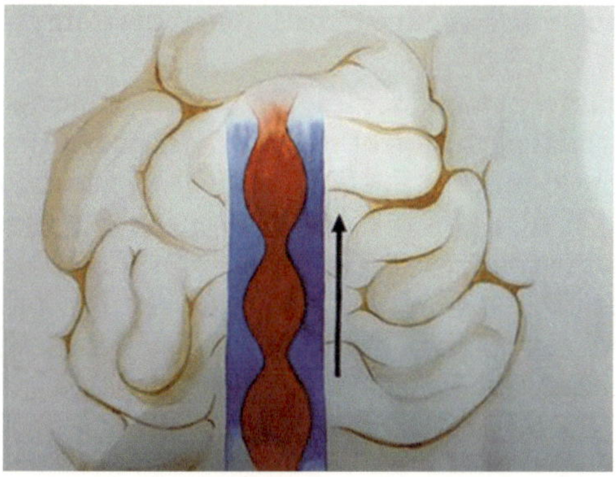

**Figure 7.**
*Graphical representation of pulsations in the artery and veins being the driving force to the CSF in the paravascular pathway.*

the brain [14]. This reciprocal movement influences the flow of fluids in the brain parenchyma to initiate a "pumping" effect of CSF around the vessels. These movements are driven by physiological oscillations of arterial and venous blood during craniospinal blood circulation, which are influenced by respiration, body activity, and posture [7].

Loss of arterial elasticity may lead to an impairment of this "pumping" effect in the paravascular system. This is classically seen in small vessel disease or as a consequence of low craniospinal compliance that impedes the expansion of the arteries, as can be seen in normal pressure hydrocephalus, gliosis [15], or post-traumatic hypertension. This would result in a decrease of CSF turnover that hinders the clearance of metabolites [16] and generates excess metabolic heat, thereby contributing to the pathogenesis of neurological diseases.

Aging is a phenomenon that leads to a decline in the exchange efficiency between CSF in the paravascular spaces, and ISF occurs. This can be related to a reduction in the vessel wall pulsatility of intracortical arterioles and the widespread loss of perivascular AQP4 channels [17]. This "hardening" of vessel walls, as a consequence of aging, decreases the drainage of amyloid peptides, which may deposit in the paravascular pathways as cerebral amyloid angiopathy (CAA). These deposits further impede the drainage of ISF along the paravascular spaces, resulting in loss of homeostasis of the neuronal environment that may contribute to neuronal malfunction [15, 18]. The concurrent loss of localized thermal regulation by the paravascular pathway may add to the cascade of damage by modification of proteinaceous components, which are very sensitive to subtle changes in temperature. These structural changes in molecular geometries might disturb solubility and thus the drainage of this metabolic waste, giving rise to a vicious circle.

## 5. Alterations in the glymphatic system: impaired brain cleaning and cooling

The functional impairment of the paravascular system appears to be an underlying condition of the aging human brain [19], which has also been related to various CNS disorders, such as neurodegenerative disorders that are brought on by the accumulation of misfolded, prion-like proteins (e.g., Alzheimer's or amyloid angiopathy) [17, 20, 21], normal pressure hydrocephalus [19, 22, 23], post-traumatic encephalopathy [24, 25], or neuroinflammatory disorders, such as multiple sclerosis. Furthermore, the presence of the paravascular system would explain the advantages of cisternostomy over decompressive craniectomy, in the treatment of acute brain trauma [8, 26].

Decreased intracranial compliance leads to increased intraparenchymal pressure, affecting the arterial perfusion of the brain and promoting venous congestion. On the whole, the kinetics of the fluid in the paravascular spaces is impaired. Should there be a loss of AQP4 localization, as seen in reactive astrogliosis and the aging brain, or following trauma or ischemia, or if the CSF outflow is reduced as a consequence of either CSF flow obstruction, cerebral artery pulsatility inefficiency, cerebrospinal venous insufficiency, or lymphatic disorders [27], the localized perivascular CSF recirculation may be impaired.

## 5.1 Clinical implication

### *5.1.1 Cisternostomy: the clinical implementation of CSF-shift reversal in TBI*

The corresponding author serendipitously uncovered the fact that opening cisterns in severe head trauma had the effect of abating severe brain swelling while drastically reducing the requirement for decompressive hemicraniectomies [24, 28]. His decade-long work on this led him to believe that CSF was ingressing to the brain through the Virchow Robin spaces, producing a condition which has been recently termed as CSF shift edema. Experimental studies on the glymphatic system by Iliff et al. categorically proved the communication of the CSF with the brain through the Virchow Robin spaces, or paravascular spaces, and that this pathway was critical for clearing the brain of metabolites [5, 6]. Perhaps the biggest clinical implication of this finding is the microsurgical opening of the cisterns: cisternostomy, in cases of moderate to severe head injury in order to reverse CSF shift edema, which is the mainstay of the cascade of the TBI damage. This procedure has been discussed in detail in previous publications and prevents progression to diffuse axonal damage or cortical stretch as otherwise seen in decompressive procedures. The phenomenal prognosis in the patients undergoing cisternostomy led the author to investigate the paravascular system in further depth, as well as CSF shifts, and subsequently the likely functionality of the paravascular system (**Figure 8**).

Today, cisternostomy has shown to be efficacious as a primary surgical intervention in moderate to severe traumatic brain injury. While following the principles of reversal of CSF shift edema, cisternostomy has proven to help in the prognosis by decreasing the rates of morbidities and mortalities [22]. It is now being practiced in many neurosurgical centers around the world [25] and has also been accepted

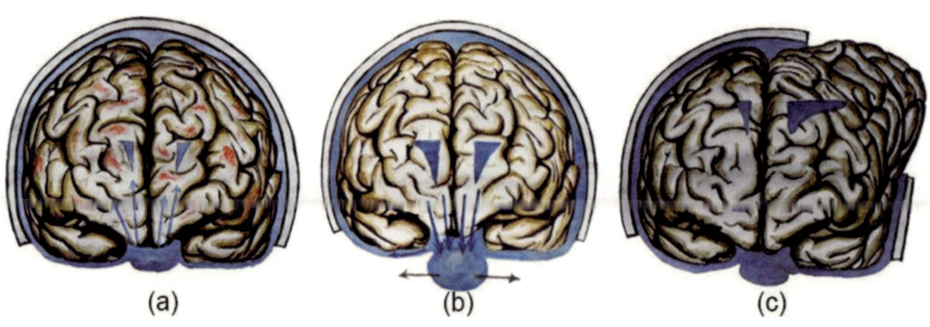


**Figure 8.**
*(a) Raised cisternal pressure due to the traumatic subarachnoid hemorrhage shifts cerebrospinal fluid into the brain, causing raised intracerebral pressure. (b) Opening of the cisterns reverses the cisternal pressure gradient, causing cerebrospinal fluid to flow back into the cisterns, thus decreasing the brain pressure. (c) Decompressive hemicraniectomy allows extracalvarial herniation, leading to further deterioration due to axonal stretch and altered blood flow dynamics. Courtesy: Cherian et al. [24].*

as one of the options of surgical intervention in the ongoing Global Neurotrauma Outcomes Study [29].

### *5.1.2 Road to further research*

The paravascular system, its cleaning and cooling properties, and the consequent pathophysiological conditions secondary to the impedance of this system as well as potential treatment measures have not yet been investigated in detail. Reports of an experiment where a bacteriophage is being introduced into the olfactory system of a mouse resulted in the reversal of Alzheimer's symptoms. This could be due to the clearance of the obstructed paravascular system as the phage traveled into the cisterns through the perineural space of the olfactory. This observation opens doors for a paradigm shift in the management of neurodegenerative diseases and warrants extensive research. Further experimental work in this area will include the injection of paramagnetic nanoparticles into the suprasellar cisterns of mice, porcine, or baboon models, where the movement of these nanoparticles may be observed with a T1 W3T MRI.

## 6. Conclusion

The paravascular system is a branching structure that extensively connects the cells and vessels within the brain. The intricacy of the system and the challenges in performing studies have been a hurdle in exploring this system. However, an in-depth analysis of brain fluid dynamics and its relationship to the cardiopulmonary mechanisms can provide a game changing pathway to the preventive and therapeutic measures of various pathophysiological brain disorders.

## Author details

Hira Burhan and Iype Cherian*
Institute of Neurosciences, Nobel Medical College and Teaching Hospital, Biratnagar, Nepal

*Address all correspondence to: drrajucherian@gmail.com

## References

[1] Cherian I, Beltran M. A unified physical theory for CSF circulation, cooling and cleaning of the brain, sleep, and head injuries in degenerative cognitive disorders. In: Opris I, Casanova M, editors. The Physics of the Mind and Brain Disorders. Springer Series in Cognitive and Neural Systems. Vol. 11. Cham: Springer; 2017

[2] Kress BT et al. Impairment of paravascular clearance pathways in the aging brain. Annals of Neurology. 2014;**76**(6):845-861

[3] Papadopoulos MC, Verkman AS. Aquaporin water channels in the nervous system. Nature Reviews. Neuroscience. 2013;**14**(4):265-277

[4] Agre P. The aquaporin water channels. Proceedings of the American Thoracic Society. 2006;**3**(1):5-13

[5] Iliff JJ et al. A paravascular pathway facilitates CSF flow through the brain parenchyma and the clearance of interstitial solutes, including amyloid. Science Translational Medicine. 2012;**4**(147):147ra111

[6] Iliff JJ et al. Brain-wide pathway for waste clearance captured by contrast-enhanced MRI. The Journal of Clinical Investigation. 2013;**123**(3):1299-1309

[7] Oreškovi'c D, Klarica M. A new look at cerebrospinal fluid movement. Fluids and Barriers of the CNS. 2014;**11**:16

[8] Cherian I, Beltran M. Cisternostomy—Introducing the concept of "CSF-shift edema". International Journal of Psychology and Neuroscience. 2016;**2**(1):15-29

[9] Cherian I, Yi G, Munakomi S. Cisternostomy: Replacing the age old decompressive hemicraniectomy? Asian Journal of Neurosurgery. 2013;**8**(3):132-138

[10] Hutchings M, Weller RO. Anatomical relationships of the pia mater to cerebral blood vessels in man. Journal of Neurosurgery. 1986;**65**(3):316-325

[11] Xie L et al. Sleep drives metabolite clearance from the adult brain. Science. 2013;**342**(6156):373-377

[12] Lee H et al. The effect of body posture on brain glymphatic transport. The Journal of Neuroscience. 2015;**35**(31):11034-11044

[13] Linninger AA, Tangen K, Hsu CY, David FD. Cerebrospinal fluid mechanics and its coupling to cerebrovascular dynamics. Annual Review of Fluid Mechanics. 2016;**48**(1):219-257

[14] Yamada S et al. Influence of respiration on cerebrospinal fluid movement using magnetic resonance spin labeling. Fluids and Barriers of the CNS. 2013;**10**(1):36

[15] Kida S. Progress in diagnosis of and therapy for idiopathic normal-pressure hydrocephalus—Lymphatic drainage of CSF and ISF from the brain: Recent concept and hypothesis. Rinsho Shinkeigaku (Clinical Neurology). 2014;**54**(12):1187-1189

[16] Kiefer M, Unterberg A. The differential diagnosis and treatment of normal-pressure hydrocephalus. Deutsches Ärzteblatt International. 2012;**109**(1-2):15-25

[17] Simka M. Recent advances in understanding the lymphatic and glymphatic systems of the brain. Phlebological Review. 2015;**23**(3):69-71

[18] Weller RO, Djuanda E, Yow HY, Carare RO. Lymphatic drainage of the brain and the pathophysiology

of neurological disease. Acta Neuropathologica. 2009;**117**(1):1-14

[19] Silverberg GD, Mayo M, Saul T, Rubenstein E, McGuire D. Alzheimer's disease, normal-pressure hydrocephalus, and senescent changes in CSF circulatory physiology: A hypothesis. Lancet Neurology. 2003;**2**(8):506-511

[20] Iliff JJ et al. Impairment of glymphatic pathway function promotes tau pathology after traumatic brain injury. The Journal of Neuroscience. 2014;**34**(49):16180-16193

[21] Gallina P, Scollato A, Conti R, Di Lorenzo N, Porfirio B. A clearance, "hub" of multiple deficiencies leading to Alzheimer disease. Frontiers in Aging Neuroscience. 2015;**7**:200

[22] Cherian I, Burhan H. Outcomes of severe head injury patients undergoing cisternostomy from a tertiary care hospital in Nepal. Indonesian Journal of Neurosurgery. 2019;**2**(3). DOI: 10.15562/ijn.v2i3.58

[23] Greitz D. Radiological assessment of hydrocephalus: New theories and implications for therapy. The Neuroradiology Journal. 2006;**19**(4):475-495

[24] Cherian I, Grasso G, Bernardo A, Munakomi S. Anatomy and physiology of cisternostomy. Chinese Journal of Traumatology. 2016;**19**(1):7-10

[25] Levi V, Vetrano IG. May cisternostomy and glymphatic system be considered the Deus ex Machina of refractory posttraumatic intracranial hypertension? World Neurosurgery. 2018;**117**:471-472. DOI: 10.1016/j.wneu.2018.05.231

[26] Cherian I, Munakomi S. Review article and surgical technique surgical technique for cisternostomy: A review. International Journal of Student's Research. 2013;**3**(1):147-148

[27] Brinker T, Stopa E, Morrison J, Klinge P. A new look at cerebrospinal fluid circulation. Fluids and the Barriers of the CNS. 2014;**11**:10

[28] Cherian I, Bernardo A, Grasso G. Cisternostomy for traumatic brain injury: Pathophysiologic mechanisms and surgical technical notes. World Neurosurgery. 2016;**89**:51-57

[29] Global Neurotrauma Outcomes Study. Retrieved from: https://globalneurotrauma.com/

Chapter 13

# Calcium Channel Blockers

*Yaser Alahamd, Hisham Ab Ib Swehli, Alaa Rahhal, Sundus Sardar, Mawahib Ali Mohammed Elhassan, Salma Alsamel and Osama Ali Ibrahim*

## Abstract

Vasospasm refers to a condition in which an arterial spasm leads to vasoconstriction. This can lead to tissue ischemia and necrosis. Coronary vasospasm can lead to significant cardiac ischemia associated with symptomatic ischemia or cardiac arrhythmia. Cerebral vasospasm is an essential source of morbidity and mortality in subarachnoid hemorrhage patients. It can happen within 3–15 days with a peak incidence at 7 days after aneurysmal subarachnoid hemorrhage (SAH). Calcium channel blockers are widely used in the treatment of hypertension, angina pectoris, cardiac arrhythmias, and other disorders like SAH vasospasm related and Migraine. The specific treatment of cerebral vasospasm helps improving cerebral blood flow to avoid delayed ischemic neurologic deficit by reducing ICP, optimizing the rate of cerebral oxygen demand, and enhancing cerebral blood flow with one of the following approaches: indirect pharmacological protection of brain tissue or direct mechanical dilation of the vasospastic vessel. Nimodipine is the standard of care in aneurysmal SAH patients. Nimodipine 60 mg every 4 hours can be used for all patients with aneurysmal SAH once the diagnosis is made for 21 days.

**Keywords:** coronary vasospasm, cerebral vasospasm, calcium channel blockers, cerebral blood flow, nimodipine

## 1. Introduction

Vasospasm is a condition which is associated with an arterial spasm and vasoconstriction, which may lead to tissue ischemia and necrosis. Coronary vasospasm can lead to significant cardiac ischemia associated with symptomatic ischemia or cardiac arrhythmia. Cerebral vasospasm may arise as a complication of subarachnoid hemorrhage (SAH). The most common cause of delayed cerebral ischemia after SAH is assumed to be vasospasm; delayed cerebral ischemia contributes substantially to morbidity and mortality after SAH especially aneurysmal SAH. Calcium channel blockers are widely used in the treatment of hypertension, angina pectoris, cardiac arrhythmias, and other disorders like SAH vasospasm related and migraine. Data is suggesting that their use reduces the risk of subsequent cardiovascular events [1, 2]. Besides, some meta-analyses have suggested that calcium channel blockers may be more effective than other drugs in reducing stroke risk [3, 4]. Fleckenstein's work in the 1960s led to the concept that drugs alter cardiac and smooth muscle contraction by blocking the entry of $Ca^{2+}$ into myocytes. Godfraind and associates showed that the effect of the diphenylpiperazine analogs in the prevention of agonist-induced vascular smooth muscle contraction could be overcome by raising the concentration of $Ca^{2+}$ in the extracellular medium. Hass and Hartfelder reported in 1962 that verapamil, a coronary vasodilator, possessed negative inotropic and chronotropic effects that were not seen with other vasodilatory agents, such as GTN. In 1967, Fleckenstein suggested that the negative inotropic effect resulted from an inhibition of excitation-contraction coupling and that the mechanism involved reduced movement of $Ca^{2+}$ into cardiac myocytes. Verapamil was the first clinically available $Ca^{2+}$ channel blocker; it is a congener of papaverine. Many other $Ca^{2+}$ entry blockers with a wide range of structures are now available [5].

## 2. Mechanism of action and effects

Calcium is an essential element for excitation-contraction coupling in muscle cells. The increase in the cytosolic $Ca^{2+}$ concentration leads to an increased contraction in both cardiac and vascular smooth muscle cells [6]:

1. In smooth muscle and cardiac muscle cells, $Ca^{2+}$ can enter cells through transmembrane voltage-gated and ligand-gated channels (**Figures 1** and **2**).

2. In striated and cardiac muscle cells, a rise in intracellular free $Ca^{2+}$ promotes the release of further $Ca^{2+}$ from the sarcoplasmic reticulum (SR) through actions at ryanodine receptors (**Figures 1** and **2**).

3. Ligand-gated channels linked to G-protein-coupled receptors promote the release of $Ca^{2+}$ from intracellular stores in the sarcoplasmic reticulum.

4. $Ca^{2+}$ leaves striated and cardiac muscle cells in exchange for Na + via the Na+/$Ca^{2+}$ exchanger (**Figure 1**).

Therefore, in striated muscle, free $Ca^{2+}$ in the cytosol comes only from the sarcoplasmic reticulum, while in smooth muscle, it must enter the cell through transmembrane $Ca^{2+}$ channels. Cardiac muscle uses both mechanisms.

Four types of transmembrane calcium channels, differing in location and function, have been identified:

**A.** L type, located in skeletal, cardiac, and smooth muscles, causing contraction of muscle cells.

**B.** T type, found in pacemaker cells, causing $Ca^{2+}$ entry, inactivated at more negative potentials and more rapid than the L type.

**C.** N type is available in neurons and acting in transmitter release.

**D.** P type is in Purkinje cells whose function is unknown currently.

5- Voltage-gated L-type $Ca^{2+}$ channels (long-acting, high threshold-activated, slowly inactivated) are found in the cell membranes of a large number of excitable cells, including cardiac and vascular smooth muscle. $Ca^{2+}$ enters the cell through these channels when the cell membrane is depolarized. The cardiac and vascular smooth muscle L-type $Ca^{2+}$ channels have different subunit structures. L-type channels are essential therapeutically. The L-type calcium channel, acted on by calcium channel blockers, consists of five different subunits ($\alpha1$, $\alpha2$, $\beta$, $\delta$, $\gamma$). **Figure 3** represents the L type of $Ca^{2+}$ channel [7].

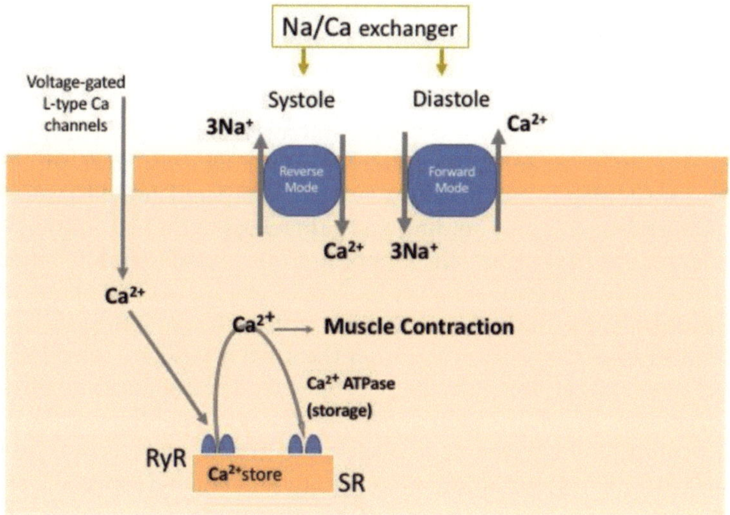


**Figure 1.**
*Regulation of calcium in cardiac myocytes and blood vessels.*

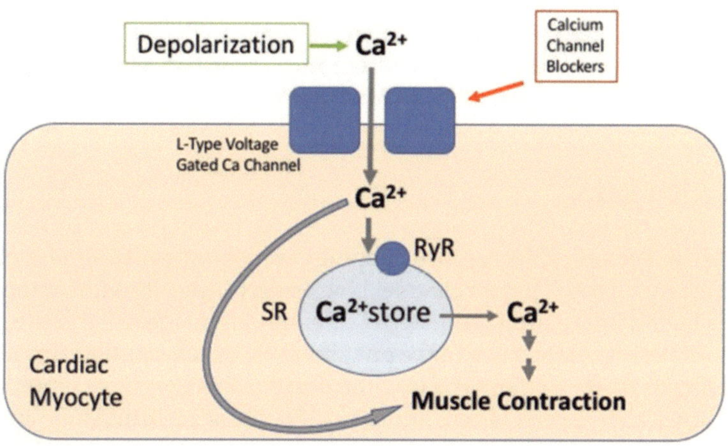


**Figure 2.**
*Mechanism of contraction of the cardiac myocyte by L-type voltage-gated Ca channel.*

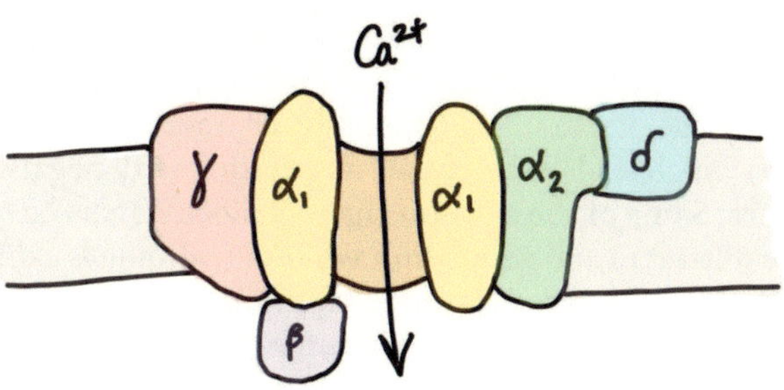


**Figure 3.**
*Subunits of the L-type calcium channel.*

6- Voltage-gated T-type $Ca^{2+}$ channels (transient, low threshold-activated, fast inactivated) are found in pacemaker cells of the sinoatrial and atrioventricular nodes and are also present in vascular smooth muscle. Calcium channel blockers have different chemical structures, but their standard action is to reduce $Ca^{2+}$ influx through voltage-gated L-type $Ca^{2+}$ channels in smooth cardiac muscle (**Figure 2**).

There are clinically significant differences among the different types of calcium channel blockers, which bind to discrete receptors on the L-type $Ca^{2+}$ channel. The receptor for verapamil is intracellular, while diltiazem and the dihydropyridines (e.g., nifedipine, amlodipine) have extracellular binding sites; however, the receptor domains for verapamil and diltiazem overlap. Verapamil and diltiazem exhibit frequency-dependent receptor binding and gain access to the $Ca^{2+}$ channel when it is in the open state; in contrast, the dihydropyridines preferentially bind to the channel in its inactivated state. As more $Ca^{2+}$ channels are in the inactive state, dihydropyridines selectively bind to $Ca^{2+}$ channels in vascular smooth muscle. These receptor binding characteristics account for the relative vascular selectivity of the dihydropyridines and the antiarrhythmic properties of verapamil and diltiazem [6].

Calcium concentrations in cardiac cells and vascular smooth muscles are under the influence of different mechanisms. Calcium entry through voltage-gated L-type $Ca^{2+}$ channels stimulates ryanodine receptors (RyR) in the sarcoplasmic reticulum, releasing stored $Ca^{2+}$ (a process known as $Ca^{2+}$ –induced calcium release, CICR). Intracellular $Ca^{2+}$ is also regulated by exchange with Na + via the Na+/$Ca^{2+}$ exchangers (NCX) in the cell membrane.

The depolarization phase during the action potential activates the voltage-gated channels, and the influx of $Ca^{2+}$ into the cell results in myosin phosphorylation and muscle contraction. It also promotes further $Ca^{2+}$ release from the sarcoplasmic reticulum by stimulation of ryanodine receptors. L-type $Ca^{2+}$ channels can, therefore, be reduced directly by calcium channel blockers.

## 3. Pharmacokinetics

Most calcium channel blockers are lipophilic compounds with similar pharmacokinetic properties. Calcium channel blockers are typically administered in oral dosage forms, but orally administered calcium channel blockers undergo significant first-pass metabolism in the gut and liver, which can significantly reduce bioavailability to 10–30%. Most oral calcium channel blockers have a rapid onset of action between 20 minutes and 2 hours like nifedipine resulting in reflex tachycardia, which can worsen myocardial ischemia due to shortening diastolic phase of the cardiac cycle. Most of the agents typically have short elimination half-lives (2–10 hours), necessitating short dosing intervals or extended-release formations. Amlodipine was developed in an attempt to overcome the pharmacokinetic limitations of nifedipine. This drug has an increased oral bioavailability of 60%. The time of onset is 6 hours, and prolonged elimination half-life is 40 hours. These kinetic properties are likely due, in part, to its lipophilic character and its positive charge at physiologic pH, which leads to increased association with negatively charged plasma membranes. Some of the calcium channel blockers also have intravenous formulations like diltiazem and verapamil, while clevidipine is a dihydropyridine agent that is available only as an intravenous formulation. All calcium channel blockers are metabolized by the liver. Diltiazem is primarily excreted by the liver, while dihydropyridines and verapamil are mainly excreted in the urine [6–8].

## 4. Pharmacological actions

The main targets of calcium channel blockers are vascular tissue and cardiac cells. $Ca^{2+}$ channel blockers inhibit the voltage-dependent $Ca^{2+}$ channels in vascular smooth muscle and decrease $Ca^{2+}$ entry. All $Ca^{2+}$ channel antagonists relax arterial smooth muscle and thereby reduce arterial resistance, blood pressure, and cardiac afterload. $Ca^{2+}$ channel blockers do not influence cardiac preload significantly when given at regular doses, suggesting that capacitance veins that determine venous return to the heart are resistant to the relaxing effect of $Ca^{2+}$ channel antagonists. Depolarization in the SA and AV nodes depends mainly on the movement of $Ca^{2+}$ through the slow channel. The impact of a $Ca^{2+}$ channel blocker on AV conduction and the rate of the sinus node pacemaker depend on whether the agent delays the recovery of the slow channel.

Diltiazem and verapamil decrease the rate of the SA node pacemaker and slow AV conduction at clinically used doses; the latter effect is the basis for their use in the treatment of supraventricular tachyarrhythmias [6–8].

## 5. Cardiovascular effects of different $Ca^{2+}$ channel blockers

The hemodynamic profiles of the $Ca^{2+}$ channel blockers approved for clinical use differ and depend mainly on the ratio of vasodilating and negative inotropic and chronotropic effects on the heart (**Table 1**, **Figures 4** and 5). Although all calcium channel blockers are vasodilators, dihydropyridine derivatives such as nifedipine and amlodipine are the most potent and have the most significant vascular selectivity. Arterial dilation reduces peripheral resistance and lowers blood pressure, which reduces the work of the left ventricle and therefore reduces myocardial oxygen demand. Most dihydropyridines have a rapid onset of action. A rapid reduction in blood pressure can lead to reflex sympathetic nervous system activation and tachycardia. Amlodipine or modified-release formulations of short-acting dihydropyridines are more slowly absorbed and gradually reduce blood pressure with little reflex tachycardia. But generally, the differences between the relatively vaso-selective dihydropyridines and the much less-selective diltiazem and verapamil have essential consequences because the decrease in arterial blood pressure elicits reflex sympathetic activation, resulting in the stimulation of heart rate, AV conduction velocity, and myocardial force, just the opposite of the direct effect of $Ca^{2+}$ channel blockers. While direct and indirect impacts usually balance each other in the case of verapamil and diltiazem, sympathetic stimulation often prevails in dihydropyridines, causing an increase in heart rate and contractility. Cardiac depressant effects

| Comparative Cardiovascular Effects of Calcium Channel Blockers | | | | |
|---|---|---|---|---|
| Example (Drug class) | Vasodilation | Decreased cardiac contractility | Decreased automaticity (SA node) | Decreased conduction (AV node) |
| Verapamil (phenylalkylamine) | 4 | 4 | 5 | 5 |
| Diltiazem (benzothiazepine) | 3 | 2 | 5 | 4 |
| Amlodipine (dihydropyridine) | 5 | 1 | 1 | 0 |
| Nifedipine (dihydropyridine | 5 | 1 | 1 | 0 |

**Table 1.**
*Comparative cardiovascular effects of calcium channel blockers graded from 0 (no effect) to 5 (prominent effect).*

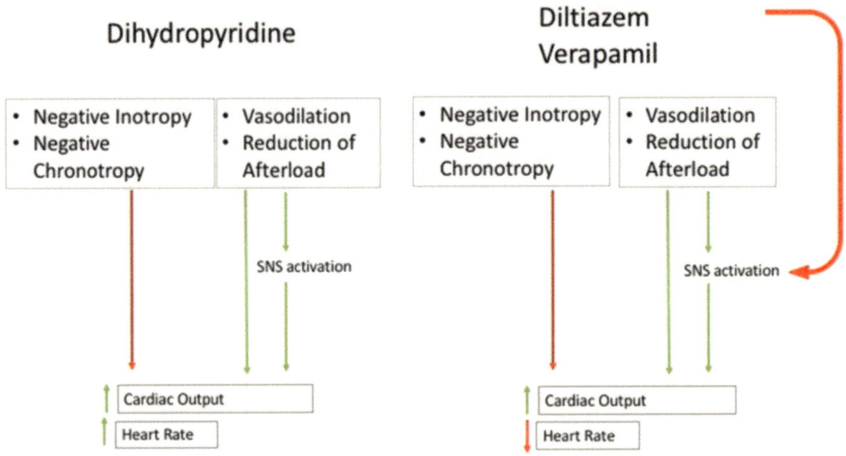


**Figure 4.**
*Effects of calcium channel blocker agents.*

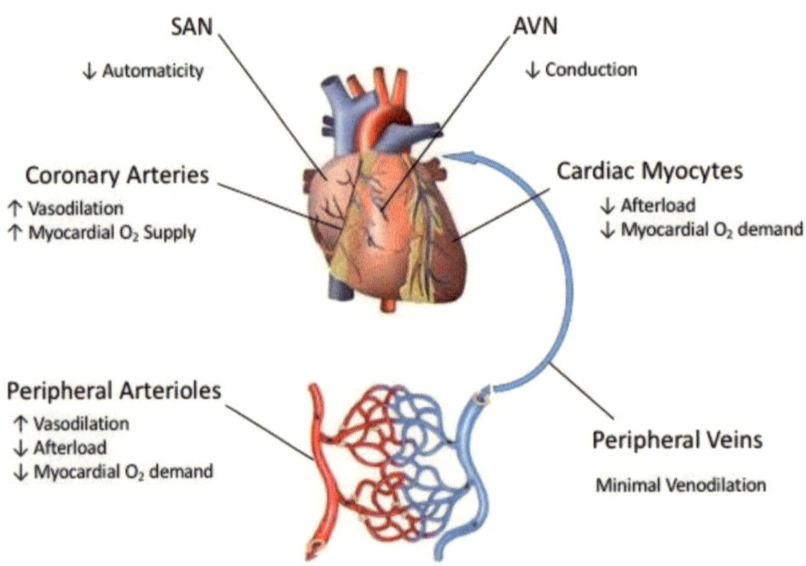


**Figure 5.**
*Calcium channel blocker sites of action.*

of dihydropyridines may be unmasked, though, in the presence of β blockers and patients with heart failure.

Also, they can have a significant impact on coronary artery dilation; for this reason, CCB can prevent or relieve coronary vasospasm and improve myocardial blood flow. On the other hand, CCBs have negative chronotropic effect. Verapamil and diltiazem (but not the dihydropyridines) slow the rate of firing of the sinoatrial node and slow the conduction of the electrical impulse through the atrioventricular node. Reflex tachycardia does not occur with these drugs, and they also slow the rate of rising in heart rate during exercise. CCBs play an essential role in reducing cardiac contractility as most calcium channel blockers (particularly verapamil) have some negative inotropic effects. Amlodipine does not impair myocardial contractility.

## 6. Calcium channel blocker agents

There are two types of CCBs:

**A.** Dihydropyridines: amlodipine, clevidipine, felodipine, isradipine, lercanidipine, nicardipine, nifedipine, nimodipine, and nisoldipine

Dihydropyridines exhibit much higher arterial vasodilation than non-dihydropyridines while having relatively little impact on cardiac tissue (i.e., there is less depression on myocardial contractility, less impairment on SA node automaticity, and less slowing on AV node conduction velocity) (**Table 1**, **Figure 4**).

**B.** Non-dihydropyridines:

- Benzothiazepines (diltiazem)

- Phenylalkylamines (verapamil)

Non-dihydropyridines are more effective in tissue with frequent channel openings (i.e., SA node, AV node, and cardiac myocytes), and channel inhibition increases in proportion to heart rate. The negative chronotropic and inotropic effects on non-dihydropyridine agents appear greater for verapamil than diltiazem. The phenylalkylamine verapamil and the benzothiazepine diltiazem have both cardiac and vascular actions (**Table 1**, **Figure 4**). These drugs have antiarrhythmic, antianginal, and antihypertensive activity.

### 6.1 Nifedipine

It is a dihydropyridine that does not resemble the other calcium antagonists in chemical structure. Although it is not a nitrate, its nitro group is essential for its antianginal effect. Also, it has peripheral vasodilatory effects. It works by inhibiting the voltage-dependent calcium channel in the vascular smooth muscles and has little or no direct suppressant effect on the SA or AV nodes. Nifedipine is thought to be more effective in patients with coronary vasospasm, and it is usually used for vasospastic angina along with angina pectoris.

Additionally, it is used in selected patients to treat hypertension because of its vasodilatory properties. Nifedipine has efficient absorption with buccal or oral administration. Around 90% of nifedipine is protein-bound. The bioavailability of an oral dose reaches 65%. Nifedipine gets metabolized into two inactive metabolites which are found in equilibrium with each other. Only a limited amount of unchanged nifedipine is found in the urine [7].

### 6.2 Amlodipine

Similar to second-generation dihydropyridines, it has a higher selectivity for the vascular smooth muscles than the myocardial tissue. It has a longer half-life (34 hours) but less negative inotropic effect than nifedipine. It is used in the treatment of chronic stable angina and essential hypertension [7]. Amlodipine increases exercise duration, decreases anginal attacks, and reduces the consumption of **nitroglycerin.** It is given once daily (at a dose of 5 or 10 mg). Common side effects of the dihydropyridines are less likely with amlodipine.

### 6.3 Nicardipine

It is a short-acting dihydropyridine with a side effect profile similar to nifedipine; it has also been shown to be useful in angina. It is remarkably effective in vasospastic angina.

### 6.4 Felodipine

It is a second-generation dihydropyridine channel blocker of the nifedipine type. It is more selective for vascular smooth muscles than myocardial tissue. And it serves as an effective vasodilator. It is usually used in the treatment of angina and essential hypertension. Additionally, it exhibits a high degree of protein binding and has a half-life ranging from 10 to 18 hours.

### 6.5 Nimodipine

It is a dihydropyridine calcium channel blocker that differs from other dihydropyridines as it dilates the cerebral blood vessels more than other dihydropyridines do. It is indicated in the treatment of subarachnoid hemorrhage-associated neurological deficits.

### 6.6 Verapamil

It is a phenylalkylamine. It was introduced in 1962 as a coronary vasodilator. It is used for the treatment of angina pectoris, arrhythmias due to ischemic cardiac syndromes, and supraventricular arrhythmias as well. Verapamil's primary effect is on the slow $Ca^{2+}$ channel, which results in a slowing of AV conduction and the sinus rate. It has a rapid absorption following oral administration. However, it is metabolized quickly and, therefore, has low bioavailability. Its main site of first-pass metabolism is the liver, forming several products. Yet, its metabolites have no significant biological effects. Verapamil has an elimination half-life of around 5 hours. Verapamil, like the dihydropyridines, causes little impact on venous return and preload but has more direct negative inotropic and chronotropic effects than the dihydropyridines at doses that produce arteriolar dilation and afterload reduction (**Figure 4**). Thus, the consequences of a reflex increase in adrenergic tone are generally offset by the direct cardio depressant effects of the drug. In patients without heart failure, oral administration of verapamil reduces peripheral vascular resistance and blood pressure with minimal changes in heart rate. Ventricular performance is not impaired and may improve, especially if ischemia limits performance. In contrast, in patients with heart failure, intravenous verapamil can cause a marked decrease in contractility and left ventricular function. The antianginal effect of verapamil, like that of all $Ca^{2+}$ channel blockers, is due primarily to a reduction in myocardial $O_2$ demand [7].

### 6.7 Diltiazem

It was introduced in Japan as a cardiovascular agent for the treatment of angina pectoris. It was detected to dilate peripheral arteries and arterioles. By relieving coronary artery spasm, diltiazem increases myocardial oxygen supply, and by decreasing heart rate, it reduces myocardial oxygen demand. It is used in patients with variant angina as well. Additionally, it has electrophysiological properties similar to those of verapamil and, therefore, is used as an antiarrhythmic agent, but it is less potent than verapamil. It has a rapid oral absorption through the digestive tract, and it reaches peak plasma levels within 1 hour of administration. Nevertheless, the sustained-release preparations provide peak plasma levels within 3–4 hours of oral administration.

Diltiazem is metabolized extensively by the first-pass metabolism after oral administration. Hence, its bioavailability is about 40%. It undergoes several biotransformations, including deacetylation, oxidative O- and N-demethylations, and conjugation of the phenolic metabolites. Although it has various metabolites, only deacetyldiltiazem is pharmacologically active, which has about 40–50% of the potency of the parent drug [7].

### 6.8 Side effects

- Headache, flushing, and dizziness due to arterial dilation, although tolerance often occurs with continued use.
- Ankle edema probably arises from increased transcapillary hydrostatic pressure. It happens mostly with dihydropyridines, and it is frequently resistant to diuretics.
- Decompensated heart failure is due to reduced cardiac contractility, especially in patients with preexisting poor left ventricular function, particularly with verapamil, but amlodipine does not depress cardiac contractility.
- Tachycardia and palpitations can arise with dihydropyridines, especially with rapid-release formulations.
- Bradycardia and heart block can occur with verapamil and diltiazem.
- Constipation is most common with verapamil and less with diltiazem.
- Heartburn associated with Amlodipine and other dihydropyridines use is due to lower esophageal sphincter relaxation.
- Gum hyperplasia.

## 7. Calcium channel blocker indications

### 7.1 Calcium channel blockers for hypertension

CCBs are prevalent antihypertensive drugs. CCBs lower BP by causing peripheral arterial dilation, with the rank order of potency being dihydropyridines > diltiazem > verapamil. They are generally well-tolerated, do not require monitoring with blood tests, and have proven safe and effective in many large RCTs. CCBs also have antianginal and some antiarrhythmic effects and seem to provide more protection against stroke than other antihypertensive agents do.

The Antihypertensive and Lipid-Lowering Treatment to Prevent Heart Attack Trial (ALLHAT) and subsequent RCTs showed that CCBs (represented by amlodipine) prevent coronary events as effectively as diuretics and RAS blockers do.

### 7.2 Calcium channel blockers for coronary vasospasm

Coronary spasm results in transient functional occlusion of a coronary artery that is reversible with nitrate vasodilation. It occurs in the setting of coronary stenosis. Variant angina results from reduced blood flow (a consequence of transient localized vasoconstriction) rather than increased $O_2$ demand. Drug-induced causes (e.g., cocaine, amphetamines, sumatriptan, and related antimigraine drugs) should be excluded. CCBs are effective in about 90% of patients. These agents are considered first-line treatment and may be combined with nitrate. The effects of pharmacologic vasodilators on coronary flow reflect direct actions on vascular smooth muscle as well as secondary adjustments in resistance artery tone. All calcium channel blockers induce vascular smooth muscle relaxation and are to various degrees pharmacologic coronary vasodilators (**Figure 6**). In epicardial arteries, the vasodilator response is like nitroglycerin and is effective in preventing coronary vasospasm superimposed on coronary stenosis as well as in normal arteries of patients with variant angina. They also submaximally vasodilate coronary resistance vessels. In this regard, dihydropyridine derivatives such as nifedipine are particularly potent and can sometimes precipitate subendocardial ischemia in the presence of critical stenosis. This arises from a transmural redistribution of blood flow (coronary steal) as well as the tachycardia and hypotension that transiently occur with short half-life formulations of nifedipine. One study demonstrated that the use of calcium channel blocker therapy was an independent predictor of myocardial infarct-free survival in vasospastic angina patients.

### 7.3 Calcium channel blockers for stable angina

All calcium channel blockers can be used in the treatment of stable angina pectoris. They vasodilate coronary arteries, reduce coronary resistance, increase coronary blood flow, and may enhance the development of coronary collaterals. The vasodilatation and increase in coronary artery blood flow result from the blockade of calcium influx as well as an increase in the levels of nitric oxide and bradykinin; therefore, the increase in coronary artery blood flow is a result of bradykinin/nitric oxide-dependent and bradykinin/nitric oxide-independent mechanisms. They elicit a strong reflex beta-adrenergic response, making any potential negative inotropic or chronotropic effect clinically insignificant. This adrenergic response often includes

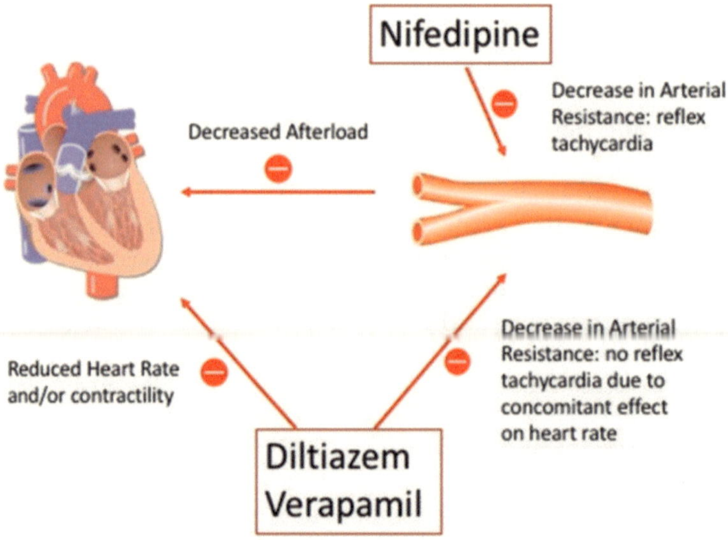


**Figure 6.**
*Sites of effects of calcium channel blockers in angina.*

a reflex tachycardia. Verapamil and diltiazem are useful in angina because they decrease myocardial oxygen demand by acting as a negative inotropic and chronotropic effect, by lowering the systemic blood pressure, and by lowering heart rate by blocking AV node (**Figure 6**). The use of short-acting dihydropyridines, such as nifedipine, can exacerbate ischemia due to reflex tachycardia, and therefore, it can be used as a monotherapy in this setting. Calcium channel blockers are used with combination therapy with beta-blockers, which can be more effective than either therapy alone. Amlodipine or felodipine could be considered before other calcium channel blockers, given their better side effect profiles when used in combination with beta-blockers. In stable angina patients with suspension of a vasoactive component, a trial of a calcium channel blocker can be added to beta blocker agents. Calcium channel blockers, particularly verapamil and diltiazem, should be used with caution in patients with left ventricular systolic dysfunction, such as those with an ejection fraction less than 40 percent or heart failure due to their negative inotropic effect.

### 7.4 Calcium channel blockers for acute coronary syndrome

Calcium channel blockers have been effective in reducing ischemia in patients with NSTE-ACS and persistent ischemia despite treatment with full-dose nitrates and beta-blockers as well as in patients with contraindications to beta-blockers and among those with hypertension. Such patients should receive non-dihydropyridine calcium channel-blocking agents that lower the heart rate [9, 10].

### 7.5 Calcium channel blockers for hypertrophic cardiomyopathy (HCM)

Verapamil improves left ventricular outflow obstruction and symptoms in patients with HCM.

### 7.6 Calcium channel blockers in the treatment of cardiac arrhythmias

Calcium channel blockers (CCBs) are useful antiarrhythmic agents in the management of certain arrhythmias, primarily supraventricular tachyarrhythmias. Verapamil is the drug of choice to terminate idiopathic fascicular ventricular tachycardia.

### 7.7 Calcium channel blockers for migraine

Verapamil can be used in the prevention of migraine headaches but is considered a second-choice drug.

### 7.8 Calcium channel blockers for aneurysmal subarachnoid hemorrhage

It is essential to review the cause behind intracranial arterial spasm, mechanisms, diagnostic tools, and management to understand the role of CCBs in vasospasm among patients with aneurysmal subarachnoid hemorrhage.

Vascular calcification is specific for arteries, which can involve all arteries, including the carotid artery and cerebral arteries. Intracranial arterial calcification (IAC) was first detected in the early 1960s. It is associated with atherosclerosis, especially in older people. Vascular calcification is an integral part of the active process of atherosclerosis, occurring in up to 90% of atherosclerotic lesions. Recent clinical studies have consistently found the intracranial internal carotid artery (IICA) to be the most common site of IAC. The incidence of IICA calcification has been reported to range from 60 to 90% according to ethnicity, age, and stroke or other risk factors. The vertebral artery is the second most common artery affected by calcification, while other arteries have been affected only by less than 5%. An unenhanced CT scan is the most accessible and direct method to evaluate IAC in patients.

The prevalence of intracranial artery calcification is:

- Internal carotid artery: 60%
- Vertebral artery: 20%
- Middle cerebral artery: 5%
- Basilar artery: 5%

Risk factors of intracranial artery calcification:

Advanced age.
Diabetes mellitus.
Hypercholesterolemia.
Hypertension.
History of cardiovascular disease.
Excessive alcohol intake.
End-stage renal disease with long duration of hemodialysis [11–13].

### *7.8.1 Hemodynamic and clinical effects of IAC*

IAC can lead to three significant hemodynamic effects: Firstly, it can lead to increase the arterial stiffness. This phenomenon is associated with aging and accelerated by other vascular risk factors. It can be measured by the pulse wave velocity (PWV) and may indicate early atherosclerotic changes. Several studies have verified the correlation between IAC and arterial stiffness, and this may increase the risk of stroke. Secondly, arterial stenosis can be linked to arterial calcification, which may lead to ischemic stroke due to direct luminal stenosis. Thirdly, IAC may lead to plaque stability. Intravascular ultrasound studies found heavily calcified plaques to be more resistant to plaque progression. Therefore, the findings for CAC suggest that substantial calcification may help stabilize atherosclerotic plaques. Also, a heavy plaque burden hidden in heavily calcified arteries may partially account for the association between severe arterial calcification and ischemic events regardless of plaque vulnerability.

### *7.8.2 Vasospasm and delayed cerebral ischemia*

Cerebral vasospasm is an essential source of morbidity and mortality in subarachnoid hemorrhage patients. Vasospasm is one of the most common acute complications. It can happen within 3–15 days with a peak incidence at 7 days after aneurysmal SAH. Symptomatic vasospasm occurs in 20–40% of subarachnoid hemorrhage cases and is considered as the least understood component in their care. The symptom severity depends upon the artery affected and the degree of collateral circulation. Strokes from vasospasm account for nearly 50% of the early deaths in patients who survive the initial subarachnoid hemorrhage treatment. It is characterized by a pathological; diffuse, affecting all layers of the involved arterial wall; and long-lasting narrowing of the lumen of the vessel of large-capacity cerebral arteries at the base of the brain either close or distal to the bleeding site. And it is associated with reduced perfusion of the territories distal to the affected vessel.

Risk factors for vasospasm include:

1. The severity of bleeding

2. The proximity to the significant intracerebral blood vessels

3. The location and extent of blood on CT scan and radiologic grading scales

4. Age less than 50 years

5. Hyperglycemia

6. Glasgow Coma Scale score < 14

*7.8.3 Mechanism*

While the underlying mechanisms causing vasospasm are not fully understood, a proliferative inflammatory arteriopathy is the pathological feature of cerebral vasospasm. The intima shows disruption of the internal elastic lamina, and the media is thickened and fibrotic, with an increased smooth muscle cell proliferation. The adventitia is infiltrated with inflammatory cells, and the neuronal endings are impaired [14]. A significant predictor of vasospasm after SAH is the volume of blood present around the cerebral arteries of the circle of Willis which can be measured by transcranial Doppler (TCD), although it has been clearly demonstrated that prolonged exposure of cerebral arteries to perivascular blood is essential for the development of vasospasm. It is not possible to identify a single causative molecule as the culprit of vasospasm. However, vasospasm is believed to be produced by spasmogenic substances generated during the lysis of subarachnoid blood such as oxyhemoglobin (a product of auto-oxidation of hemoglobin), nitric oxide, and endothelin-1. Those agents may be contributors to the pathological event of vasospasm.

Oxyhemoglobin may directly or indirectly trigger arterial vasoconstriction.

Oxyhemoglobin can also exert a scavenging effect on nitric oxide. It has been demonstrated that nitric oxide (a potent vasodilator) depleted during vasospasm and can stimulate endothelial cells to produce endothelin-1.

Endothelin-1 is the most potent and long-lasting vasoconstrictor effect, which is also associated with morphological changes, mimicking the delayed cerebral vasospasm. It has been shown that endothelin-1 levels are increased, not only in the cerebrospinal fluid during SAH and severe neuronal injury due to vasospasm or bleeding event. Moreover, endothelin levels change in neurological symptoms, but they do not predict vasospasm as assessed by transcranial Doppler. These observations suggest that endothelin-1 acts as a marker of cerebral ischemic injury [15, 16].

*7.8.4 Diagnosis*

*7.8.4.1 Transcranial Doppler*

It is a noninvasive tool and is useful for the detection and evaluation of vasospasm. It can be performed at the bedside.

It used as a screening tool in high-grade World Federation of Neurological Surgeons (WFNS) scale patients in whom a neurological examination cannot be readily followed to identify those at higher risk [17].

It is a highly specific noninvasive exam but has a low level of sensitivity, and it is operator-patient dependent, and its value is debated.

In 2004, the American Academy of Neurology conducted a systematic review of the literature and concluded that TCDs could be used reliably to screen for the presence of vasospasm in the only MCA. Their criteria for the diagnosis or exclusion of vasospasm include flow velocity > 200 or 120 cm/s, respectively, significant increase in the flow velocities from day to day (>50 cm/s), and a Lindegaard ratio (MCAvelocity/ICAvelocity) > 6 [18].

#### *7.8.4.2 CT scan*

Noninvasive angiography with CT angiography (CTA) to confirm vasospasm for patients with elevated velocities on transcranial Doppler ultrasound. The plane CT scan is useful for ruling out other causes in the event of the occurrence of a deficit or worsening of the clinical state like rebleeding or ischemia. Several prospective cohorts showed a correlation between CTA and DSA in predicting vasospasm and that many unnecessary angiograms could be avoided by using CTA as a screening test [19, 20]. A recent meta-analysis found a sensitivity and specificity for CTA of 80 and 93%, respectively [21].

#### *7.8.4.3 MRI*

MRI can help to identify and diagnose cerebral ischemia at the early stage.

#### *7.8.4.4 Cerebral angiography*

Cerebral angiography is the gold standard radiographic tool for the diagnosis of cerebral vasospasm. Angiography is used to identify patients with symptomatic vasospasm who might benefit from treatment.

In 30–70% of patients with SAH, angiographic vasospasm occurs, but it leads to clinically evident signs and symptoms in 20–30% of patients who experience delayed ischemic neurological deficits. About half of the symptomatic group of patients suffer severe permanent neurological dysfunction or death.

### *7.8.5 Treatment*

The specific treatment of cerebral vasospasm helps improving cerebral blood flow to avoid delayed ischemic neurologic deficit by reducing ICP, optimizing the rate of cerebral oxygen demand, and enhancing cerebral blood flow with one of the following approaches: indirect pharmacological protection of brain tissue or direct mechanical dilation of the vasospastic vessel.

Nimodipine is the standard of care in aneurysmal SAH patients. Nimodipine 60 mg every 4 hours can be used for all patients with aneurysmal SAH once the diagnosis is made for 21 days. Nimodipine is to be given orally or by nasogastric tube because intravenous administration causes serious adverse events, including death. The mechanism of benefit of nimodipine in SAH is unknown. Oral nimodipine is the only Class I evidence regarding cerebral vasospasm used in the publication of the AHA subarachnoid hemorrhage guidelines [22]. Early aneurysm treatment, HHH-therapy (hypertension, hypervolemia, and hemodilution), cerebral angioplasty, and selective intra-arterial vasodilator therapy were recommended based on Class II evidence.

In summary, nimodipine was initially studied in SAH to prevent vasospasm. However, despite its vasodilatory effects on cerebral vessels, the evidence of nimodipine effects on the incidence of either angiographic or symptomatic vasospasm is not convincing [23]. Nevertheless, nimodipine has been demonstrated to improve outcomes in SAH and is the agent of choice in these patients [23].

### 7.9 Calcium channel blockers for reversible cerebral vasoconstriction syndrome

Reversible cerebral vasoconstriction syndrome (RCVS) represents a group of conditions that show a reversible narrowing of the cerebral arteries with clinical manifestations that typically include thunderclap headache and less commonly neurologic deficits related to brain edema, seizure, or stroke. The clinical outcome is usually benign, although major strokes can result in severe disability and death in a minority. The pathophysiology of the abrupt-onset headache and the prolonged but reversible vasoconstriction is not known. Reversible angiographic narrowing suggests an abnormality in the control of cerebrovascular tone [24].

RCVS has been associated with a variety of conditions including pregnancy, migraine, use of vasoconstrictive drugs, neurosurgical procedures, hypercalcemia, unruptured saccular aneurysms, cervical artery dissection, and cerebral venous thrombosis. The diagnosis of RCVS is based upon the characteristic clinical, brain imaging, and angiographic features. Nimodipine and verapamil and brief courses of magnesium sulfate, serotonin antagonists, and dantrolene have been administered to relieve the vasoconstriction. Data from two prospective case series suggest that nimodipine does not affect the time course of cerebral vasoconstriction [25, 26]. However, nimodipine might relieve the number and intensity of headaches and has documented effects on the smaller vasculature not easily imaged by angiography. Calcium channel blockers can be discontinued after resolution of symptoms or angiographic abnormalities if they are used.

## Author details

Yaser Alahamd[1*], Hisham Ab Ib Swehli[2], Alaa Rahhal[3], Sundus Sardar[2], Mawahib Ali Mohammed Elhassan[1], Salma Alsamel[4] and Osama Ali Ibrahim[1]

1 Cardiology Department, Heart Hospital, Hamad Medical Corporation, Doha, Qatar

2 Internal Medicine Department, Hamad General Hospital, Hamad Medical Corporation, Doha, Qatar

3 Pharmacy Department, Heart Hospital, Hamad Medical Corporation, Doha, Qatar

4 Military Medical Specialty Center, Doha, Qatar

*Address all correspondence to: yalahmad@hamad.qa

## References

[1] Whelton PK, Carey RM, Aronow WS, et al. ACC/AHA/AAPA/ABC/ACPM/AGS/APhA/ASH/ASPC/NMA/PCNA guideline for the prevention, detection, evaluation, and management of high blood pressure in adults: A report of the American College of Cardiology/American Heart Association task force on clinical practice guidelines. Hypertension. 2017:**71**:e13

[2] James PA, Oparil S, Carter BL, et al. Evidence-based guideline for the management of high blood pressure in adults: Report from the panel members appointed to the eighth Joint National Committee (JNC 8). JAMA. 2014;**311**:507

[3] Mancia G, Fagard R, Narkiewicz K, et al. ESH/ESC guidelines for the management of arterial hypertension: The task force for the management of arterial hypertension of the European Society of Hypertension (ESH) and of the European Society of Cardiology (ESC). Journal of Hypertens. 2013;**31**:1281

[4] Hart P, Bakris GL. Calcium antagonists: Do they equally protect against kidney injury? Kidney International. 2008;**73**:795

[5] Brunton LL, Hilal-Dandan R, Knollmann BC. Goodman & Gilman's: The Pharmacological Basis of Therapeutics, 13e. New York: McGraw-Hill Education; 2018

[6] Waller D, Sampson A. Medical Pharmacology and Therapeutics. 5th ed. Amsterdam: Elsevier Limited; 2018

[7] Beale JM, Block JH. Wilson and Gisvold's Textbook of Organic Medicinal and Pharmaceutical Chemistry. 12th ed. Philadelphia: Lippincott Williams & Wilkins, a Wolters Kluwer Business; 2011

[8] Golan DE, Tashjian AH, Armstrong EJ, April W. Armstrong Principles of Pharmacology: The Pathophysiologic Basis of Drug Therapy. 4th ed. South Holland: Wolters Kluwer; 2017

[9] Hamm CW, Bassand JP, Agewall S, et al. ESC guidelines for the management of acute coronary syndromes in patients presenting without persistent ST-segment elevation: The task force for the Management of Acute Coronary Syndromes (ACS) in patients presenting without persistent ST-segment elevation of the European Society of Cardiology (ESC). European Heart Journal. 2011;**32**:2999

[10] Anderson JL, Adams CD, Antman EM, et al. 2011 ACCF/AHA focused update incorporated into the ACC/AHA 2007 guidelines for the management of patients with unstable angina/non–ST-elevation myocardial infarction: A report of the American College of Cardiology Foundation/American Heart Association task force on practice guidelines. Circulation. 2011;**123**:e426

[11] de Weert TT, Cakir H, Rozie S, Cretier S, Meijering E, Dippel DW, et al. Intracranial internal carotid artery calcifications: Association with vascular risk factors and ischemic cerebrovascular disease. AJNR. American Journal of Neuroradiology. 2009;**30**:177-184

[12] Power A, Chan K, Haydar A, Hamady M, Cairns T, Taube D, et al. Intracranial arterial calcification is highly prevalent in hemodialysis patients but does not associate with acute ischemic stroke. Hemodialysis International. 2011;**15**:256-263

[13] Bos D, van der Rijk MJ, Geeraedts TE, Hofman A, Krestin GP,

Witteman JC, et al. Intracranial carotid artery atherosclerosis: Prevalence and risk factors in the general population. Stroke. 2012;**43**:1878-1884

[14] Pluta RM. Delayed cerebral vasospasm and nitric oxide: Review, new hypothesis, and proposed treatment. Pharmacology & Therapeutics. 2005;**105**:23-56

[15] Pluta RM. Dysfunction of nitric oxide synthases as a cause and therapeutic target in delayed cerebral vasospasm after SAH. Acta Neurochirurgica. Supplement. 2008;**104**:139-147

[16] Mascia L, Fedorko L, Stewart DJ, Mohamed F, terBrugge K, Ranieri VM, et al. Temporal relationship between endothelin-1 concentrations and cerebral vasospasm in patients with aneurysmal subarachnoid hemorrhage. Stroke. 2001;**32**:1185-1190

[17] Mascia L, Fedorko L, terBrugge K, Filippini C, Pizzio M, Ranieri VM, et al. The accuracy of transcranial Doppler to detect vasospasm in patients with aneurysmal subarachnoid hemorrhage. Intensive Care Medicine. 2003;**29**:1088-1094

[18] Sloan MA, Alexandrov AV, Tegeler CH, Spencer MP, Caplan LR, Feldmann E, et al. Assessment: Transcranial Doppler ultrasonography: Report of the thera peutics and technology assessment subcommittee of the American Academy of Neurology. Neurology. 2004;**62**(9):1468-1481. DOI: 10.1212/WNL.62.9.1468

[19] Anderson GB, Ashforth R, Steinke DE. Findlay JM.CT angiography for the detection of cerebral vasospasm in patients with acute subarachnoid hemor rhage. American Journal of Neuroradiology. 2000;**21**(6):1011-1015

[20] Yoon DY, Choi CS, Kim KH, Cho B-M. Multidetector-row CT angiography of cerebral vasospasm after aneurysmal subarachnoid hemorrhage: Comparison of volume-rendered images and digital subtraction angiography. American Journal of Neuroradiology. 2006;**27**(2):370-377

[21] Greenberg ED, Gold R, Reichman M, John M, Ivanidze J, Edwards AM, et al. Diagnostic accuracy of CT angiography and CT perfusion for cerebral vasospasm: Ametaanalysis. American Journal of Neuroradiology. 2010;**31**(10):1853-1860. DOI: 10.3174/ajnr.A2246

[22] Bederson JB, Connolly ES, Batjer HH, Dacey RG, Dion JE, Diringer MN, et al. Guidelines for the management of aneurysmal subarachnoid hemorrhage: A statement for health care professionals from a special writing group of the stroke council, American heart association. Stroke. 2009;**40**(3):994-1025. DOI: 10.1161/STROKEAHA.108.191395

[23] Dorhout Mees SM, Rinkel GJE, Feigin VL, Algra A, van den Bergh WM, Vermeulen M, et al. Calcium antagonists for aneurysmal subarachnoid hemorrhage. Stroke AHA. 2008;**39**:514-515. DOI: 10.1161/STROKEAHA.107.496802

[24] Ducros A, Boukobza M, Porcher R, et al. The clinical and radiological spectrum of reversible cerebral vasoconstriction syndrome. A prospective series of 67 patients. Brain. 2007;**130**:3091

[25] Chen SP, Fuh JL, Chang FC, et al. Transcranial color doppler study for reversible cerebral vasoconstriction syndromes. Annals of Neurology. 2008;**63**:751

[26] Topcuoglu MA, Chan ST, Silva GS, et al. Cerebral vasomotor reactivity in reversible cerebral vasoconstriction syndrome. Cephalalgia. 2017;**37**:541

Section 6

# Repair

Chapter 14

# Aneurysmal Subarachnoid Hemorrhage and Resolution of Inflammation

*Geisi Saito and Rodrigo Zapata*

## Abstract

Aneurysmal subarachnoid hemorrhage (SAH) is a severe life-threatening disease and an important source of neurological disability. Therapeutic interventions over the last few decades have repeatedly failed to improve functional outcome after SAH; however, resolution of inflammation has largely been ignored as a potential therapeutic target. The omega-3 fatty acids (FAs), eicosapentaenoic acid (EPA), and docosahexaenoic acid (DHA) are the precursors of key mediators involved in resolution of inflammation and endogenous neuroprotection. EPA also plays a major role in microvascular function, and DHA accretion in the brain is crucial for normal neuronal function. Although considerable loss of brain DHA has been identified in SAH patients, the pathological significance of this process has also been overlooked. Current Western diets provide insufficient amounts of omega-3 FAs to compensate for the loss of brain DHA following SAH. Here, we review the rationale for future clinical trials of omega-3 FAs in SAH. Furthermore, the potential role of defective resolution of inflammation in the growth and rupture of intracranial aneurysms is inferred from recent findings in atherosclerosis and nutrition. The novel concepts of resolution of inflammation and endogenous neuroprotective signaling may open new avenues for public health interventions and innovative research in intracranial aneurysms and SAH.

**Keywords:** fish oil, inflammation, intracranial aneurysms, omega-3 fatty acids, pharmaconutrition, subarachnoid hemorrhage, translational approach

## 1. Introduction

Aneurysmal subarachnoid hemorrhage (SAH) is a complex condition with an intricate and poorly understood pathophysiology. Increasing evidence strongly suggests that neuroinflammation plays a critical role after SAH, but conventional anti-inflammatory treatments have failed to improve clinical outcome [1]. Clinical research on SAH has mainly focused on delayed cerebral ischemia (DCI); however, DCI does not encompass the entire spectrum of pathological and clinical manifestations of SAH [2–4]. Although cerebral infarction is associated with poor clinical outcome and death after SAH, a significant proportion of SAH patients without cerebral infarction suffer from cognitive deficits and mood disorders and a reduced ability for activities of daily living and working, even in the long term [5, 6]. The absence of a close correlation between DCI and functional recovery indicates an ongoing pathophysiological process has been overlooked in SAH. The failure of the recent major NEWTON 2 clinical trial, of sustained intraventricular release of nimodipine, is the latest in a series of unsuccessful phase 3 randomized controlled trials (RCTs) to improve clinical outcome after SAH and further reinforces the need to identify novel therapeutic strategies [7, 8].

Nutrition is essential to human health, and appropriate nutritional support is currently considered a standard of care for critically ill patients. Malnutrition—including depletion of essential micronutrients—frequently occurs among critically ill patients and is associated with an increased risk of morbimortality [9]. However, the clinical relevance of key nutrient deficiencies in acute neurological illnesses has not been thoroughly investigated. EPA and DHA are essential constituents of endothelial and neuronal membranes, respectively, and also the precursors of key mediators involved in resolution of inflammation and endogenous neuroprotection [10, 11]. Although massive loss of brain DHA in SAH patients was first reported over 15 years ago, the pathological significance of this process and the role of inflammation resolution following SAH have largely been ignored [11, 12]. Therapeutic interventions aimed at stimulating inflammation resolution and recovering the homeostasis of the brain and other vital organs after SAH could improve patients' functional outcome [13].

This chapter provides an overview of the potentially harmful consequences of selective deficiency of omega-3 FAs on brain structure and function in SAH patients. Moreover, given the possible clinical relevance to SAH and the growth and rupture of intracranial aneurysms (IAs), we provide a detailed discussion of recent findings on the role of omega-3 FAs in resolution of inflammation, with a focus on brain homeostasis.

## 2. Role of omega-3 FAs in resolution of acute inflammation

Remarkable progress in our understanding of the pathophysiology of acute inflammation has been achieved through basic science over the last 20 years. Resolution of acute inflammation is now considered to be an active biochemical process that is required to enable tissues to restore normal structure and function following an injury [14]. Interference with the resolution phase of acute inflammation may result in necrosis, chronic inflammation, fibrosis, and organ dysfunction. The resolution process is triggered at the beginning of inflammation by a temporal switch in lipid mediator classes, which is induced by cross talk between cells of the innate immune system and other cells in the inflammatory microenvironment [11].

A diverse range of biologically active pro-resolving and anti-inflammatory mediators are synthetized by complex pathways that involve several enzymes, including cyclooxygenase 2 (COX-2), cytochrome P450s and several lipoxygenases (LOX). The majority of these endogenous mediators are derived from the long-chain omega-3 fatty acids (FAs) EPA and DHA and are members of the specialized pro-resolving mediator (SPM) superfamily [15]. SPMs represent an essential biochemical interface between inflammation and tissue repair and regeneration. The resolution of inflammation is a highly orchestrated adaptive process that depends on both the availability of SPMs precursors and the efficiency of the related biosynthetic pathways.

### 2.1 Specialized pro-resolving mediators

Each endogenous lipid mediator is structurally distinct and possesses specific biological functions which have been extensively studied in diverse experimental models. EPA is the precursor of the E-series resolvins (RvEs), which contains four main mediators (RvE1-RvE3 and 18-HEPE). DHA is the precursor of the D-series resolvins (RvDs), which contains six mediators (RvD1-RvD6), as well as the protectins (PD1-PDX) and the maresins (MaR1-MaR2); DHA derivatives are also known as docosanoids [15].

SPMs are active at pico-nanogram ranges and exert pleiotropic actions at the inflammatory microenvironment. SPMs stimulate the clearance of bacteria, dead cells, and debris that is required during tissue repair. SPMs also reduce leukocyte transendothelial migration, platelet activation, and production of inflammatory cytokines, thus providing multi-organ protection. The maresins (macrophage mediators in resolving inflammation) exert potent phagocyte-directed actions that include phenotypic conversion of proinflammatory macrophages into macrophages that suppress inflammation and promote tissue regeneration [16]. Collectively, SPMs actively promote resolution of inflammation and recovery of tissue homeostasis [15]. Interestingly, resolution of systemic inflammation appears to have its counterpart in the CNS represented by different DHA-derived endogenous mediators (see Section 5.1).

The biosynthetic pathways that generate SPMs are clinically relevant and have been comprehensively studied [15, 16]. Drugs that inactivate the enzymes involved in SPM biosynthesis, such as selective COX-2 inhibitors and certain LOX inhibitors, delay the return to homeostasis and are considered resolution antagonists. Importantly, selective COX-2 inhibitors were synthesized before the identification of inflammation resolution pathways and are currently widely used as anti-inflammatory agents. Aspirin and statins also modify COX-2 by acetylation and S-nitrosylation, respectively, which results in generation of longer-acting SPM R-epimers. Thus, aspirin and statins are resolution agonists [15, 16].

## 3. Incorporation and transport of omega-3 FAs

Incorporation and transport of omega-3 FAs have been comprehensively described; here, we focus on the clinically relevant aspects [10, 17, 18]. Several studies have consistently shown that in vivo conversion of alpha linolenic acid (ALA), the short-chain omega-3 FAs from vegetable origin, to its bioactive long-chain derivatives (EPA and DHA) is very low in humans. In addition, the metabolism of omega-6 and omega-3 FAs is tightly linked, and thus a high dietary intake of omega-6 FAs further reduce the conversion of ALA to EPA and DHA and their biological effects. The body has also a limited capacity to store long-chain omega-3 FAs; only very small amounts of EPA and DHA are present in adipose tissue, and the brain retains DHA for its own function. Thus, providing preformed EPA and DHA is the most efficient method of increasing the concentrations of EPA and DHA in plasma and tissues.

EPA and DHA are incorporated into different blood lipid fractions after absorption by the gastrointestinal tract or after release from intravenously infused fish oil-based lipid emulsions (FOLE). These lipid fractions reflect the diverse means by which FAs are transported in the circulation and execute their physiological functions. The fractions incorporated in the phospholipid coat of plasma lipoproteins and plasma nonesterified FAs (NEFAs) are considered transport pools. Notably, the NEFA pool seems to be the main DHA plasma fraction that supplies the brain. The NEFA pool also represents a direct source of FAs to cells for generation of SPMs, as this pool readily transfers to inflammatory tissue via edema formation [19]. The FAs fraction incorporated in peripheral blood mononuclear cells (PBMCs) represents a functional pool due to the crucial roles of PBMCs in inflammation.

### 3.1 Omega-3 index

The EPA and DHA content of red blood cells (RBCs) membrane which can be quantified by a specific and standardized analytical procedure—the HS-Omega-3 Index® methodology—reliably reflects the omega-3 FAs content of several tissues [20]. This omega-3 index has been increasingly utilized as a surrogate marker of omega-3 status. Long-term intake of EPA and DHA is the main predictor of the omega-3 index, but other factors influence its variability. Acute supplementation of omega-3 FAs does not modify the omega-3 index, as expected given the long lifetime of RBCs (100–120 days). In terms of clinical relevance, strong inverse correlations have been observed between the omega-3 index and cardiovascular morbimortality, particularly sudden cardiac death, as well as depression [21–23].

## 4. Role of EPA in microvascular thromboinflammation

Microvascular inflammation is an early event in the pathogenesis of atherosclerosis and other inflammatory conditions and is inextricably linked to microthrombosis [24]. Eicosanoid metabolism and leukocyte-endothelial interactions are interrelated processes and in turn are major drivers of thromboinflammation [25, 26]. Inflammation stimulates eicosanoid synthesis and expression of cell-surface adhesion molecules through upregulation of the nuclear factor kappa B (NF-kB), a master transcription factor necessarily involved in the inflammatory response.

Most eicosanoids derived from the long-chain omega-6 FAs arachidonic acid (ARA), including prostaglandins, leukotrienes, and thromboxanes, are potent vasoconstrictors, platelet activators, and leukocyte chemotactic factors. Moreover, the expression of cell-surface adhesion molecules on endothelial and inflammatory cells is essential for leukocyte-endothelial interactions; rolling and adhesion on vascular surfaces are the first step in the recruitment of circulating leukocytes or platelets to sites of thromboinflammation [27].

EPA incorporated in the membrane phospholipids of inflammatory cells can modulate eicosanoid metabolism by replacing ARA as an eicosanoid precursor [25]. EPA-derived eicosanoids are significantly less potent than those derived from ARA, and nonesterified EPA can also directly inhibit the production of eicosanoids from ARA. In addition, EPA has been shown to decrease the expression of several cell-surface adhesion molecules on inflammatory cells. EPA appears to elicit these pleiotropic effects by modulating the activity of the NF-kB.

Additionally, recent mechanistic studies have shown that minor changes in the EPA content of endothelial membranes may markedly alter the biophysical properties of the membrane [28]. Furthermore, changes in membrane fluidity, thickness, and deformability induced by modifications to lipid dynamics and/or structural organization can profoundly impact endothelial function [29]. Given the intimate association between brain capillary pericytes and endothelial cells, it would not be surprising if EPA also incorporates into pericyte cell membranes and potentiates the function of these cells as regulators of brain homeostasis [30, 31].

## 5. Unique function of DHA in the brain

DHA is widely distributed throughout the human body in membrane phospholipids and is particularly abundant in neural tissues such as the brain and retina [10]. DHA represents 30–40% of the fatty acid content of the gray matter in the cortex and is absorbed into the brain by a specific transporter that is found in the endothelium of the blood-brain barrier (BBB) microvasculature [32, 33]. The functional significance of selective enrichment of DHA in neural tissues has been actively researched over the last few decades. DHA possesses unique biophysical and biochemical characteristics that make it particularly suitable for brain and retinal membranes. DHA has been highly conserved during evolution and is present throughout the entire spectrum of living organisms [34]. DHA has even been suggested to be a major determinant for evolution of the modern hominid brain due to its unique encephalization potential [35].

DHA is an essential component of neuronal membrane architecture and composition and promotes selective accumulation of phosphatidylserine (PS), a crucial phospholipid involved in intracellular signaling [36]. PS participates in the signaling events of several key enzymes, including protein kinase C, Raf-1 kinase, and Akt, which play essential roles in cell proliferation, differentiation, and survival. Thus, DHA significantly modulates the activity of essential cellular kinases in neuronal cells.

### 5.1 DHA and endogenous neuroprotective signaling

In addition to its function as a unique building block of cell membranes, DHA is also a precursor for docosanoids and other bioactive endogenous derivatives in the neural tissue [37]. The number of recently identified DHA derivatives in neural tissue is increasingly growing and includes neuroprotectin D1 (NPD1), synaptamide, endocannabinoid epoxides, and elovanoids [38–40]. Collectively, the potent bioactive properties of these DHA derivatives contribute to preservation of normal neuronal function, tissue homeostasis, and neuronal survival [37–41]. In addition, the DHA derivatives exert a range of potent neuroprotective properties that include inhibition of proinflammatory gene expression and leukocyte infiltration. A striking hallmark of the DHA derivatives is their ability to potentiate microglial polarization from a proinflammatory phenotype to a surveillance-repair state and reduce NF-kB-mediated expression of inflammatory cytokines in the brain. Moreover, DHA derivatives contribute to BBB integrity and are neurogenic and synaptogenic [38, 42]. Thus, the DHA derivatives seem to be key mediators of the resolution of inflammation and recovery of homeostasis in the CNS microenvironment.

### 5.2 DHA and neurovascular unit

The concept of neurovascular unit emphasizes the intimate relationship between the brain and its vessels, particularly the coupling between neural activity and cerebral blood flow [43]. Although the role of DHA neurolipidomics in neurovascular coupling appears to be underestimated, substantial experimental evidence suggests that the morphologic and functional integrity of the neurovascular unit largely depends on high DHA enrichment [37, 40, 43]. Moreover, the potential role of EPA in microvascular function further supports the evolutionary importance of these essential nutrients to maintain efficient functional couplings between neural and vascular networks [28, 29]. A functional neurovascular unit may be crucial not only for neurovascular coupling but also for BBB integrity and neurogenesis.

A regular dietary supply of DHA is required to preserve normal brain and retinal function. Under physiologic conditions, the net DHA incorporation rate for the entire human brain is very low and equivalent to the net rate of DHA consumption by the brain ($3.8 \pm 1.7$ mg/day) [44]. However, loss of DHA in pathological states or due to nutritional deficiency of omega-3 FAs may severely impair neurovascular integrity and have far-reaching implications on normal brain function [36].

## 6. Loss of brain DHA after SAH

To date, three clinical studies have examined the loss of DHA from the brain after SAH. Pilitsis et al. conducted the first observational study to analyze free fatty acid (FFA) concentrations in cerebrospinal fluid (CSF) [12]. The concentrations of ARA, DHA, linoleic acid, myristic acid, oleic acid, and palmitic acid were measured over the first 14 days following SAH in 20 patients. A cohort of 73 patients with no evidence of acute neurological disease served as the control group. Compared to control patients, the concentrations of all FFAs tested were significantly elevated in CSF during the first 2 days after SAH, with a significant secondary increase in FAA concentrations at 8–10 days. The concentrations of DHA exhibited a biphasic increase and remained significantly elevated (200–600%) throughout the first 14 days after SAH.

Increased levels of free DHA in CSF after SAH are likely to be the result of the cleavage of DHA from membrane phospholipids by either direct structural damage or an increase in phospholipase A2 activity in response to neuroinflammation. DHA can also be readily oxidized due to its high degree of unsaturation and excessive generation of free radicals following SAH [45]. Such nonenzymatic oxidation of DHA generates F4-neuroprostanes (F4-NPs), which represent a lipid marker of oxidative stress in the CNS. Two clinical studies confirmed that the concentrations of F4-NPs in CSF significantly increased within the first 24 hours following SAH compared to control patients [46, 47]. Hsieh et al. also showed the concentrations of F4-NPs in CSF remained significantly elevated throughout the first 10 days after SAH and suggested a positive correlation exists between F4-NP concentrations and clinical outcome at 3 months after SAH. Despite the limited number of patients analyzed, these studies provided valuable evidence that substantial loss of brain DHA occurs after SAH.

Moreover, it is highly likely that SAH may increase metabolic consumption of DHA though increased generation of neuroprotective derivatives. This potential additional source of DHA loss has not yet been evaluated but could be significant. Net cumulative DHA loss from the brain (DHA loss + DHA consumption) following SAH may be massive in some cases and is likely to impose a severe burden on the brain.

### 6.1 Selective brain malnutrition

A current Western diet may provide sufficient amounts of FAs to compensate for the loss of other FAs, but not DHA. Current Western diets are characterized by very low intakes of long-chain omega-3 FAs and high intakes of other FAs, especially omega-6 FAs such as ARA and linoleic acid [48]. Thus, a significant imbalance between brain DHA loss and inadequate nutritional intake of omega-3 FAs may persist over the long term in SAH patients, hindering the recovery of DHA accretion in the brain required for normal neuronal function [35, 36].

Loss of EPA after SAH has not yet been examined; however, it is reasonable to assume that depletion of EPA from cerebral endothelial membranes may play a significant role in microvascular dysfunction after SAH. Indeed, EPA seems to have a more potent effect than DHA in the treatment of mood disorders, though the underlying mechanisms remain elusive [22].

We coined the term "selective brain malnutrition" to describe the pathological consequences of EPA and DHA loss following SAH on the structure and function of the brain. This novel hypothesis of selective brain malnutrition offers a plausible explanation for some of the intriguing clinical features of SAH, including diffuse cerebral atrophy and the frequently observed long-lasting functional sequelae, such as cognitive dysfunction and mood disorders, that occur even in the absence of focal injury [5, 49]. Importantly, a higher omega-3 index has been associated with larger total brain and hippocampal volumes in observational studies in humans [50].

## 7. Roles of EPA and DHA in resolution of inflammation after SAH

Consensus has emerged on the pressing need to find a multipronged therapeutic intervention to address the various deleterious effects of early brain injury (EBI) after SAH [51]. Nonetheless, the loss of brain DHA after SAH is likely to be an unrecognized effect of EBI, and in turn loss of DHA may represent a critical event in the pathogenesis of secondary brain injury after SAH. Depending on the severity of SAH, the cumulative burden of brain DHA loss may be massive and decreases endogenous neuroprotective capacity in the short term [12, 36]. Thus, unresolved homeostatic disturbances within the cerebral microenvironment may lead to neurovascular uncoupling, which may spread over the cerebral cortex in the most severe cases [52]. The loss of an entire series of signaling events required for maintenance of neurovascular network integrity may further increase the risk of focal injury, diffuse cerebral atrophy, and functional sequelae [37]. In this context, it is reasonable to assume that large-artery vasospasm may paradoxically be a compensatory mechanism to preserve tissue oxygen availability in the presence of progressive microvascular failure, i.e., when capillary transit time heterogeneity substantially increases [3, 31]. Unresolved inflammation may also induce hyperproliferation of arachnoid cap cells, which increases the risk of hydrocephalus [4]. Uncontrolled systemic complications, such as severe cardiopulmonary dysfunction, may further aggravate homeostatic disturbances and have devastating consequences on brain function [53].

Theoretically, EPA, DHA, and their respective SPMs possess the bioactive capacity to counteract the major homeostatic disturbances that occur after SAH. EPA-RvEs could reduce thromboinflammation at the cerebral microvasculature by inhibiting vasoconstriction, leukocyte transendothelial migration, and platelet aggregation [15, 26]. DHA and its derivatives may trigger the critical signals required to maintain functional neurovascular coupling and cell survival [16, 36, 37]. DHA-induced upregulation of the enzyme heme oxygenase 1 (HO-1) may accelerate the clearance of subarachnoid clots and thus decrease heme-induced cerebral inflammation [54]. SMPs may attenuate inflammation-induced hyperproliferation of arachnoid cap cells, further contributing to diminish the risk of hydrocephalus. SPMs may also provide multi-organ protection and enhance the immune response against infections.

Furthermore, the promising role of DHA derivatives in reducing microglial polarization toward an inflammatory phenotype may offer a novel approach to reduce the brain inflammation induced by neurosurgical trauma in surgically treated SAH patients [55]. Neurogenesis has also been identified in SAH patients, and thus DHA could represent a novel therapeutic strategy to improve neurological recovery by stimulating neurogenesis [56]. Moreover, subtle changes on microvascular function and synaptogenesis induced by EPA and DHA may improve cognitive function and mood and thus increase the likelihood of complete functional recovery of SAH patients.

### 7.1 Clinical rationale for omega-3 FAs therapy in SAH

The theoretical framework described above provides scientific rationale for future clinical trials of omega-3 FAs in SAH patients. The disappointing results of RCTs of isolated pharmaceutical interventions in SAH could be overcome if a translational approach is correctly implemented [8]. In support of this notion, the recently published phase 3 REDUCE-IT trial provided a robust demonstration of the clinical efficacy and therapeutic potential of EPA to reduce cardiovascular events in chronic cardiovascular (CV) patients with hypertriglyceridemia [57]. Obviously, there are major differences between patients with chronic CV disease and hypertriglyceridemia and patients with SAH. Nevertheless, the considerable clinical benefits of EPA observed in patients with CV disease (who were already on statin therapy) may be due not only to the triglyceride-lowering effect of EPA. Interestingly, the results of the REDUCE-IT trial resemble those of the GISSI-Prevenzione trial conducted 20 years ago, in which a low-dose oral treatment of EPA plus DHA significantly reduced CV morbimortality in patients who had suffered a recent myocardial infarction and were already on aspirin treatment [58].

Minor changes in overall membrane FAs composition and the increase in local production of longer-acting SPM R-epimers after combined treatment with omega-3 FAs and aspirin or statins are likely to mediate a wide variety of biological effects and have a profound impact on cellular and multi-organ function [15]. Indeed, emerging evidence clearly indicates a strong association between a higher omega-3 index and major health benefits (reduced risk of both CV and all-cause mortality) over the long term [21]. However, the acute and critical nature of SAH imposes a particularly demanding therapeutic challenge as the homeostatic disturbances in the brain and other vital organs must be effectively addressed in the short term. An intervention based exclusively on oral supplementation with omega-3 FAs is unlikely to be fully effective on its own in the clinical context of SAH. However, the superiority of parenteral administration over oral or enteral administration of omega-3 FAs has been reliably demonstrated in short-term interventions [17, 59]. Parenteral administration of omega-3 FAs allows rapid delivery of higher doses of EPA and DHA without bioavailability issues and does not depend on the patient's clinical condition. Indeed, the incorporation profiles of EPA and DHA in the transport and functional pools after a single parenteral dose are equivalent to up to several weeks of oral supplementation. EPA and DHA appear in PBMCs as rapidly as 6 hours after a single parenteral dose, thus highlighting the ability of parenterally administered omega-3 FAs to easily reach the innate immune system [59]. The concentration of omega-3 FAs in the main plasmatic fraction that supplies the brain and other vital organs (the NEFA pool) also increases rapidly after a single parenteral dose [17, 60]. Thus, the SPM precursors EPA and DHA seem to be rapidly and widely available to activate resolution of inflammation on demand in different organs after parenteral administration. Therefore, parenteral administration may be the most efficient way to deliver omega-3 FAs during the acute stage of SAH. This novel therapy is in accordance with the concept of pharmaconutrition, in which key nutrients are utilized as pharmacological agents and delivered in appropriate doses via the most efficient administration route [61]. Oral or enteral administration may be suitable for medium- or long-term treatment when the patient's gastrointestinal function has completely recovered.

## 8. Omega-3 FAs dosage for clinical use

A regular supplementation dose for healthy subjects defined by several health associations worldwide is around 500–750 mg/day of EPA plus DHA and can be achieved by consuming a regular diet that contains two portions of fatty fish per week [62]. Therapeutic anti-inflammatory doses of EPA plus DHA are usually considered to be above 2 g/day [25]. A daily dose of at least 1 g EPA plus DHA/day (EPA > 60% DHA) has been shown to be effective in patients with depressive disorders [22]. EPA doses above 1.8 g/day seem to be required to produce clinically meaningful effects on endothelial and vascular function [63]. In patients with age-related cognitive decline, 900 mg DHA/day improved learning and memory function [64]. Importantly, omega-3 FAs doses can be significantly reduced by decreasing the dietary intake of omega-6 FAs. This fact likely explains the notably different dosages of EPA required to obtain beneficial outcomes in patients with chronic CV disease in a Japanese trial (1.8 g/day) and the REDUCE-IT trial (4 g/day) conducted in 11 Western countries [48, 57, 63].

The therapeutic dose of parenteral fish oil (FO) to complement total parenteral nutrition (TPN) is of 0.1–0.2 g of FO/kg/day [59]. This dosage is equivalent to 1–2 ml/kg/day of a specific FOLE that contains 10 g of FO/100 ml.

### 8.1 Bioavailability of omega-3 FAs oral formulations

Bioavailability refers to both the speed of absorption and the quantity of the substance absorbed in the gastrointestinal tract. The bioavailability of omega-3 FAs oral formulations should be carefully considered as it may have direct clinical implications [65]. The bioavailability of EPA and DHA depends on the chemical form in which they are bound (phospholipids > triglycerides > free fatty acids > ethyl esters) as well as their Galenic form (i.e., microencapsulation, emulsification) and also matrix effects (capsule ingestion with concomitant content of food, fat content in food). Galenic form and matrix effects are the most important factors that influence the bioavailability of EPA and DHA. Thus, administration of high-quality pharmaceutical formulations with fatty meals is necessary to ensure the effectiveness of oral therapy.

## 9. Experimental models and clinical interventional studies of omega-3 FAs in SAH

### 9.1 Experimental models

To date, only two preclinical studies of omega-3 FAs in experimental models of SAH have been published. Yin et al. suggested that pre-treatment with omega-3 FAs by oral gavage elicited anti-inflammatory and anti-apoptotic effects in a rat model of SAH [66]. Zhang et al. showed intravenous administration of DHA may prevent oxidative stress-induced apoptosis by improving mitochondrial dynamics in a rat model of SAH induced by endovascular perforation [67]. However, the scarcity of preclinical studies on omega-3 FAs in SAH contrasts with the large number of experimental studies on ischemic stroke. The effects of omega-3 FAs (or specific derivatives) in neural tissue have been widely examined in experimental ischemia-reperfusion models [55, 68, 69]. These studies have consistently shown that omega-3 FAs significantly reduce cerebral infarction volume by around 40–50% and are associated with a drastic decrease in the neuroinflammatory response [70, 71]. Interestingly, the long-term neurobehavioral recovery in experimental models of ischemic stroke is associated with neuroprotective effects of DHA on both gray and white matter [55]. It is noteworthy that one of these studies used a specific FOLE that is widely approved for clinical use [70].

### 9.2 Clinical studies

A limited number of omega-3 FAs interventional studies have been performed in SAH patients [13, 72–74]. The main characteristics and findings of these studies are summarized in **Table 1**. Two studies utilized EPA and DHA, and only one study included a parenteral regimen. In total, 229 patients with SAH have received an omega-3 FAs intervention; most patients were surgically treated (*n* = 223). Although two studies were published as RCTs, one study had significant methodological shortcomings in the randomization process that conferred a high risk of selection bias [74]. While these preliminary clinical studies reported encouraging results (see **Table 1**), high-quality RCTs are needed to confirm the benefits of omega-3 FAs in SAH patients.

### 9.3 Safety considerations

Evidence obtained over more than two decades in other clinical fields indicates omega-3 FAs interventions are unlikely to lead to serious clinical harm in SAH patients [25, 59]. Nevertheless, parenteral administration of omega-3 FAs may raise some safety concerns. Total parenteral nutrition is associated with an increased risk of complications in critically ill patients [9]. Furthermore, administration of lipid emulsions (LEs) may cause fat overload syndrome; the amount of fat administered and LE infusion rate are the primary risk factors. In this regard, it should be emphasized that the therapeutic dose of FO (0.1–0.2 g of FO/kg/day) is about one order of magnitude lower than that of regular LE (0.7–1.5 g of fat/kg/day) [59]. Additionally, the plasma clearance rate is faster for FAs administered in FOLE than soybean oil-based LEs. These unique features contribute to the good safety profile of FOLE. Fish oil has been widely used as a component of total parenteral nutrition and is associated with reduced rates of infection, shorter hospital stay, and decreased mortality, particularly in surgically treated patients [59].

Furthermore, isolated parenteral administration of FO has increasingly been used in pediatric patients with parenteral nutrition-associated liver disease (PNALD). Several case series published since 2006 have reported parenteral FO monotherapy (PFOM) remarkably improved clinical outcome of patients with PNALD [75]. Importantly, PFOM has demonstrated a good safety profile in these

| Reference | Type of study | Population, *n* | Intervention | Main result |
|---|---|---|---|---|
| Yoneda et al. [73] | Prospective, non-randomized | *n* = 101<br>EPA = 73 | Oral EPA: 1800 mg/day × 10 postoperative (PO) days | Reduction in vasospasm and cerebral infarction |
| Yoneda et al. [74] | RCT | *n* = 162<br>EPA = 81 | Oral EPA: 2700 mg/day × 30 PO days | Reduction in vasospasm and cerebral infarction |
| Nakagawa et al. [72] | Retrospective study | *n* = 100<br>EPA + DHA = 55 | Oral EPA: 1860 mg/day + oral DHA: 750 mg/day × 90 PO days | Reduction in vasospasm and cerebral infarction |
| Saito et al. [13] | Pilot RCT | *n* = 11<br>EPA + DHA = 20 | Parenteral perioperative: 5 days<br>Oral EPA: 1840 mg/day + oral DHA: 1520 mg/day × 8 weeks | No postoperative intracranial bleeding complications<br>Easy-to-implement intervention |

**Table 1.**
*Summary of the features and outcomes of clinical interventional studies in SAH patients.*

critically ill patients, even at FO doses up to 1.5 g FO/kg/day and overextended treatments beyond 4 weeks, well beyond the manufacturer's recommendations.

The aim of replacement FO therapy in PNALD is obviously different to SAH patients. Parenteral administration of FO is intended to address key nutrient deficiencies during the acute stage after SAH, and thus only short-term administration of a regular FO dose should be necessary. In fact, a 5-day parenteral perioperative regimen did not increase the occurrence of major postoperative complications in 19 surgically treated SAH patients [13]. Thus, there is good quality evidence to warrant further clinical trials of parenteral pharmaconutrition as an integral component of interventions with omega-3 FAs in SAH patients.

## 10. Role of inflammation resolution in the growth and rupture of intracranial aneurysms

The role of inflammation in the growth and rupture of intracranial aneurysms (IAs) has been increasingly recognized over the last few decades; however, the specific role of resolution of inflammation in IAs has not yet been considered [76]. Although the pathophysiology of atherosclerosis and the growth and rupture of IAs are distinct, both conditions are mediated by an underlying inflammatory process [77]. The progression of atherosclerotic plaques determines plaque morphology and the risk of rupture. The degree of macrophage infiltration plays a crucial role in the progression of atherosclerotic plaques. Interestingly, IAs have also been recently regarded as a macrophage-mediated inflammatory disease in which prostaglandin E2 and the master transcription factor NF-kB may be crucial drivers of inflammatory signals [78, 79]. It should be remembered that prostaglandin E2 is derived from the long-chain omega-6 FAs ARA and that EPA can inhibit the generation of eicosanoids from ARA and also downregulates the activity of NF-kB [25].

Atherosclerotic plaques readily incorporate omega-3 FAs, and a higher plaque EPA content is associated with a reduced number of foam cells and macrophages, as well as increased plaque stability, as determined by a well-formed fibrous cap [80]. Additionally, signs of defective resolution of inflammation have been identified in atherosclerotic plaques [81]. One major function of SPMs (particularly maresins) is to induce phenotypic conversion of macrophages, which decrease inflammation and promote tissue regeneration [16]. In animal models of atherosclerosis, a traditional Western high-fat diet disrupts the homeostasis of inflammation resolution by nutrigenetic modulation of the 12/15-LOX pathways, thereby inhibiting the generation of protective SPMs [81, 82]. These recent findings in atherosclerosis, particularly the involvement of docosanoids in vascular inflammation, provide biological plausibility that defective resolution of inflammation is implicated in the pathogenesis of IA growth and rupture.

Human beings evolved, and their genetic patterns were established on a diet with an omega-6/omega-3 FAs ratio of 1/1, whereas in current Western diets, this ratio is around 16/1 [83]. Thus, this extreme nutritional imbalance in current Western diets should be seriously considered as a potential aggravating factor for the growth and rupture of IAs [48, 82]. This suggestion may appear somewhat counterintuitive considering the high prevalence of IAs with increased risk of rupture in the Japanese population, which has one of the highest dietary intakes of omega-3 FAs worldwide [48, 84]. However, nutritional deficiency of long-chain omega-3 FAs may not be the only factor associated with defective resolution of inflammation. Inter-individual and ethnic variations in the susceptibility to IA growth and rupture could be related to tissue-specific enzymatic deficiencies in the biosynthetic routes that regulate the resolution of inflammation. However, while defective resolution has already been associated with other chronic inflammatory diseases, it is not yet known whether enzymatic deficiencies contribute to IA growth and rupture, and this novel hypothesis requires further investigation [85, 86].

## 11. Final remarks

The vital roles of EPA and DHA in the human body emphasize the evolutionary importance of maintaining efficient functional couplings between chemical and biological systems as well as between the vasculature and the brain [87]. Resolution of inflammation and endogenous neuroprotective signaling are interrelated processes that largely depend on EPA and DHA derivatives. This novel concept may open new avenues for public health interventions and innovative research in IAs and SAH.

Although nutrition has been traditionally viewed as a supportive measure, increasing evidence strongly suggests that a more balanced dietary intake of omega-6 and omega-3 FAs may represent the most efficient means of improving the status of inflammation resolution at the population level [48, 82, 83]. This specific dietary recommendation could contribute to decrease the risk of IAs growth and rupture and the devastating consequences of SAH, along with other important health benefits.

The pathological significance of the loss of brain DHA after SAH has been widely ignored, even though strong preclinical evidence supports the hypothesis that the integrity of the neurovascular unit largely depends on high DHA enrichment. This previously unrecognized pathophysiological process may significantly increase the risk of secondary brain injury following SAH.

The robust demonstration of the clinical efficacy of EPA in patients with chronic CV disease supports the encouraging results obtained in preliminary clinical studies of omega-3 FAs in SAH and warrants a large-scale RCT. It needs to be emphasized that DHA should always be included in neuroprotective interventions, as DHA plays an essential role in neural tissue and is the cornerstone for docosanoid generation. Parenteral pharmaconutrition with FO offers major clinical advantages for the treatment of SAH patients and should also be an integral component of omega-3 FAs interventions during the acute stage of the disease.

The design of future RCTs of omega-3 FAs in SAH should bear in mind a potentially important factor. Clinical approaches that mainly focus on large-artery vasospasm may actually counteract the beneficial effects of omega-3 FAs and other neuroprotective interventions. The main rationale behind this seemingly paradoxical notion is based on both theoretical models and clinical perspectives [3, 31]. An unpublished subgroup analysis of our pilot pharmaconutrition trial of omega-3 FAs showed unexpected differences in the occurrence of cerebral infarction due to DCI between study centers, each of which had different clinical approaches to large-artery vasospasm [13]. In addition, a recently published observational study performed in the UK showed centers that screened for large-artery vasospasm using transcranial Doppler ultrasound (TCD) had poorer inhospital outcomes and similar rates of DCI diagnosis compared to centers that did not [88]. These results support the dissociation between large-artery vasospasm and clinical outcome that has been observed in major phase 3 RCTs in SAH [8]. Therefore, reliance on a surrogate clinical endpoint such as large-artery vasospasm may lead to the adoption of useless or even harmful clinical approaches [88–91]. Indeed, some research centers in Europe do not include TCD ultrasound or endovascular rescue therapy in their treatment protocols for SAH patients [92].

Moreover, it would be clinically meaningful to determine if correlations exist between the omega-3 index and the concentrations of EPA and DHA as well as the status of inflammation resolution in the wall of ruptured and non-ruptured IAs. There may be a real opportunity for a readily implementable and low-cost therapy if the walls of IAs are as responsive to omega-3 FAs as atherosclerotic plaques.

The interplay between omega-3 FAs and widely used drugs (aspirin and statins) that lead to the generation of longer-acting SPM R-epimers provides ample opportunities for future translational approaches in IAs and SAH. Indeed, combined therapies with omega-3 FAs and aspirin or statins could represent a viable, easy-to-implement therapeutic strategy for patients with unruptured IAs.

Parenteral pharmaconutrition with FO could also be a clinically effective intervention for perioperative neuroprotection for patients subjected to other surgeries at high risk of neurological injury, such as carotid endarterectomy, cardiac surgery, or diverse neurosurgical procedures.

In the future, new drug delivery systems capable of carrying synthetic analogues of SPMs could become a viable therapeutic strategy for patients with tissue-specific enzymatic deficiencies in the resolution pathways [93].

## Conflict of interest

The authors have no conflicts of interest to declare.

## Notes/thanks/other declarations

We express our appreciation to our patients from whom we have learned so much.

## Author details

Geisi Saito[1] and Rodrigo Zapata[2]*

1 Department of Anaesthesiology, Asenjo Neurosurgery Institute, Santiago, Chile

2 Neurosurgery Service, Regional Hospital of Rancagua, Hospital Regional Libertador Bernardo O'Higgins, Rancagua, Chile

*Address all correspondence to: rzapata.barra@gmail.com

## References

[1] Miller BA, Turan N, Chau M, Pradilla G. Inflammation, vasospasm, and brain injury after subarachnoid hemorrhage. BioMed Research International. 2014;**2014**:384342

[2] Veldeman M, Hollig A, Clusmann H, Stevanovic A, Rossaint R, Coburn M. Delayed cerebral ischaemia prevention and treatment after aneurysmal subarachnoid haemorrhage: A systematic review. British Journal of Anaesthesia. 2016;**117**(1):17-40

[3] Ostergaard L, Aamand R, Karabegovic S, Tietze A, Blicher JU, Mikkelsen IK, et al. The role of the microcirculation in delayed cerebral ischemia and chronic degenerative changes after subarachnoid hemorrhage. Journal of Cerebral Blood Flow and Metabolism. 2013;**33**(12):1825-1837

[4] Massicotte EM, Del Bigio MR. Human arachnoid villi response to subarachnoid hemorrhage: Possible relationship to chronic hydrocephalus. Journal of Neurosurgery. 1999;**91**(1):80-84

[5] Al-Khindi T, Macdonald RL, Schweizer TA. Cognitive and functional outcome after aneurysmal subarachnoid hemorrhage. Stroke. 2010;**41**(8):e519-e536

[6] Haug Nordenmark T, Karic T, Roe C, Sorteberg W, Sorteberg A. The post-aSAH syndrome: A self-reported cluster of symptoms in patients with aneurysmal subarachnoid hemorrhage. Journal of Neurosurgery. 2019:1-10

[7] Hanggi D, Etminan N, Mayer SA, Aldrich EF, Diringer MN, Schmutzhard E, et al. Clinical trial protocol: Phase 3, multicenter, randomized, double-blind, placebo-controlled, parallel-group, efficacy, and safety study comparing EG-1962 to standard of care oral nimodipine in adults with aneurysmal subarachnoid hemorrhage [NEWTON-2 (nimodipine microparticles to enhance recovery while reducing toxicity after subarachNoid hemorrhage)]. Neurocritical Care. 2019;**30**(1):88-97

[8] Etminan N, Vergouwen MD, Ilodigwe D, Macdonald RL. Effect of pharmaceutical treatment on vasospasm, delayed cerebral ischemia, and clinical outcome in patients with aneurysmal subarachnoid hemorrhage: A systematic review and meta-analysis. Journal of Cerebral Blood Flow and Metabolism. 2011;**31**(6):1443-1451

[9] Ziegler TR. Parenteral nutrition in the critically ill patient. The New England Journal of Medicine. 2009;**361**(11):1088-1097

[10] Arterburn LM, Hall EB, Oken H. Distribution, interconversion, and dose response of n-3 fatty acids in humans. The American Journal of Clinical Nutrition. 2006;**83**(6):1467S-1476S

[11] Serhan CN, Chiang N, Van Dyke TE. Resolving inflammation: Dual anti-inflammatory and pro-resolution lipid mediators. Nature Reviews Immunology. 2008;**8**(5):349-361

[12] Pilitsis JG, Coplin WM, O'Regan MH, Wellwood JM, Diaz FG, Fairfax MR, et al. Free fatty acids in human cerebrospinal fluid following subarachnoid hemorrhage and their potential role in vasospasm: A preliminary observation. Journal of Neurosurgery. 2002;**97**(2):272-279

[13] Saito G, Zapata R, Rivera R, Zambrano H, Rojas D, Acevedo H, et al. Long-chain omega-3 fatty acids in aneurysmal subarachnoid hemorrhage: A randomized pilot trial of pharmaconutrition. Surgical Neurology International. 2017;**8**:304

[14] Serhan CN, Savill J. Resolution of inflammation: The beginning programs the end. Nature Immunology. 2005;**6**(12):1191-1197

[15] Serhan CN, Levy BD. Resolvins in inflammation: Emergence of the pro-resolving superfamily of mediators. The Journal of Clinical Investigation. 2018;**128**(7):2657-2669

[16] Serhan CN, Dalli J, Colas RA, Winkler JW, Chiang N. Protectins and maresins: New pro-resolving families of mediators in acute inflammation and resolution bioactive metabolome. Biochimica et Biophysica Acta. 2015;**1851**(4):397-413

[17] Hall TC, Bilku DK, Neal CP, Cooke J, Fisk HL, Calder PC, et al. The impact of an omega-3 fatty acid rich lipid emulsion on fatty acid profiles in critically ill septic patients. Prostaglandins, Leukotrienes, and Essential Fatty Acids. 2016;**112**:1-11

[18] Spector AA. Plasma lipid transport. Clinical Physiology and Biochemistry. 1984;**2**(2-3):123-134

[19] Kasuga K, Yang R, Porter TF, Agrawal N, Petasis NA, Irimia D, et al. Rapid appearance of resolvin precursors in inflammatory exudates: Novel mechanisms in resolution. Journal of Immunology. 2008;**181**(12):8677-8687

[20] von Schacky C. Omega-3 index and cardiovascular health. Nutrients. 2014;**6**(2):799-814

[21] Harris WS, Tintle NL, Etherton MR, Vasan RS. Erythrocyte long-chain omega-3 fatty acid levels are inversely associated with mortality and with incident cardiovascular disease: The Framingham heart study. Journal of Clinical Lipidology. 2018;**12**(3):718-727

[22] Grosso G, Pajak A, Marventano S, Castellano S, Galvano F, Bucolo C, et al. Role of omega-3 fatty acids in the treatment of depressive disorders: A comprehensive meta-analysis of randomized clinical trials. PLoS One. 2014;**9**(5):e96905

[23] Bigornia SJ, Harris WS, Falcon LM, Ordovas JM, Lai CQ, Tucker KL. The omega-3 index is inversely associated with depressive symptoms among individuals with elevated oxidative stress biomarkers. The Journal of Nutrition. 2016;**146**(4):758-766

[24] Levi M, van der Poll T, Buller HR. Bidirectional relation between inflammation and coagulation. Circulation. 2004;**109**(22):2698-2704

[25] Calder PC. Omega-3 polyunsaturated fatty acids and inflammatory processes: Nutrition or pharmacology? British Journal of Clinical Pharmacology. 2013;**75**(3):645-662

[26] McBride DW, Blackburn SL, Peeyush KT, Matsumura K, Zhang JH. The role of thromboinflammation in delayed cerebral ischemia after subarachnoid hemorrhage. Frontiers in Neurology. 2017;**8**:555

[27] Albelda SM, Smith CW, Ward PA. Adhesion molecules and inflammatory injury. The FASEB Journal. 1994;**8**(8):504-512

[28] Mason RP, Jacob RF, Shrivastava S, Sherratt SCR, Chattopadhyay A. Eicosapentaenoic acid reduces membrane fluidity, inhibits cholesterol domain formation, and normalizes bilayer width in atherosclerotic-like model membranes. Biochimica et Biophysica Acta. 2016;**1858**(12):3131-3140

[29] Morioka T, Emoto M, Imamura S, Kakutani Y, Yamazaki Y, Motoyama K, et al. Plasma polyunsaturated fatty acid profile is associated with vascular endothelial function in patients with

type 2 diabetes. Diabetes & Vascular Disease Research. 2018;**15**(4):352-355

[30] Fisher M. Pericyte signaling in the neurovascular unit. Stroke. 2009;**40**(3):S13-S15

[31] Hall CN, Reynell C, Gesslein B, Hamilton NB, Mishra A, Sutherland BA, et al. Capillary pericytes regulate cerebral blood flow in health and disease. Nature. 2014;**508**(7494):55-60

[32] Lauritzen L, Hansen HS, Jorgensen MH, Michaelsen KF. The essentiality of long chain n-3 fatty acids in relation to development and function of the brain and retina. Progress in Lipid Research. 2001;**40**(1-2):1-94

[33] Nguyen LN, Ma D, Shui G, Wong P, Cazenave-Gassiot A, Zhang X, et al. Mfsd2a is a transporter for the essential omega-3 fatty acid docosahexaenoic acid. Nature. 2014;**509**(7501):503-506

[34] Bradbury J. Docosahexaenoic acid (DHA): An ancient nutrient for the modern human brain. Nutrients. 2011;**3**(5):529-554

[35] Crawford MA, Bloom M, Broadhurst CL, Schmidt WF, Cunnane SC, Galli C, et al. Evidence for the unique function of docosahexaenoic acid during the evolution of the modern hominid brain. Lipids. 1999;**34**:S39-S47

[36] Kim HY, Akbar M, Kim YS. Phosphatidylserine-dependent neuroprotective signaling promoted by docosahexaenoic acid. Prostaglandins, Leukotrienes, and Essential Fatty Acids. 2010;**82**(4-6):165-172

[37] Bazan NG, Musto AE, Knott EJ. Endogenous signaling by omega-3 docosahexaenoic acid-derived mediators sustains homeostatic synaptic and circuitry integrity. Molecular Neurobiology. 2011;**44**(2):216-222

[38] Park T, Chen H, Kevala K, Lee JW, Kim HY. N-Docosahexaenoylethanolamine ameliorates LPS-induced neuroinflammation via cAMP/PKA-dependent signaling. Journal of Neuroinflammation. 2016;**13**(1):284

[39] McDougle DR, Watson JE, Abdeen AA, Adili R, Caputo MP, Krapf JE, et al. Anti-inflammatory omega-3 endocannabinoid epoxides. Proceedings of the National Academy of Sciences of the United States of America. 2017;**114**(30):E6034-E6043

[40] Bazan NG. Docosanoids and elovanoids from omega-3 fatty acids are pro-homeostatic modulators of inflammatory responses, cell damage and neuroprotection. Molecular Aspects of Medicine. 2018;**64**:18-33

[41] Belayev L, Mukherjee PK, Balaszczuk V, Calandria JM, Obenaus A, Khoutorova L, et al. Neuroprotectin D1 upregulates Iduna expression and provides protection in cellular uncompensated oxidative stress and in experimental ischemic stroke. Cell Death and Differentiation. 2017;**24**(6):1091-1099

[42] Rashid MA, Katakura M, Kharebava G, Kevala K, Kim HY. N-Docosahexaenoylethanolamine is a potent neurogenic factor for neural stem cell differentiation. Journal of Neurochemistry. 2013;**125**(6):869-884

[43] Iadecola C. The neurovascular unit coming of age: A journey through neurovascular coupling in health and disease. Neuron. 2017;**96**(1):17-42

[44] Umhau JC, Zhou W, Carson RE, Rapoport SI, Polozova A, Demar J, et al. Imaging incorporation of circulating docosahexaenoic acid into the human brain using positron emission tomography. Journal of Lipid Research. 2009;**50**(7):1259-1268

[45] Ayer RE, Zhang JH. Oxidative stress in subarachnoid haemorrhage:

Significance in acute brain injury and vasospasm. Acta Neurochirurgica. Supplement. 2008;**104**:33-41

[46] Hsieh YP, Lin CL, Shiue AL, Yin H, Morrow JD, Hsu JC, et al. Correlation of F4-neuroprostanes levels in cerebrospinal fluid with outcome of aneurysmal subarachnoid hemorrhage in humans. Free Radical Biology & Medicine. 2009;**47**(6):814-824

[47] Corcoran TB, Mas E, Barden AE, Durand T, Galano JM, Roberts LJ, et al. Are isofurans and neuroprostanes increased after subarachnoid hemorrhage and traumatic brain injury? Antioxidants & Redox Signaling. 2011;**15**(10):2663-2667

[48] Hibbeln JR, Nieminen LR, Blasbalg TL, Riggs JA, Lands WE. Healthy intakes of n-3 and n-6 fatty acids: Estimations considering worldwide diversity. The American Journal of Clinical Nutrition. 2006;**83**(6):1483S-1493S

[49] Bendel P, Koivisto T, Aikia M, Niskanen E, Kononen M, Hanninen T, et al. Atrophic enlargement of CSF volume after subarachnoid hemorrhage: Correlation with neuropsychological outcome. American Journal of Neuroradiology. 2010;**31**(2):370-376

[50] Pottala JV, Yaffe K, Robinson JG, Espeland MA, Wallace R, Harris WS. Higher RBC EPA + DHA corresponds with larger total brain and hippocampal volumes: WHIMS-MRI study. Neurology. 2014;**82**(5):435-442

[51] Hou J, Zhang JH. Does prevention of vasospasm in subarachnoid hemorrhage improve clinical outcome? No. Stroke. 2013;**44**(6):S34-S36

[52] Eriksen N, Rostrup E, Fabricius M, Scheel M, Major S, Winkler MKL, et al. Early focal brain injury after subarachnoid hemorrhage correlates with spreading depolarizations. Neurology. 2019;**92**(4):e326-e341

[53] Wartenberg KE, Mayer SA. Medical complications after subarachnoid hemorrhage. Neurosurgery Clinics of North America. 2010;**21**(2):325-338

[54] Zhang M, Wang S, Mao L, Leak RK, Shi Y, Zhang W, et al. Omega-3 fatty acids protect the brain against ischemic injury by activating Nrf2 and upregulating heme oxygenase 1. The Journal of Neuroscience. 2014;**34**(5):1903-1915

[55] Jiang X, Pu H, Hu X, Wei Z, Hong D, Zhang W, et al. A post-stroke therapeutic regimen with omega-3 polyunsaturated fatty acids that promotes white matter integrity and beneficial microglial responses after cerebral ischemia. Translational Stroke Research. 2016;**7**(6):548-561

[56] Sgubin D, Aztiria E, Perin A, Longatti P, Leanza G. Activation of endogenous neural stem cells in the adult human brain following subarachnoid hemorrhage. Journal of Neuroscience Research. 2007;**85**(8):1647-1655

[57] Bhatt DL, Steg PG, Miller M, Brinton EA, Jacobson TA, Ketchum SB, et al. Cardiovascular risk reduction with icosapent ethyl for hypertriglyceridemia. The New England Journal of Medicine. 2019;**380**(1):11-22

[58] Hopper L, Ness A, Higgins JP, Moore T, Ebrahim S. GISSI-prevenzione trial. Lancet. 1999;**354**(9189):1557

[59] Klek S. Omega-3 fatty acids in modern parenteral nutrition: A review of the current evidence. Journal of Clinical Medicine. 2016;**5**(3):e34

[60] Chen CT, Kitson AP, Hopperton KE, Domenichiello AF, Trepanier MO, Lin LE, et al. Plasma non-esterified docosahexaenoic acid is the major pool

supplying the brain. Scientific Reports. 2015;**5**:15791

[61] Jones NE, Heyland DK. Pharmaconutrition: A new emerging paradigm. Current Opinion in Gastroenterology. 2008;**24**(2):215-222

[62] Harris WS, Pottala JV, Sands SA, Jones PG. Comparison of the effects of fish and fish-oil capsules on the n 3 fatty acid content of blood cells and plasma phospholipids. The American Journal of Clinical Nutrition. 2007;**86**(6):1621-1625

[63] Nosaka K, Miyoshi T, Iwamoto M, Kajiya M, Okawa K, Tsukuda S, et al. Early initiation of eicosapentaenoic acid and statin treatment is associated with better clinical outcomes than statin alone in patients with acute coronary syndromes: 1-year outcomes of a randomized controlled study. International Journal of Cardiology. 2017;**228**:173-179

[64] Yurko-Mauro K, McCarthy D, Rom D, Nelson EB, Ryan AS, Blackwell A, et al. Beneficial effects of docosahexaenoic acid on cognition in age-related cognitive decline. Alzheimer's & Dementia. 2010;**6**(6):456-464

[65] Cholewski M, Tomczykowa M, Tomczyk M. A comprehensive review of chemistry, sources and bioavailability of omega-3 fatty acids. Nutrients. 2018;**10**(11):e1662

[66] Yin J, Li H, Meng C, Chen D, Chen Z, Wang Y, et al. Inhibitory effects of omega-3 fatty acids on early brain injury after subarachnoid hemorrhage in rats: Possible involvement of G protein-coupled receptor 120/beta-arrestin2/TGF-beta activated kinase-1 binding protein-1 signaling pathway. The International Journal of Biochemistry & Cell Biology. 2016;**75**:11-22

[67] Zhang T, Wu P, Zhang JH, Li Y, Xu S, Wang C, et al. Docosahexaenoic acid alleviates oxidative stress-based apoptosis via improving mitochondrial dynamics in early brain injury after subarachnoid hemorrhage. Cellular and Molecular Neurobiology. 2018;**38**(7):1413-1423

[68] Belayev L, Khoutorova L, Atkins KD, Eady TN, Hong S, Lu Y, et al. Docosahexaenoic acid therapy of experimental ischemic stroke. Translational Stroke Research. 2011;**2**(1):33-41

[69] Yin P, Wei Y, Wang X, Zhu M, Feng J. Roles of specialized pro-resolving lipid mediators in cerebral ischemia reperfusion injury. Frontiers in Neurology. 2018;**9**:617

[70] Berressem D, Koch K, Franke N, Klein J, Eckert GP. Intravenous treatment with a long-chain omega-3 lipid emulsion provides neuroprotection in a murine model of ischemic stroke-A pilot study. PLoS One. 2016;**11**(11):e0167329

[71] Belayev L, Hong SH, Menghani H, Marcell SJ, Obenaus A, Freitas RS, et al. Docosanoids promote neurogenesis and angiogenesis, blood-brain barrier integrity, penumbra protection, and neurobehavioral recovery after experimental ischemic stroke. Molecular Neurobiology. 2018;**55**(8):7090-7106

[72] Nakagawa I, Yokoyama S, Omoto K, Takeshima Y, Matsuda R, Nishimura F, et al. Omega-3 fatty acids ethyl esters suppress cerebral vasospasm and improve clinical outcome following aneurysmal subarachnoid hemorrhage. World Neurosurgery. 2017;**99**:457-464

[73] Yoneda H, Shirao S, Kurokawa T, Fujisawa H, Kato S, Suzuki M. Does eicosapentaenoic acid (EPA) inhibit cerebral vasospasm in patients after aneurysmal subarachnoid hemorrhage?

Acta Neurologica Scandinavica. 2008;**118**(1):54-59

[74] Yoneda H, Shirao S, Nakagawara J, Ogasawara K, Tominaga T, Suzuki M. A prospective, multicenter, randomized study of the efficacy of eicosapentaenoic acid for cerebral vasospasm: The EVAS study. World Neurosurgery. 2014;**81**(2):309-315

[75] de Meijer VE, Gura KM, Meisel JA, Le HD, Puder M. Parenteral fish oil monotherapy in the management of patients with parenteral nutrition-associated liver disease. Archives of Surgery. 2010;**145**(6):547-551

[76] Signorelli F, Sela S, Gesualdo L, Chevrel S, Tollet F, Pailler-Mattei C, et al. Hemodynamic stress, inflammation, and intracranial aneurysm development and rupture: A systematic review. World Neurosurgery. 2018;**115**:234-244

[77] Libby P. Inflammation in atherosclerosis. Arteriosclerosis, Thrombosis, and Vascular Biology. 2012;**32**(9):2045-2051

[78] Shimizu K, Kushamae M, Mizutani T, Aoki T. Intracranial aneurysm as a macrophage-mediated inflammatory disease. Neurologia Medico-Chirurgica. 2019;**59**(4):126-132

[79] Aoki T, Frosen J, Fukuda M, Bando K, Shioi G, Tsuji K, et al. Prostaglandin E2-EP2-NF-kappaB signaling in macrophages as a potential therapeutic target for intracranial aneurysms. Science Signaling. 2017;**10**(465):eaah6037

[80] Borow KM, Nelson JR, Mason RP. Biologic plausibility, cellular effects, and molecular mechanisms of eicosapentaenoic acid (EPA) in atherosclerosis. Atherosclerosis. 2015;**242**(1):357-366

[81] Fredman G, Spite M. Specialized pro-resolving mediators in cardiovascular diseases. Molecular Aspects of Medicine. 2017;**58**:65-71

[82] Merched AJ, Serhan CN, Chan L. Nutrigenetic disruption of inflammation-resolution homeostasis and atherogenesis. Journal of Nutrigenetics and Nutrigenomics. 2011;**4**(1):12-24

[83] Simopoulos AP. The importance of the omega-6/omega-3 fatty acid ratio in cardiovascular disease and other chronic diseases. Experimental Biology and Medicine. 2008;**233**(6):674-688

[84] Investigators UJ, Morita A, Kirino T, Hashi K, Aoki N, Fukuhara S, et al. The natural course of unruptured cerebral aneurysms in a Japanese cohort. The New England Journal of Medicine. 2012;**366**(26):2474-2482

[85] Tabas I. Macrophage death and defective inflammation resolution in atherosclerosis. Nature Reviews Immunology. 2010;**10**(1):36-46

[86] de Gaetano M, McEvoy C, Andrews D, Cacace A, Hunter J, Brennan E, et al. Specialized pro-resolving lipid mediators: Modulation of diabetes-associated cardio-, reno-, and retino-vascular complications. Frontiers in Pharmacology. 2018;**9**:1488

[87] Ruiz-Mirazo K, Briones C, de la Escosura A. Chemical roots of biological evolution: The origins of life as a process of development of autonomous functional systems. Open Biology. 2017;7(4):170050

[88] Hollingworth M, Jamjoom AAB, Bulters D, Patel HC. How is vasospasm screening using transcranial Doppler associated with delayed cerebral ischemia and outcomes in aneurysmal subarachnoid hemorrhage? Acta Neurochirurgica. 2019;**161**(2):385-392

[89] Temple R. Are surrogate markers adequate to assess cardiovascular disease drugs? Journal of the American Medical Association. 1999;**282**(8):790-795

[90] Adami D, Berkefeld J, Platz J, Konczalla J, Pfeilschifter W, Weidauer S, et al. Complication rate of intraarterial treatment of severe cerebral vasospasm after subarachnoid hemorrhage with nimodipine and percutaneous transluminal balloon angioplasty: Worth the risk? Journal of Neuroradiology. 2019;**46**(1):15-24

[91] Yao Z, Hu X, You C. Endovascular therapy for vasospasm secondary to subarachnoid hemorrhage: A meta-analysis and systematic review. Clinical Neurology and Neurosurgery. 2017;**163**:9-14

[92] Cremers CH, Vos PC, van der Schaaf IC, Velthuis BK, Vergouwen MD, Rinkel GJ, et al. CT perfusion during delayed cerebral ischemia after subarachnoid hemorrhage: Distinction between reversible ischemia and ischemia progressing to infarction. Neuroradiology. 2015;**57**(9):897-902

[93] Dasa SSK, Suzuki R, Mugler E, Chen L, Jansson-Lofmark R, Michaelsson E, et al. Evaluation of pharmacokinetic and pharmacodynamic profiles of liposomes for the cell type-specific delivery of small molecule drugs. Nanomedicine. 2017;**13**(8):2565-2574

Chapter 15

# Post Stroke Depression

*Rena D. Sukhdeo Singh, Abhi Pandhi and Andrei V. Alexandrov*

## Abstract

Depression is the most common neuropsychiatric disorder affecting over one third of all stroke patients. The presence of depression after a stroke greatly affects the ability of patients to participate in rehabilitation and can even affect their long-term mortality. Poststroke depression is a well-documented and studied aspect of stroke management because of the implications it has on morbidity, mortality and recovery. Despite post stroke depression being a well-studied phenomenon, it remains underdiagnosed. The development of poststroke depression is multifactorial and has been evaluated from the cellular, genetic, and environmental perspective. Using numerous studies this chapter will review facets of post stroke depression such as epidemiology, etiology and treatment, while evaluating how this phenomena effects patient recovery and rehabilitation.

**Keywords:** stroke, depression, post stroke depression, elderly, serotonin, anxiety, recovery, rehabilitation, function, rehab, acute stroke, ischemic, hemorrhagic, mood

## 1. Introduction

Stroke is one of the leading causes of long-term disability in the United States and is the third leading cause of mortality [1]. Brain parenchyma is densely packed with millions of neurons, where any assault such as an ischemic or hemorrhagic stroke can leave a patient with debilitating deficits [2]. A few of these deficits include the inability to speak or understand language; loss of vision, complete paralysis of one side of the body, quadriplegia, persistent balance issues, and loss of the ability swallow independently. Neuropsychological changes are also very common and well documented in poststroke patients; however, the number of patients that suffer from these changes are grossly underestimated [3].

More than one-third of all stroke survivors experience some form of depression [4]. Depression after a stroke can manifest in many different ways including feelings of anger, frustration, hopelessness, guilt, mental slowing, fatigue, irritability, changes in appetite, social withdrawal, loss of interest in activities they once found enjoyable (also known as anhedonia), or even suicidal thoughts [2]. Patients that suffer from poststroke depression, often have these symptoms missed or undertreated. Recovery and rehabilitation can be adversely affected if post stroke depression is not adequately treated. This can result in increased length of stay at postacute care facilities, increased morbidity, decreased quality of life and even increased mortality [5]. Numerous depression scales have been used to define poststroke depression including the Beck Depression Inventory (BDI), Montgomery-Åsberg Depression Rating Scale (MADRS), Centre for Epidemiologic Studies Depression scale (CES-D), Zung self-rating depression scale and the Hamilton Depression Rating Scale (HDRS) [5]. Post stroke depression has a great impact on the health-care system as well as on the individual patient. In this chapter, we will examine all aspect of depression as it relates to stroke by using these scales and large meta-analyses to define post-stroke depression, and assess how it relates to stroke and recovery.

## 2. Epidemiology

Advancements in acute medical therapies have led to the reduction of mortality due to acute ischemic or hemorrhagic stroke [5]. Studies have shown that 10% of patients recover without any residual deficits, a quarter have mild residual deficits, while 50% are severely disabled or require skilled nursing care within a medical facility able to manage their needs [6]. Along with severe physical disability, patients that suffer from a stroke also experience neuropsychiatric changes. The most common neuropsychiatric sequelae, post-stroke, are depression and anxiety [7]. Patients that survive stroke often experience anxiety and depression related to making adjustments to their new reality [7]. With more patients surviving stroke, quality of life becomes an area of focus. Poststroke depression has been regarded as one of the most important measures for quality of life after an acute stroke. The presence of depression after stroke results in impaired recovery, decreased participation in rehab efforts, impaired cognition, and even increased mortality. The majority of the expressed concern from patients is related to their ability to work and provide financial stability for themselves/their families, the ability to manage their activities of daily living, and the loss of their functional independence [7].

The term poststroke depression puts a focus on ischemic rather than hemorrhagic strokes, which is mostly due to the fact that ischemic strokes have been studied more in the literature, and thus will be the focus of this chapter [8]. Poststroke depression can occur anywhere from days to years after an acute ischemic event with the peak incidence of poststroke depression occurring between 3 months and 2 years, even if the patient's symptoms are improving [9]. Patients that experience the onset of poststroke depression at or after 7 weeks from the acute event are less likely to have a spontaneous remission of this depression [9]. In the acute phase, patients that had a longer inpatient hospital stay were seen to score higher on the Beck Depression Inventory than those that were in the community or in a rehabilitation facility. However, many of these studies have excluded patients that are aphasic, have cognitive impairment, or experienced pre-stroke depression. This may be one of the main reasons that poststroke depression may be underdiagnosed and undertreated [10].

### 2.1 Demographics associated with poststroke depression

Patients younger than 60 are seen to have higher depression scores poststroke. In the general population, major depression is more prevalent in patients younger than 65 years old [11]. In multiple studies that adjusted for pre-stroke depression it was found that more than 30% of the patients younger than 65 could be diagnosed as having clinical depression using the Center for Epidemiologic Studies Depression Scale (CES-D). It was found that within this younger age group there was a higher rate of depression associated with lower socioeconomic status, familial stress, and the ability to provide financial stability [7, 11]. However, having good social support has been found to be protective against poststroke depression [7, 11]. Adults over the age of 65 represent the majority of stroke patients, which can skew the data.

However, multiple meta-analyses have shown that when controlling for other variables such as sex, patients younger than 65 experienced more poststroke depression, and more obvious depressive phenotype [6, 11].

Biologic sex and poststroke depression is a controversial issue. Numerous meta-analyses have looked at the relationship between 'gender' and how it affects or predicts poststroke depression. The results were mixed when looking at data from across the globe. In some studies, women have been found to experience double the risk of poststroke depression compared to men [12, 38]. The gender disparity may be related to how each sex reacts to stressful life events. Women have been demonstrated to have more stress in reaction to negative life events, such as a stroke, which results in feelings of depression [12]. On self-reported survey, women were seen to indicate they have more depressive symptoms, compared to men, when age was controlled for [12]. The risk factors for women developing depression after an acute stroke were: pre-stroke psychiatric comorbidity, age younger than 65, and impairment in cognition [13]. Similarly, men with higher level of physical disability after a stroke had more depressive symptoms than women, or men with less physical disability. In multicenter analysis from China, and India, these studies found that male sex had a higher correlation with poststroke depression [10, 15]. However, there may be confounding factors when evaluating sex differences and poststroke depression. For example, in China there may be a higher number of men in the general population [14]. In the Indian study there were more men in the study [10]. In the USA, it is possible that there is a higher rate of self-reporting by women, as well as under reporting of depressive symptoms in men, based on their level of physical disability [14]. Therefore, more studies need to be done in this area to determine if gender is a definitive predictor of poststroke depression.

Socioeconomic status and education related to poststroke depression is also difficult to measure, due to multiple confounders and conflicting data. However, reviewing the meta-analysis of patient demographics and poststroke depression has shown that patients with lower overall education levels have an increased risk for poststroke depression with mild depressive symptoms [13]. A large meta-analysis of the literature found that there is an association between more years of education and lower risk for depression after a stroke. This study demonstrated that on average the participants in the study without poststroke depression had 0.32 years of education more than those that did have depressive symptoms after their stroke [16]. The symptoms that were seen in this data set were defined as mild depressive symptoms, but could not be classified as clinically depressed. However, this may also have confounding factors in this category. Patients that have lower socioeconomic status have been shown to have lower levels of education [16]. They may also be exposed to environmental factors that put them at increased risk for stroke, such as unhealthy diet, unhealthy lifestyle, more perceived stress, exposure to second hand smoke, and pollution in urban areas [10, 13, 16]. These factors may increase their risk of stroke, and thus their risk for poststroke depression.

## 3. Comorbidities associated with poststroke depression

Comorbid conditions prior to a stroke can affect the development of depression after an acute ischemic event. Conditions such as diabetes, and preexisting psychiatric disorders like depression, anxiety, and bipolar disorder can all have an effect on poststroke depression [17, 18]. One meta-analysis has demonstrated that patients that have vascular risk factors such as diabetes are at a higher risk for developing poststroke depression [17]. This is not thought to be related to the vascular depression theory, which will be discussed later in this chapter. In a Chinese study, it was shown that at 3 months after an acute stroke, patients with diabetes were more likely to develop poststroke depression. This was an independent risk factor for the development of poststroke depression at or after 3 months [17]. The hypothesis behind this is based on the pathophysiology behind both diabetes and poststroke depression, which involves the inflammatory pathway, and the hypothalamic pituitary access. This will be discussed later in the chapter.

Preexisting psychiatric disorders such as depression, anxiety, and bipolar disorder can also predispose patients to worse poststroke depression in the subacute phase, which is within 3 months [17]. One meta-analysis that looked at predictors of poststroke depression found that of the patients that had a preexisting mood disorders such as dysthymia, major depression, minor depression, anxiety, agoraphobia and adjustment disorder were all associated with increased risk of worsening depression after a stroke. Of 1058 patients with reported depression prior to their stroke, 27% had worse depressive symptoms after the acute ischemic event [18]. Premorbid anxiety was also predictive of worsening anxiety after the stroke. Anxiety poststroke results in impaired response to adverse events increased perceived stress and more depressive symptoms [18].

## 4. Poststroke depression etiology

Poststroke depression has been defined as a mood disorder resulting from a general medical condition, by the Diagnostic and Statistical Manual of Mental Disorders (DSM) IV, meaning it does not carry with it the same definition of major depression [16]. There has been some debate about the etiology of poststroke depression, where multiple hypotheses exist, including but not limited to disruption to monoamine pathways, inflammatory cytokines, and hypothalamic–pituitary axis within the brain that modulates mood. The other belief is based on a psychosocial model, where depression develops after a stroke due to inability to adjust to new life circumstances, inability to care for oneself, fear of recurrence, financial insecurity and carrying a new diagnosis [7].

### 4.1 Localization of poststroke depression

One question that has been analyzed extensively with no definite answers is the location of a stroke as a predictor of poststroke depression. These studies used techniques such as voxel-based symptom lesion mapping, diffusion tensor imaging (DTI), functional magnetic resonance imaging (MRI), and positron emission tomography (PET) scans [19]. Functional neuroimaging has sought to determine neuronal circuitry to discover how damage to these circuits results in mood or personality changes. These imaging modalities demonstrate that there is less activity in the frontal cortex, anterior cingulate, dorsolateral and caudate nucleus, in patients that are experiencing depression. In pilot studies using DTI, there has been some data demonstrating that damage to the fronto-striato thalamic pathway and pathways involving emotional control, reward systems and decision making can lead to increased risk of poststroke depression [19]. DTI changes were seen in stroke patients that had damage to the genu and splenium of the corpus callosum, frontal lobe white matter and anterior left corona radiata, resulting in increased levels of apathy [20]. A few theories about lesion location and depressive symptoms include-anhedonia as associated with the stroke volume affecting the hypothalamic-pituitary-adrenal axis, and increased risk for depression in patients with basal ganglia, and frontal lobe strokes [20]. A study by Paradiso and colleagues demonstrated that patients who had left hemispheric strokes were likely to have more depressive symptoms [19]. They proposed that right hemispheric strokes experience fewer depressive symptoms due to anosognosia. If the patient is unaware of his or her deficits, they will less likely feel depression related to their loss of function. Left hemispheric strokes have also been seen to have an earlier onset of poststroke depression, usually in the first 6 months poststroke [13].

One of the models that have been proposed is that subcortical strokes like those in the basal ganglia, and strokes in the frontal lobes can result in disrupted serotoninergic and norepinephrinergic pathways that can be associated with poststroke depression [21]. The belief is that strokes that affected the amine-containing axons between the brainstem and specifically the left cerebral cortex would result in decreased production of serotonin (5-HT) and norepinephrine [22]. A reduction of these neurotransmitters in the frontal and temporal lobe limbic structures, and in the basal ganglia could result in difficulty with mood regulation [19]. This theory was supported by the finding that there were low levels of the 5-HT metabolite, 5-hydroxyindoleacetic acid in the cerebrospinal fluid (CSF).

### 4.2 Biomarkers associated with poststroke depression

Inflammatory cytokines were also thought to be related to the development of poststroke depression [23, 24]. Jioa and colleagues found that interleukin (IL)-6 was elevated in patients with post-stroke depression, even after controlling for confounders, with a confidence interval of 95% [23]. The elevation of IL-6 in patients that have strokes could possibly predict the development of poststroke depression [23, 24]. In another meta-analysis, brain-derived neurotrophic factor (BDNF) was found to be involved in the development of depression and poststroke depression [25, 26]. In these studies, a low serum level of BDNF in the acute phase after a stroke was associated with the development of poststroke depression. BDNF is inherently involved in hippocampal plasticity and memory [27]. One study found a significant negative relationship between BDNF and NIHSS [25–27]. In rodent models, low levels of BDNF in the hippocampus that had an acute stroke exhibited depressed behavior, however if BDNF was overexpressed there was a marked decrease in depressed behavior [21]. Increased BDNF in the rodent model also resulted in reduced infarct size and improved functionality of the rodent [25].

Increased serum level of C-reactive protein (CRP), neopterin, ferritin, and glutamate could also be related to poststroke depression [24]. Proinflammatory markers such as tumor necrosis factor (TNF)-α, interleukins (IL)-1β, IL-6, IL-1, and interferon gamma (IFN-γ) were associated with the development of poststroke depression [23, 24]. Additionally, inflammatory cytokines can activate the hypothalamic pituitary adrenal axis [24]. Activation of the HPA access can also lead to the downstream release of glucocorticoids, which can also result in increased blood glucose levels, and potentially diabetes if this is a chronic process. After an acute stroke, patients often exhibit increased levels of serum adrenocorticotropic hormone, and cortisol. These hormones result in higher mortality and worse neurologic outcome [23]. Increased cytokine activity could also result in greater expression of genes involved in the metabolism of tryptophan such as indoleamine 2,3 dioxygenase (IDO) [27]. If IDO expression increases, tryptophan will be converted to kynurenine and not 5-HT. The downstream effect could result in decreased levels of 5-HT in the limbic system, temporal lobes, frontal lobes, and basal ganglia, which could potentially result in depression [27].

### 4.3 Genetic association with poststroke depression

There have also been studies that have shown a genetic contribution to poststroke depression. Multiple studies have evaluated the 5-HT gene located on chromosome 17q11.1-17q12, which encodes the serotonin transporter [25–27]. In a meta-analysis of 7 studies, there was a significant relationship between 5-HTTLPR polymorphism and the development of poststroke depression symptoms. 5-HTTLPR is an exon of the 5-HT transporter gene polymorphism [25, 26]. The hypothesis is that this gene polymorphism responds to the increased activity of the amygdala when responding to negative stimuli. An increase in 5-HTTLPR serum level has been positively associated with threefold increased risk of developing poststroke depression [25–28]. Another 5-HT polymorphism that has been analyzed is the STin2 VNTR, which is located within intron 2. It has variable number tandem repeats 9, 10, or 12. Repeats of the 9-allele have been well documented to be associated with multiple psychiatric disorders such as bipolar disorder, and major depression [25–28]. Repeats of the twelfth allele have been linked to the development of schizophrenia and bipolar affective disorder. It has been demonstrated that patients with variable tandem repeats of 9/12 and 12/12 were likely to have more depression after a stroke [25–28].

### 4.4 Psychosocial association with poststroke depression

Lastly, psychosocial factors must be considered when assessing who is at risk for poststroke depression. After suffering a life-altering event such as a stroke, even if there are no severe deficits, patients can undergo an adjustment period. They may feel depressed about the new diagnosis of a stroke. There is also the concern of getting back to their normal life routine such as working, caring for dependents, and caring for their own activities of daily living (ADLS) [11, 12]. Patients that do not have good social support tend to experience more depression after a stroke due to feeling helpless, and alone. Patients may also experience anxiety, related to the fear that another stroke may occur. Financial costs of health care also play a role in postacute stroke depression. If a patient is unable to work there may be a concern about medication compliance, affording medication, affording postacute special services like physical therapy or occupational therapy [11, 12].

## 5. Poststroke depression in elderly

Although there is a growing prevalence of stroke in patients aged 65 and younger, the majority of strokes affect patients that are elderly. With the prolonged life expectancy, there is an increased risk for stroke in the aging population, with 70% risk being after the age of 65 [29]. In patients older than 80 years old that suffer from strokes, there is a greater risk of fatality, prolonged hospitalization, complications, and increased postacute care needs [30]. In elderly patients that suffer from stroke, depression may be difficult to diagnose. This is largely due to the symptoms being a vegetative phenotype. It is also confounded because depression is the most common psychiatric disorder among the elderly—with 1% of the elderly population having a formal diagnosis of major depression, and 15% with depressive symptoms according to the National Institutes of Health Consensus development conference [31]. This poses a challenge that practitioners face in distinguishing between premorbid depression, inherent stroke symptoms and poststroke depression, given that many of the features overlap. Some such features include cognitive impairment, psychomotor retardation, and social withdrawal [29]. One measure used to assess poststroke depression in the elderly is the geriatric depression scale (GDS) [32]. This is a self-reported scale where patients answer yes and no questions to determine if a patient is experiencing some form of depression. A score greater than 6 indicates that the patient is likely experiencing some form of depression.

This scale is highly sensitive and predictive of poststroke depression in the geriatric population [32]. However, the GDS cannot be used by aphasic stroke patients or those with cognitive impairments caused by a stroke.

### 5.1 Vascular dementia and poststroke depression

Alexopoulos and colleagues found that elderly stroke patients that suffered ischemic strokes demonstrated increased encephalomalacia and MRI hyperintensities that would predispose these patients to develop depression [33]. Their study suggested that these changes were not seen in elderly patients that had depression without vascular risk factors. Elderly patients that have been observed to have signs of depression, but do not have any vascular risk factors were found to have less white matter hyperintensities on MRI, which were similar to the nondepressed controls [31]. It has also been demonstrated that patients that suffered from depression without vascular insult had phenotypically different depression with features of more agitation, aggression, feelings of guilt and dysphoria. This is the theory of vascular depression in the elderly [33]. The hypothesis behind vascular depression states that chronic small vessel changes or non-symptomatic cerebrovascular events accumulate over time, resulting in the disruption of cortico-striato-pallido-thalamo-cortical (CSPTC) pathways [31]. Vascular dementia is described as a subcortical phenomenon. This type of depression differs from poststroke depression, in that they are silent, and the patient is not aware that they have suffered a stroke [31]. In a Japanese sample, greater than 80% of the patients that had major depression had MRI evidence of multiple silent infarcts [32]. Up to 75% of these depressed patients had lesions in the basal ganglia and thalamus [31, 33].

Three pathways associated with CSPTC were proposed in the way that vascular depression can present phenotypically. Within the CSPTC are the orbitofrontal pathway, the cingulate pathway, and the dorsolateral pathway. Injury over time to the orbitofrontal pathway can result in irritability and disinhibition [31]. The cingulate pathway can cause apathy, and lack of initiative if injured, and lastly, injury to the dorsolateral pathway can result in poor speech productions, and inability to learn. These symptoms can all be seen in elderly depression. Prefrontal dysfunction has shown to have a poor or delayed response to antidepressants in elderly patients [31, 33]. However, early administration of antidepressants, particularly selective serotonin reuptake inhibitors have been shown to improve neuropsychological rehabilitation in elderly stroke patients.

Lacunar infarcts have been seen to result in more depression among Alzheimer patients especially basal ganglia strokes and cortical strokes were found to have more cognitive impairment [31]. Severe cognitive impairment was also seen to be one of the leading causes of depression in the elderly. There are some questions of whether cognitive impairment or dementia can increase the risk of stroke, and thus poststroke depression among the elderly, or do strokes result in cognitive decline and vascular depression [31]. Dementia and depression can be difficult to differentiate. In the elderly, pseudodementia can be secondary to depression however, the opposite is also true. This is a "what came first" type of scenario with dementia, stroke and vascular depression [31].

Although vascular depression and poststroke depression are different in the way they affect a patient, they likely lay on a continuum. Both are secondary to a vascular event, and both result in depression. Vascular depression has a higher incidence in elderly patients as they have an accumulation of more subcortical white matter changes that are seen as hyperintensities on MRI FLAIR. Poststroke depression is less subtle since the patient is usually aware that they have had a stroke [31, 33]. There may be a growing incidence of vascular depression among young patients, due to poorly controlled hypertension, tobacco, diabetes, drug use, and poor diet and lifestyle choices causing small vessel disease. These risk factors put all patients at risk for an acute stroke, and chronic small vessel disease.

## 6. Large strokes and the effect on poststroke depression

In patients that suffer from large ischemic or hemorrhagic strokes, they are often left with a serious physical disability [2]. A proximal middle cerebral artery occlusion can result in severe expressive, or receptive aphasias, hemiparesis, facial weakness, sensory loss inability to swallow, neglect, apraxia, and a propensity toward developing seizures [34]. If the patient is relatively young, the probability of cerebral edema is high, which could result in complications such as brain herniation if a hemicraniectomy is not performed. Intracerebral hemorrhage in these vascular territories can result in similar findings that may necessitate an extra ventricular drain to remove blood from the ventricles, or a decompressive hemicraniectomy to evacuate the hemorrhage [34]. A patient with a large stroke in the posterior circulation can result in the patient being obtunded, having chronic balance issues, hemiparesis, vision loss, and ataxia [3].

Patients that survive these large strokes often experience the most debility, with the majority becoming bedbound, requiring a percutaneous endoscopic gastrostomy tube for nutrition and tracheostomy tube for assistance with breathing. Due to the severity of their disability, these patients require 24-hour care, by their families or nursing professionals. The majority of these patients experience severe depression and guilt, due to feeling like a financial or physical burden on their loved ones [35]. They also experience loss of autonomy due to their deficits. They are no longer able to manage their own activities of daily living, which results in feelings of inadequacy, and resentment for those that are doing the caregiving. Depression has also seen to be positively correlated with the national institute of health stroke scale (NIHSS) which measures stroke severity, wherein the higher the stroke scale, the more severe the depressive symptoms [36].

Patients with large strokes and increased debility often require management in a skilled nursing facility (SNF). At SNF, the patients do not participate in as much rehabilitation activities, as compared to other stroke patients in an inpatient rehabilitation setting [32]. These patients are therefore at disadvantage because their exposure to rehabilitation is limited. The combination of decreased functionality, less access to rehabilitation, and depression impairs the recovery for these patients. They too lose the desire to participate in meaningful interaction due to their disability [32].

## 7. Challenges in diagnosing depression after stroke

Diagnosing depression after a stroke may be difficult for practitioners given that stroke patients can have complex symptoms. The physicians that treat stroke patients should be aware that over a third of patients experience depression after a stroke, and to note that even subtle changes in behavior could represent an aspect of poststroke depression [17]. Small changes like irritability, frustration, extreme fatiguability, and refusing to partake in physical therapy and occupational therapy. Another challenge is that many symptoms of stroke and depression overlap, such as fatigue, pain, decreased motor activity, and decreased verbal output [7]. Only a few of the depression scales used to assess poststroke depression include somatic symptoms in their evaluation. The Beck Depression Inventory is one such scale. However, again some somatic symptoms from the stroke itself can be mistaken as a positive finding on a depression scale. It is important to be able to tease apart what symptoms are due to a stroke and what symptoms are related to depression. If a diagnosis of poststroke depression is missed, it can negatively affect how the patient recovers, and even affect their mortality.

The symptoms that make the diagnosis of poststroke depression the most difficult are aphasia, anosognosia, neglect, abulia and cognitive disabilities that result from their stroke [37]. Unfortunately, the majority of studies that evaluate poststroke depression exclude patients with these symptoms. This is largely due to their inability to answer questions, fill out questionnaires, or because it is difficult for medical staff to assign a score to the patient based on their daily interactions. Aphasia is independently associated with an increased risk of developing poststroke depression [37]. However, three scales have been developed to assess depression in aphasic patients. These scales include the Stroke Aphasic Depression Questionnaire-10 (SADQ-10), the Aphasia Depression Rating Scale (ADRS), and the Perceived Stress Scale (PSS). The (SADQ/SADQ-10/SADQH-10) and the Aphasia Depression Rating Scale are based on the observation of other people to determine if the patient being assessed is in fact depressed or not. The SADQ-10 used caregivers as the observers, with non-aphasic patients as the controls [37]. A value of 14/30 or higher was correlated with the development of depression and depressive symptoms with a sensitivity of 70% and specificity of 77%. The ADRS scoring system used external signs that could be observed such as fatigue, insomnia, changes in weight, and signs of anxiety. A score of 9/30 or higher was associated with the development of depression with a sensitivity of 83% and specificity of 71% [37]. After a comparative analysis, it was determined that either one of these tools could be used for assessing depression in aphasic patients. A review of the current studies could be more generalizable if aphasic patients were included and analyzed with these scales.

## 8. Poststroke depression effect on morbidity and mortality

Poststroke depression was found to be an independent predictor of symptom severity after a stroke, and difficulty with managing activities of daily living [35]. In a meta-analysis of seven studies, poststroke depression was found to have an association with increased mortality [39]. Specifically, patients that experienced early poststroke depression as defined to be within 3 months of stroke onset, were found to have 1.5 increased risk of death. A literature review by Robinson and colleagues, found that using the Hospital Anxiety and Depression scale (HADS), patients that had a score greater than 7 at 3 months had increased mortality than those with a score less than 7 [38]. These scores were evaluated up to 5 years poststroke, and the hazard ratio was found to be 1.41. It was seen that mortality was increased in patients with poststroke depression that were younger than 65 years old [38]. Their study also demonstrated that in greater than 50,000 veterans that suffered an ischemic stroke, those that developed poststroke depression had higher rates of mortality within 3 years of that acute event. The hypothesis behind this being that early poststroke depression can occur in a patient with a severe disability such as neurocognitive decline, paralysis, aphasia, or dysphagia [38]. Due to the severity of their post-stroke symptoms these patients may be at increased risk of death due to complications like pneumonia secondary to dysphasia or infection from decubitus ulcers. Another hypothesis is that patients that are suffering from poststroke depression may be less likely to be compliant with medical recommendations, such as healthy diet, avoiding tobacco, alcohol, drug use, scheduled follow up appointments and medication compliance [37, 38]. These factors can increase the risk of mortality. Another theory states that mortality associated with poststroke depression may be related to cardiovascular mortality [38, 39]. There is an association between depression and myocardial infarction, where it was found that depressed patients had less heart rate variability. This finding was also seen in patients with poststroke depression. This could put these patients at risk for myocardial infarction and subsequently, death. This meta-analysis also highlighted the idea that pharmacologic antidepressants have a mixed response in poststroke depression [38].

## 9. Treatment of poststroke depression

In order to treat poststroke depression, it needs to be accurately diagnosed. Currently the DSM IV is used to diagnose this disorder, along with multiple depression rating scales such as the Hamilton Rating Scale for Depression, Beck Depression Inventory, Montgomery-Åsberg Depression Rating Scale, Center for Epidemiological Studies Depression Scale, Zung self-rating depression scale and the Post-Stroke Depression Rating Scale [5]. There are many challenges in diagnosing depression in a patient after an acute stroke. Many of these patients have a somatic component to their symptoms, like pain, fatigue, or limited speech after a cerebrovascular event. These symptoms can confound a depression scale that account for somatic symptoms—like the Beck Depression Index [5]. Depending on which scale is used to measure depression in these patients, there may be an overestimation or underestimation of depression. Since the hypothesis that stroke results in disruption of the monoamine pathways, there has been a focus on antidepressants like selective serotonin reuptake inhibitors, or tricyclic antidepressants to target poststroke depression. However, the role of antidepressants has been debated. There are some studies that show efficacy and reduction in mortality, and some that show a minimal effect or even adverse side effects [38–40]. Selective serotonin reuptake inhibitors (SSRIs) are well tolerated and can lead to fewer symptoms of depression at 3 weeks of use [40]. It is one therapy that is thought to work well in all age groups, regardless of comorbid conditions. SSRIs are better tolerated in all populations, compared to tricyclic antidepressants (TCA) [39, 40]. One endpoint found that patients that were started on SSRI early had decreased risk of myocardial infarction and recurrent stroke [40]. In a meta-analysis by Robinson and colleagues, the use of nortriptyline or fluoxetine demonstrated improvement in activities of daily living in poststroke depression compared to patients on placebo [38]. This study also demonstrated that the continued use over 12 weeks resulted in improved cognition in patients with poststroke depression, where the effect could last up to 2 years. Not only do SSRI inhibit reuptake of serotonin, but it was demonstrated in rodent models that SSRIs can decrease infarct volumes, reduced inflammation and increase neuroplasticity by modulating BDNF expression [38]. SSRI was also found to increase neurogenesis in the hippocampus, and improve cerebral blood flow autoregulation which is thought to be related to the upregulation of BDNF [27, 38].

In the fluoxetine in motor recovery of patients with acute ischemic stroke (FLAME) trial, fluoxetine use for 3 months was tested to see if it would improve motor recovery in patients with hemiparesis [41]. This trial was used to assess if the use of fluoxetine would change the Fugl-Meyer motor scale (FMMS) score which is an index used to test motor recovery, with a score of 100 representing complete motor function without any deficit. Two groups were analyzed a fluoxetine dose of 20 mg was the placebo and a 40 mg dose was used as the test treatment. At 3 months there was a significant improvement in motor function among the patients in the treatment arm [41]. At 90 days modified rankin scale (MRS) scores were better in the treatment arm as well. The frequency of depression was lower in the treatment arm when assessed with the MADRS score at 90 days. Even in patients that did not receive intravenous thrombolysis, their FMMS scores at 90 days were higher in the treatment arm. Patients that were assessed to be depressed at the onset of the trial, based on MADRS score, were excluded from this trial [41]. Pretreatment with SSRI prior to stroke was also an exclusion criterion. Although the FLAME trial seemed to be promising for improving motor function in poststroke patients and reducing depression within that 3-month period, newer studies have shown the use of SSRI prior to stroke, was negatively associated with ambulation poststroke [8].

In a study by Etherton et al., it was found that the use of SSRI prior to an acute stroke was associated with a decrease in discharges back to the patient's home, and increasing need for ambulatory aids [8]. When examining the patients in the two groups: pre-SSRI/spread vs. non antidepressant, there were no significant difference in admission NIHSS or length of hospital stay. The authors thought this may be due to the possibility that patients that were on SSRI or antidepressants prior to admission for their stroke event may have suffered a stroke before or TIA, resulting in a larger stroke burden. Another ischemic event could cause recrudescence of old stroke symptoms due to an increased burden on that area that was receiving adequate blood flow, which could lead to the patient having more needs such as rehabilitation at discharge. Pre-SSRI use was also associated with increased mortality at 30 days, and worse stroke severity in patients with hemorrhagic stroke [8].

Another criticism for the use of SSRIs was due to the increase in the risk of major bleeding or death. In a meta-analysis of 31 case-controlled studies, it was found that SSRI use was associated with risk of major bleeding events, with the increased risk being 41% [40, 42]. This meta-analysis also examined cohort studies that evaluated the use of SSRI vs. non-SSRI in association with major bleeding risk of 36%. The pooled data from the meta-analysis found that SSRI was associated with major bleeding risk with an odds ratio of 1.41. Gastrointestinal bleeding accounted for the majority of these major bleeding events, with a few intracerebral hemorrhage cases [42]. The hypothesis behind the increased bleeding risk is that platelet activity is inhibited by serotonin. This hypothesis is strengthened by the idea that patients taking SSRI have less myocardial infarctions and fewer strokes. The major bleeding risk associated with SSRI are amplified with adjunct use of non-steroidal anti-inflammatory drugs (NSAIDS) [42].

Overall, antidepressants such as SSRI and TCA have been thought to be the best initial treatment for post-stroke depression. SSRI are overall better tolerated in all populations [40]. These antidepressants can help patients combat poststroke depression enough to allow them to participate in rehabilitation efforts. Psychotherapies such as cognitive behavioral therapy (CBT) have been studied to assess if it would be beneficial in the treatment of poststroke depression. Due to the small sample size of the studies, and other limitations there was no real effect seen with CBT [5]. It may be an area of adjunct therapy for patients with severe poststroke depression that need more than pharmaceutical treatment. However, the use of CBT should not delay the initiation of treatment with antidepressants.

## 10. Depression and stroke rehabilitation

Depression after stroke strongly affects the way patients participate in and respond to rehabilitation. Depression has been linked with decreased participation in rehabilitation efforts which in turn results in more increased morbidity and mortality and decreased quality of life. In a Japanese study that evaluated poststroke depression in patients admitted to a rehabilitation center, their results demonstrated that the patients that were identified as having poststroke depression had less response to rehab and minimal improvement in activities of daily living and functional independence measures [32]. This study found that the level of independence in the activities of daily living at the time of discharge from rehab was related to the severity of poststroke depression at the time of admission. Poststroke depression had a negative 5-year correlation with the ADL. Psychological factors accounted for a large part of how patients responded to rehabilitation [32]. This study found that patients with poststroke depression experience feelings of hopelessness and were thus not motivated to participate in rehabilitation. Depression in these patients also leads to listlessness and inattention, which predisposed the patients with poststroke depression to falls. Thus, another reason why mortality is higher in patients with poststroke depression. Falling was also correlated with a decreased ability to manage their ADL [32].

Another study on depression and rehabilitation found that patients with hemiparesis and poststroke depression had 51% less participation in rehabilitation activities [43]. This study showed that any amount of depression after a stroke can affect a patient's quality of life despite the severity of the stroke. This is because each patient has a unique response to acute stress. The perceived stress score is valuable in rehabilitation because it helps practitioners identify which patients are more at risk of developing depression. If they are identified early, treatment of depression can be initiated, and rehabilitation does not need to be adversely affected. Some of the indexes used to measure the quality of life in patients with poststroke depression include the Stroke Specific Quality of Life Scale SS-QOL, stroke impact scale, Barthel index of ADL as well as the multiple depression rating scales [43]. The Scandinavian Stroke Scale (SSS) and Bergman Balance Scale (BBS) are measures used to assess the progress of rehabilitation, which is more encompassing than the Modified Rankin Score [10]. If patients are able to meaningfully participate in rehabilitation, studies have proven that symptoms of depression can improve, and their quality of life scores increase as well [43]. This coupled with the use of antidepressants can help patients with depression poststroke manage their symptoms of depression and improve their functional outcome. It could also help prevent a subsequent ischemic event [43].

Depression has also been found to be a risk factor for stroke [44]. This has been demonstrated even when controlling for confounders like tobacco use or substance use. Patients with psychosocial stressors put patients at an increased risk of stroke [11, 12, 44, 45]. Not only do these patients have an increased risk of hypertension, and diabetes, but also have an increased prevalence of tobacco use and substance use that also put them at greater risk for an ischemic stroke [44]. A meta-analysis by Dong and colleagues, looked at 17 prospective studies that included greater than 200,000 patients [45]. Of this subset of patients, greater than 6000 had a positive association between depression and a second stroke. A depressed patient had 34% higher risk of developing stroke, even when age and sex were controlled for [45]. Thus, stroke and depression may be a part of a vicious cycle where a stroke results in depression and then depression results in another stroke. This process repeats and, in turn, hinders recovery and rehabilitation. Thus, proving again why it is important to diagnose depression after a stroke, and treat it adequately.

## 11. Poststroke depression and effect on the health care system

Poststroke depression can increase the burden on the healthcare system. In two literature reviews the effect of depression after a stroke was assessed by looking at large veteran populations [46, 47]. These studies demonstrated that patients that suffered from poststroke depression had on average a longer hospital stay, as well as increased outpatient and inpatient physician visits over 1 year. These patients also had a higher likelihood of having significant deficits such as dysphagia after their stroke, and complex comorbidities that required frequent hospital visits, or prolonged stays in nursing facilities/rehabilitation centers [47]. They were also noted to have higher risk of a subsequent stroke within 1 year of their first stroke, and readmissions for complications related to their strokes such as aspiration pneumonia, or falls [47]. In Husaini and colleague's analysis of 17,010 patients from Tennessee, their study demonstrated that patients with stroke and depression had higher average health care costs than patients with only stroke, or stroke with another comorbid psychiatric disorder, even while controlling for age, sex and race [48]. On average stroke patients with depression had a healthcare cost of $77,864, compared to $47,790 in patients with stroke only these costs are due to increase use of diagnostic tests, increased pharmacologic interventions, and addition therapist and physician consultations [47, 48]. If poststroke depression could be identified early, and treated it could reduce the total cost to the patient, and could decrease the overall healthcare burden (**Figure 1**).

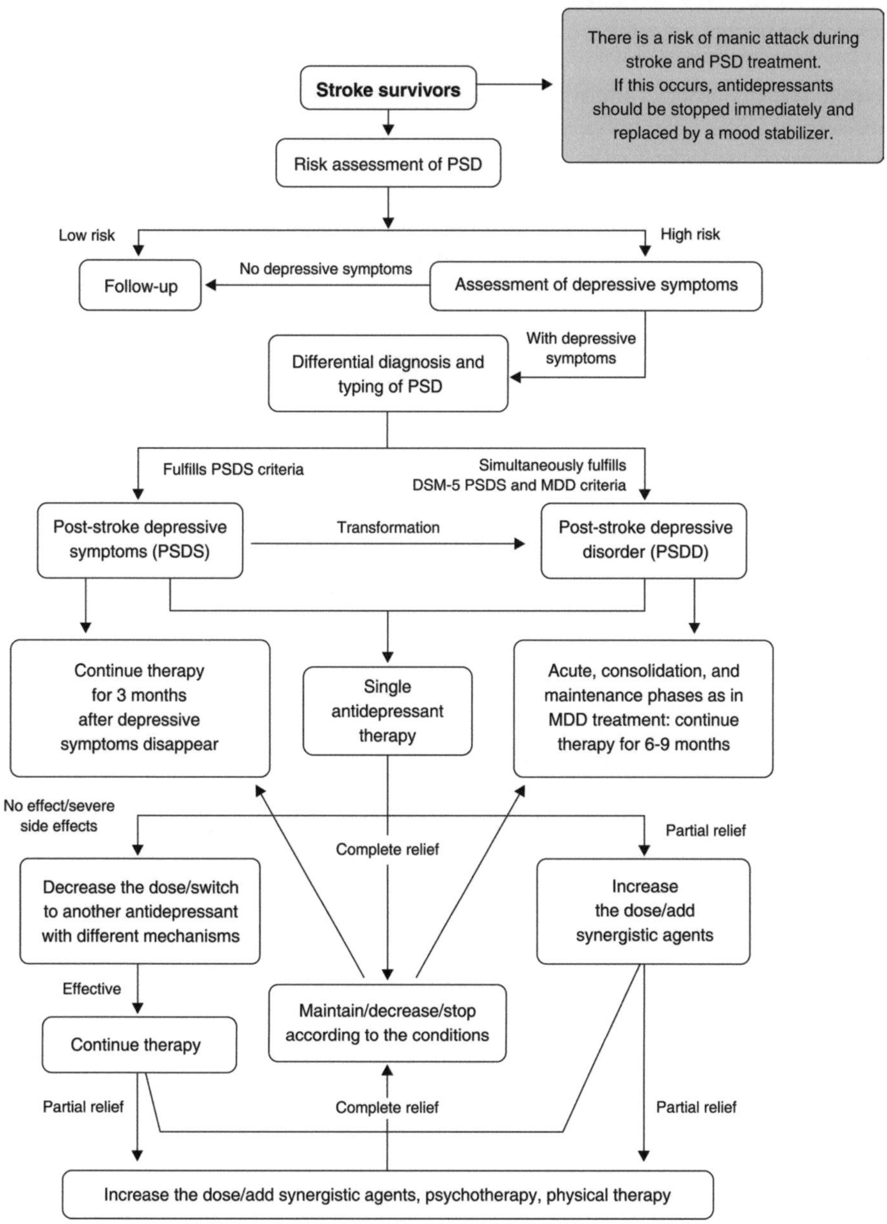


**Figure 1.**
*The diagnostic and treatment procedures of PSD. MDD = major depressive disorder; PSD = poststroke depression [49].*

## 12. Conclusion

Depression and stroke have a bidirectional relationship where one acts as a risk for the other. Poststroke depression is an area of study that has evolved over the years. New studies on its etiology have been discovered, and continued research efforts are providing more insight on the questions we still have, such as the associations of lesion location, the role of inflammation, neuroplasticity, and even genetics. Some patients are more at risk than others for developing poststroke depression, but the main goal is detection, management, and rehabilitation. Detecting poststroke depression is important, so treatment can be initiated as soon as possible, thus reducing morbidity, mortality, and assisting these patients with participating in rehabilitation efforts. Rehabilitation not only improves function in these patients, but also has beneficial effects on depression as well. If patients can effectively partake in rehabilitation efforts, their quality of life scores have been shown to improve (with quality of life being a measure for depression in these patients). Improvements in perceived quality of life can have downstream effects resulting in a reduction of readmissions to the hospital, and outpatient visits, and thus a reduction in the healthcare burden caused by this disease process. If depression can be effectively managed, patients will be more likely to have meaningful participation in poststroke rehabilitation, and reduce the risk of morbidity and mortality associated with their stroke.

## Author details

Rena D. Sukhdeo Singh*, Abhi Pandhi and Andrei V. Alexandrov
University of Tennessee Health Science Center, USA

*Address all correspondence to: r.sukhdeo@hotmail.com

## References

[1] CDC. Stroke facts [Internet]. 2019. Available from: https://www.cdc.gov/stroke/facts.htm [Accessed: 02 April 2019]

[2] Johns Hopkins Medicine. Effects of stroke [Internet]. 2019. Available from: https://www.hopkinsmedicine.org/health/conditions-and-diseases/stroke/effects-of-stroke [Accessed: 20 March 2019]

[3] Bartoli F, Lillia N, Lax A, Crocamo C, Mantero V, Carra G, et al. Depression after stroke and risk of mortality: A systematic review and meta-analysis. Stroke Research and Treatment. Article ID 862978. 2013;**2013**:11. DOI: 10.1155/2013/862978. Available from: https://www.ncbi.nlm.nih.gov/pmc/articles/PMC3606772/ [Accessed: 12 March 2019]

[4] National Stroke Association. Depression [Internet]. 2019. Available from: https://www.stroke.org/we-can-help/survivors/stroke-recovery/post-stroke-conditions/emotional/depression/ [Accessed: 03 April 2019]

[5] Paolucci S. Epidemiology and treatment of post-stroke depression. Neuropsychiatric Disease and Treatment. 2008;**4**(1):145-154. Available from: https://www.ncbi.nlm.nih.gov/pmc/articles/PMC2515899/ [Accessed: 20 March 2019]

[6] Alajbegovic A, Djelilovic-Vranic J, Alajbegovic S, Nakicevic A, Todorovic L, Tiric-Campara M. Post stroke depression. Medical Archives – Journal of the Academy of Medical Sciences in Bosnia and Herzegovina. 2014;**68**(1):47-50. DOI: 10.5455/medarh.2014.68.47-50. Available from: https://www.ncbi.nlm.nih.gov/pmc/articles/PMC4272477/ [Accessed: 15 March 2019

[7] Oni O, Olagunju A, Olisah V, Aina O, Ojini F. Post-stroke depression: Prevalence, associated factors and impact on quality of life among outpatients in a Nigerian hospital. South African Journal or Psychiatry. 2018;**24**. DOI: 10.4102/sajpsychiatry.v24i0.1058. Available from: https://www.ncbi.nlm.nih.gov/pmc/articles/PMC6138133/ [Accessed: 22 March 2019]

[8] Etherton M, Siddiqui K, Schwamm L. Prestroke selective serotonin reuptake inhibitor use and functional outcomes after ischemic stroke. Stroke and Vascular Neurology. 2017;**3**(1). DOI: 10.1136/svn-2017-000119. Available from: https://svn.bmj.com/content/3/1/9 [Accessed: 30 March 2019]

[9] Robinson RG, Bolduc PL, Price TR. Two-year longitudinal study of poststroke mood disorders: Diagnosis and outcome at one and two years. Stroke. 1987;**18**(5):837-843. Available from: https://www.ncbi.nlm.nih.gov/pubmed/3629640 [Accessed: 11 March 2019]

[10] Srivastava A, Taly AB, Guptra A, Murali T. Post-stroke depression: Prevalence ad relationship with disability in chronic stroke survivors. Annals of Indian Academy of Neurology. 2010;**13**(2)123-127. DOI: 10.4103/0972-2327.64643. Available from: https://www.ncbi.nlm.nih.gov/pmc/articles/PMC2924510/. [Accessed: 01 April 2019]

[11] McCarthy M, Sucharew H, Alwell K, Moomaw C, Woo D, et al. Age, subjective stress, and depression after ischemic stroke. Journal of Behavioral Medicine. 2015;**39**(1):55-64. DOI: 10.1007/s10865-015-9663-0. Available from: https://www.ncbi.nlm.nih.gov/pmc/articles/PMC4724284/ [Accessed: 30 March 2019]

[12] Mazure CM, Weinberger AH, Pittman B, Sibon I, Swendsen J. Gender and stress in predicting

depressive symptoms following stroke. Cerebrovascular Disease. 2014;**38**: 240-246. DOI: 10.1159/000365838. Available from: https://www.karger.com/Article/FullText/365838 [Accessed: 01 April 2019]

[13] Paradiso S, Robinson RG. Gender differences in poststroke depression. The Journal of Neuropsychiatry and Clinical Neurosciences. 1998;**10**:41-47. DOI: 10.1176/jnp.10.1.41. Available from: https://neuro.psychiatryonline.org/doi/pdf/10.1176/jnp.10.1.41 [Accessed: 29 March 2019]

[14] Poynter B, Shuman M, Diaz-Granados N, Kapral M, Grace S, Stewart D. Sex differences in the prevalence of post-stroke depression: A systematic review. Psychosomatics. 2009;**50**(6):563-569. DOI: 10.1016/S0033-3182(09)70857-6. Available from: https://www.ncbi.nlm.nih.gov/pubmed/19996226 [Accessed: 28 March 2019]

[15] Wang Z, Zhu M, Su Z, Guan B, Wang A, Wang Y, et al. Post-stroke depression: Different characteristics based on follow-up stage and gender-a cohort perspective study from Mainland China. Neurological Research. 2017;**39**(11):996-1005. DOI: 10.1080/01616412.2017.1364514. Available from: https://www.ncbi.nlm.nih.gov/pubmed/28828931 [Accessed: 26 March 2019]

[16] Backhouse E, Mchutchison C, Cvoro V, Shenkin S, Wardlaw J, Priller J. Cognitive ability, education and socioeconomic status in childhood and risk of post-stroke depression in later life: A systematic review and meta-analysis. PLOS One. 2018;**13**(7). DOI: 10.1371/journal.pone.0200525. Available from: https://www.ncbi.nlm.nih.gov/pmc/articles/PMC6047794/ [Accessed: 19 March 2019]

[17] Zhang Y, He JR, Liang HB, et al. Diabetes mellitus is associated with late-onset post-stroke depression. Journal of Affective Disrorders. 2017;**221**:222-226. DOI: 10.1016/j.jad.2017.06.045. Available from: https://www.ncbi.nlm.nih.gov/pubmed/28654846 [Accessed: 23 March 2019]

[18] Mitchell AJ, Sheth B, Gill J, Yadegarfar M, Stubbs B, Yadegarfar M, Meader N. Prevalence and predictors of post stroke mood disorders: A meta-analysis and meta-regression of depression, anxiety and adjustment disorder. General Hospital Psychiatry. 2017;**47**:48-60. DOI: 10.1016/j.genhosppsych.2017.04.001. Available from: https://www-sciencedirect-com.ezproxy.uthsc.edu/science/article/pii/S0163834317301433?via%3Dihub . [Accessed: 28 March 2019]

[19] Gozzi SA, Wood AG, Chen J, Vaddadi K, Phan TG. Imaging predictors of poststroke depression: methodological factors in voxel-based analysis. British Medical Journal. 2014;**4**(7). DOI: 10.1136/bmjopen-2014-004948. Available from: https://www.ncbi.nlm.nih.gov/pmc/articles/PMC4091263/ [Accessed 28 March 2019]

[20] Pasi M, VanUden I, Tuladhar AM, de Leeuw FE, Pantoni L. White matter microstructural damage on diffusion tensor imaging in cerebral small vessel disease clinical consequences. Stroke. 2016;**47**(6). DOI: 10.1161/STROKEAHA.115.012065. Available from: https://www.ahajournals.org/doi/10.1161/STROKEAHA.115.012065. [Accessed: 28 March 2019]

[21] Villa RF, Ferrari F, Moretti A. Post-stroke depression: Mechanisms and pharmacological treatment. Pharmacology & Therapeutics. 2018;**184**:131-144. DOI: 10.1016/j.pharmthera.2017.11.005. Available from: https://www-sciencedirect-com.ezproxy.uthsc.edu/science/article/pii/S0163725817302899?via%3Dihub [Accessed: 28 March 2019]

[22] Nickel A, Thomalla G. Post-stroke depression: Impact of lesion location and methodological limitations—A topical review. Frontiers in Neurology. 2017;**8**:498. DOI: 10.3389/fneur.2017.00498. Available from: https://www.ncbi.nlm.nih.gov/pmc/articles/PMC5613107/ [Accessed: 16 March 2019]

[23] Jiao J, Cheng C, Ma Y, Huang J, Dai M, Jiang C, et al. Association between inflammatory cytokines and the risk of post-stroke depression, and the effect of depression on outcomes of patients with ischemic stroke in a 2-year prospective study. Experimental and Therapeutic Medicine. 2016(3):1591-1598. DOI: 10.3892/etm.2016.3494. Available from: https://www.ncbi.nlm.nih.gov/pmc/articles/PMC4998048/ [Accessed: 24 March 2019]

[24] Levada O, Troyan A. Poststroke depression biomarkers: A narrative review. Frontiers in Neurology. 2018;**9**:577. DOI: 10.3389/fneur.2018.00577. Available from: https://www.ncbi.nlm.nih.gov/pmc/articles/PMC6055004/ [Accessed: 03 April 2019]

[25] Guo WY, Zhang ZH, Mu JL, Liu D, Zhao L, Yao ZY, et al. Relationship between 5-HTTLPR polymorphism and post-stroke depression. Genetics and Molecular Research. 2016;**15**(1):1-6. DOI: 10.4238/gmr.15017460. Available from: http://www.funpecrp.com.br/gmr/year2016/vol15-1/pdf/gmr7460.pdf [Accessed: 17 March 2019]

[26] Zhao Q, Guo WY, Yang D, Yang T, Meng X. Serotonin transporter gene 5-HTTLPR polymorphism as a protective factor against the progression of post stroke depression. Molecular Neurobiology. 2016;**53**:1699-1705. DOI: 10.1007/s12035-015-9120-7. Available from: https://link-springer-com.ezproxy.uthsc.edu/content/pdf/10.1007%2Fs12035-015-9120-7.pdf. [Accessed: 01 April 2019]

[27] Lobinoux I, Kronenberg G, Endres M, Schumann-Bard P, Freret T, Filikowski R, et al. Post-stroke depression: Mechanisms, translation and therapy. Journal of Cellular and Molecular Medicine. 2012;**16**(9): 1961-1969. DOI: 10.1111/j.1582-4934.2012.01555.x. Available from: https://www.ncbi.nlm.nih.gov/pmc/articles/PMC3822966/. [Accessed 01 April 2019]

[28] Kohen R, Cain KC, Mitchell PH, Becker K, Buzaitis A, Millard SP, et al. Association of serotonin transporter gene polymorphisms with poststroke depression. Archives of General Psychiatry. 2008;**65**(11):1296-1302. DOI: 10.1001/archpsyc.65.11.1296. Available from: https://www.ncbi.nlm.nih.gov/pmc/articles/PMC2679964/. [Accessed: 01 April 2019]

[29] Kelly-Hayes M. Influence of age and health behaviors on stroke risk: Lessons from longitudinal studies. Journal of American Geriatric Society. 2010;**58**:325-328. DOI: 10.1111/j.1532-5415.2010.02915.x. Available from: https://www.ncbi.nlm.nih.gov/pmc/articles/PMC3006180/ [Accessed: 07 April 2019]

[30] Saposnik G, Cote R, Phillips S, Gubitz G, Bayer N, Minuk J, et al. SORCan Working Group. Stroke outcome in those over 80. Stroke. 2008;**39**(8). DOI: 10.1161/STROKEAHA.107.511402. Available from: https://www.ahajournals.org/doi/10.1161/strokeaha.107.511402 [Accessed: 04 April 2019]

[31] Alexopoulos G, Bruce M, Silbersweig D, Kalayam B, Stern E. Vascular depression: A new view of late-onset depression. Dialogues in Clinical Neuroscience. Sep 1999;**1**(2):68-80. Available from: https://www.ncbi.nlm.nih.gov/pmc/articles/PMC3181568/ [Accessed: 22 March 2019]

[32] Tsuchiya K, Fujita T, Tozato F, Sato D, Midorikawa M, Mariyama Y

et al. Post-stroke depression inhibits improvement in activities of daily living in patients in a convalescent rehabilitation ward. Journal of Physical Therapy Science. 2016;**28**(8):2253-2259. DOI: 10.1589/jpts.28.2253. Available from: https://www.ncbi.nlm.nih.gov/pmc/articles/PMC5011572/ [Accessed: 01 April 2019]

[33] Alexopoulos GS, Meyers BS, Young RC, Kakuma T, Silbersweig D, Charlson M. Clinically defined vascular depression. American Journal of Psychiatry. 1997;(4):562-565. DOI: 10.1176/ajp.154.4.562. Available from: https://www.ncbi.nlm.nih.gov/pubmed/9090349 [Accessed: 21 March 2019]

[34] Gupta R. Hemicraniectomy in malignant middle cerebral artery infarction. Stroke. 2011;**42**(2). DOI: 10.1161/STROKEAHA.110.605642. Available at: https://www.ahajournals.org/doi/10.1161/STROKEAHA.110.605642. [Accessed: 01 April 2019]

[35] Ostwald, S, Turner, I, Bernal, M, Cron, S, Godwin, K. Stress experienced by stroke survivors and spousal caregivers during the first year after discharge from inpatient rehabilitation. Top Stroke Rehabilitation. 2009;**16**(2):93-104. DOI: 10.1310/tsr1602-93. Available from: https://www.ncbi.nlm.nih.gov/pmc/articles/PMC2748854/ [Accessed: 02 April 2019]

[36] Ilut S, Stan A, Blesneag A, Vacaras V, Fonforeanu VS. Factors that influence the severity of post stroke depression. Journal of Medicine and Life;**10**(3):167-171. Available from: https://www.ncbi.nlm.nih.gov/pmc/articles/PMC5652262/. [Accessed: 01 April 2019]

[37] Laures-Gore J, Farina M, Moore E, Russell S. Stress and depression scales in aphasia: relation between the aphasia depression rating scale, stroke aphasia depression questionnaire-10, and the perceived stress scale. Top Stroke Rehabilitation. 2016;**24**(2):114-118. DOI: 10.1080/10749357.2016.1198528. Available from: https://www.ncbi.nlm.nih.gov/pubmed/27348232

[38] Robinson R, Jorge R. Post-stroke depression: A review. American Journal of Psychiatry. 2015;**173**(3):221-231. DOI: 10.1176/appi.ajp.2015.15030363. Available from: https://ajp.psychiatryonline.org/doi/10.1176/appi.ajp.2015.15030363 [Accessed: 14 March 2019]

[39] Bartoli F, Brita C, Crocamo C, Clerici M, Carra G. Early post-stroke depression and mortality: Meta-analysis and meta-regression. Frontiers in Psychiatry. 2018;**9**:530. DOI: 10.3389/fpsyt.2018.00530. Available from: https://www.ncbi.nlm.nih.gov/pmc/articles/PMC6221899 [Accessed 25 March 2019]

[40] Mortense J, Larsson H, Johnsen S, Andersen G. Post stroke use of selective serotonin reuptake inhibitors and clinical outcome among patients with ischemic stroke: A nationwide propensity score-matched follow-up study. Stroke. 2013;**44**(2):420-426. DOI: 10.1161/STROKEAHA.112.674242. Available from: https://www.ncbi.nlm.nih.gov/pubmed/23306326 [Accessed: 17 March 2019]

[41] Chollet F, Tardy J, Albucher J, Thalamas C, Berard E, et al. Fluoxetine for motor recovery after acute ischemic stroke (FLAME): A randomized placebo-controlled trial. Lancet Neurology. 2011;**10**(2):123-130. DOI: 10.1016/S1474-4422(10)70314-8. Available from: https://www.ncbi.nlm.nih.gov/pubmed/21216670 [Accessed: 29 March 2019]

[42] Laporte S, Chapelle C, Caillet P, Beyens M, Bellet F, Delavenne X, et al. Bleeding risk under selective serotonin reuptake inhibitor (SSRI)

antidepressants: A meta-analysis of observational studies. Pharmacological Research. 2017;**118**:19-32. DOI: 10.1016/j.phrs.2016.08.017. Available from: https://www.sciencedirect.com/science/article/abs/pii/S1043661816307769 [Accessed: 24 March 2019]

[43] Micaela Silva S, Carlos Ferrari Corrêa J, da Silva Mello T, Rodrigues Ferreira R, Fernanda da Costa Silva P, Ishida Corrêa F. Impact of depression following a stroke on the participation component of the international classification of functioning, disability and health. Disability and Rehabilitation [s. l.]. 2016;**38**(18):1830-1835. Available from: http://search.ebscohost.com.ezproxy.uthsc.edu/login.aspx?direct=true&db=cmedm&AN=26728302&site=eds-live [cited 1 April 2019]

[44] Pan A, Sun Q, Okereke O, Rexrode, KM, Hu FB. Depression and the risk of stroke morbidity and mortality: A meta-analysis and systematic review. The Journal of the American Medical Association. 2011;**306**(11):1241-1249. DOI: 10.1001/jama.2011.1282. Available at: https://www.ncbi.nlm.nih.gov/pmc/articles/PMC3242806/ [Accessed: 05 April 2019]

[45] Dong J, Zhang YH, Tong J, Qin LQ. Depression and risk of stroke. Stroke. 2011;**43**(1). DOI: 10.1161/STROKEAHA.111.630871. Available at: https://www.ahajournals.org/doi/10.1161/STROKEAHA.111.630871. [Accessed: 02 April 2019]

[46] Towfighi, A, Ovbiagele, B, Husseini, N, et al. Poststroke depression: A scientific statement for healthcare professionals from the American Heart Association/American Stroke Association. Stroke. 2016;**48**(2). DOI: 10.1161/STR.0000000000000113. Available from: https://www.ahajournals.org/doi/10.1161/STR.0000000000000113 [Accessed: 18 March 2019]

[47] Jia H, Damush TM, Qin H, et al. The impact of poststroke depression on healthcare use by veterans with acute stroke. Stroke. 2006;**37**(11). DOI: 10.1161/01.STR.0000244783.53274.a4. [Accessed: 23 April 2019]

[48] Husaini B, Levine R, Sharp L, et al. Depression increases stroke hospitalization cost: An analysis of 17010 stroke patients in 2008 by race and gender. Stroke Research and Treatment. 2013;**2013**:7. DOI: 10.1155/2013/846732. Available from: https://www.ncbi.nlm.nih.gov/pmc/articles/PMC3608101/ [Accessed: 23 April 2019]

[49] Zhao FY, Yue YY, Li L, Lang SY, Wang MW, et al. Clinical practice guidelines for post stroke depression in China. Brazilian Journal of Psychiatry. 2018;**40**(3). DOI: 10.1590/1516-4446-2017-2343. Available from: http://www.scielo.br/scielo.php?script=sci_arttext&pid=S1516-44462018000300325 [Accessed: 04 April 2019]

Section 7

# Healing

Chapter 16

# Available Therapeutics after a Stroke: Current and Promising Options

*María Yolanda Cruz Martínez,*
*Karla Alejandra Cantú Saldaña and*
*José Juan Antonio Ibarra Arias*

## Abstract

Morbidity and mortality after a cerebrovascular event have increased during the past few years, even after extensive efforts have been made concerning research in prevention, acute treatment, pharmacotherapy, revascularization, and rehabilitation. The functional deficits that arise from an ischemic event are related to the increasing chronic disability that results from lower mortality rates. More people are becoming chronically disabled; currently, as much as 90% of survivors are affected and face difficulties to continue with daily life activities. In this chapter, we briefly review the pathophysiology of ischemia and immediate clinical attention to the event. We argue about the need to seek new pharmacological and non-pharmacological alternatives and discuss the most representative in the field of neuroprotection and neurorestoration. In addition, we review the most relevant dietetic strategies and physical rehabilitation therapies, all aimed at improving the survivors' quality of life.

**Keywords:** cerebral ischemia, neuroprotection, neuroregeneration, rehabilitation, immunomodulation

## 1. Introduction

Acute ischemic stroke (AIS) remains the second cause of death worldwide [1], despite showing a mortality rate reduction of 1.19% [2]; only in 2017, there were 6 million 167, 291 deaths; 1, 291,000 more with respect to 1997. During the same period, the survival rate increased by 0.02%; this caused an increment in the disability-adjusted life years percentage (DALYs), which went from 4.17 to 5.29% [2].

Data from the World Health Organization (WHO) indicate that stroke represents the third cause of permanent adult disability worldwide [3], and is present in 90% of survivors. Motor deficits after stroke account for the high rates of long-lasting disability. The most common impairments are related to speech, or language and communication disorders (aphasia and dysphasia), apraxia [4], swallowing, depression, cognitive impairment, and hemiparesis of the contralateral limb [5] characterized by muscle weakness or spasticity in distal rather than proximal muscles [6]. These deficits ultimately cause chronic disability, affecting the ability to


IntechOpen

work and the patient's independence and autonomy for performing daily life activities such as dressing or eating, ensuring they will require long-lasting care, which also deteriorates their quality of life and that of the patients' caregivers.

Stroke complications represent a considerable economic burden both individually and as a society; such complications are associated with a substantial increase in household expenses related to a higher requirement of medical attention, medication, lost workdays, and payment to external or additional caregivers, and in several cases, physical rehabilitation. It is estimated that the United States alone had an annual expenditure of 45.5 billion dollars during the 2014–2015 period, which is only expected to increase through 2035, according to estimations of RTI international [7].

It is therefore fundamental to revisit the procedures regarding basic and clinical research points of view, as well as the most recent recommendations issued by the American Heart Association/American Stroke Association (AHA/ASA), which endorse multiple-component quality improvement initiatives including emergency department education and multidisciplinary teams with neurological management experience, thus increasing the application of fibrinolytic treatment IV.

The strategies that are currently being studied in search of treatments for cerebral ischemia can be categorized into four areas: clinical care, neuroprotection, neurorestoration strategies, and rehabilitation therapy.

The term neuroprotection is defined as the intentional intervention, either inhibition or modulation, that takes place at a certain point during the ischemic cascade, to intervene in a specific mechanism of damage to prevent tissue injury from increasing during the acute phase of ischemia [8]. The neurorestoration is developed through the stimulation of neurogenesis and neuroplasticity to restore the tissue and functional integrity of the neural tissue.

In the clinical setting, several recanalization strategies have been explored to restore blood flow to the injured area of tissue as soon as possible, to assure the lesser damage and decrease secondary sequelae to the original lesion. Finally, physical therapy has become a rehabilitation tactic that has positively impacted the recovery of patients' independence, autonomy, and quality of life, which is worth reviewing.

## 2. Pathophysiology of stroke

Cerebral ischemia is caused by an abrupt and sustained occlusion of blood flow to a large artery that unties a series of biochemical alterations that are known as the ischemic cascade, **Figure 1** [9]; during the development of such changes, a set of mechanisms that lead to cell death occurs: ionic imbalance and excitotoxicity, oxidative stress, and inflammation [10].

The reduction of blood flow leads to a depletion in levels of glucose and $O_2$, which alters aerobic metabolism, increasing lactic acid accumulation. Simultaneously, astrocytes use stored glycogen to provide energy to the neurons in the form of lactate [11]; but, because aerobic metabolism is interrupted at this time, lactic acid continues to accumulate, causing lactic acidosis, which causes ionic dysfunction [12]. Ionic alterations, together with $Na^+/K^+$ pump inactivity, give rise to neuronal depolarization, which leads to the opening of the $Ca^{2+}$ channels and the subsequent release of excitatory neurotransmitters such as glutamate, causing increased activation of ionotropic receptors, especially NMDA, increasing the $Ca^{2+}$ flux into the cell [13].

$Ca^{2+}$ is an essential protagonist within the ischemic cascade since it is capable of activating a significant amount of proteins that lead to cell death, and

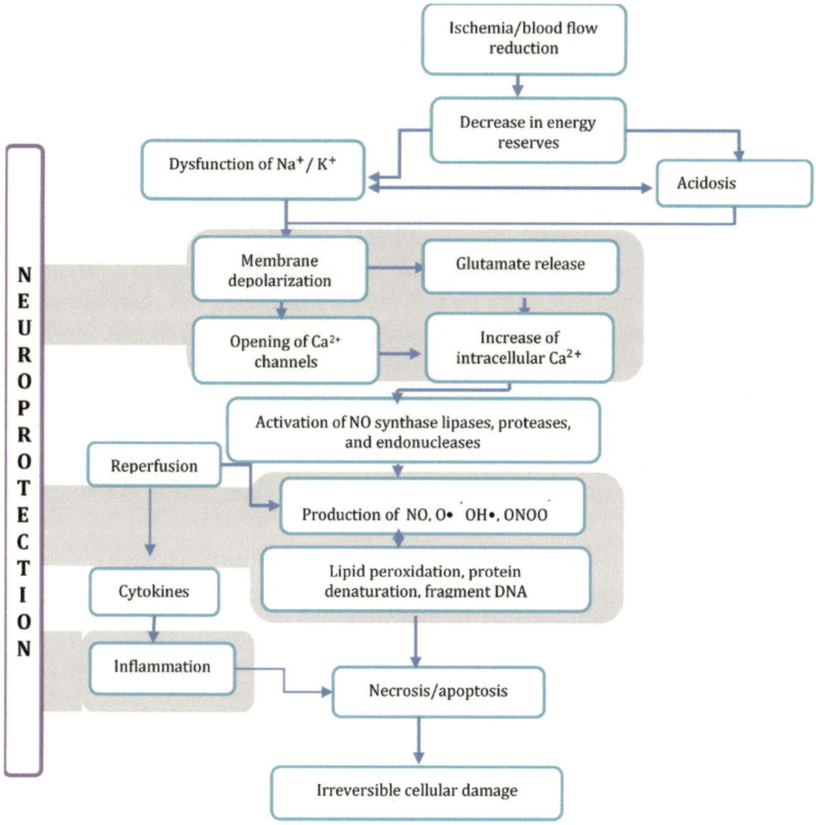


**Figure 1.**
*Key points to the pathophysiology of stroke.*

overproduction of free radicals; such proteins are calpains [14], endonucleases [15], calmodulin [16], and A2 phospholipase (**Figure 1**) [17]. Activation of these proteins leads to a further increase in free radical production and other oxidant species that directly damage structural molecules and activate inflammatory processes [18].

The mitochondria are where the highest production of free radicals takes place; under normal conditions, superoxide anion ($O_2^-$) and hydrogen peroxide ($H_2O_2$) are produced continuously and eliminated by antioxidant enzymes such as superoxide dismutase (SOD), catalase, and glutathione peroxidase [19]. Alternatively, under ischemic conditions, reperfusion provides sufficient substrate for different enzymatic oxidation reactions to take place, causing an overproduction of free oxygen radicals (ROS) and the inactivation of antioxidant enzymes [20]. Concurrently, nitric oxide (NO) increases due to the activation of endothelial and neuronal nitric oxide synthases as a result of increased $Ca^{2+}$ concentration, NO reacts with ROS and forms a highly toxic peroxynitric acid (ONOOH) [21].

Free radicals promote mitochondrial membrane permeability and allow for cytochrome c to be released into the cytosol, where the intrinsic pathway of apoptosis becomes activated, the concentration of free radicals also increases lipid peroxidation and protein denaturalization [22], DNA fragmentation, and activate several signaling pathways that lead to neural death, such as PI3K/AKT [23], Bcl2, p53 [24] and others. From the moment of the occlusion, endothelial cells express damage-associated molecular patterns (DAMPs), produce ROS and adhesion molecules that allow for their activation and that of surrounding mast cells and macrophages, which, as a consequence, release histamine, proteases, TNF-a, and chemokines [25]. The production and release of these molecules promote the blood-brain barrier (BBB) rupturing, thus causing peripheral leukocyte invasion into the injured brain parenchyma [26].

Microglial cells are then activated in the non-perfused region of the brain parenchyma [27], microglial cells acquire phagocytic characteristics and a predominantly pro-inflammatory phenotype (M1), which in turn increases the release of interleukin-6 (IL-6), interleukin 1β (IL-1β), tumor necrosis factor-alpha (TNF-α), NO molecules, and prostanoids [28]. Peripheral immune cells such as neutrophils, B lymphocytes, T lymphocytes, and NK are recruited into the injured tissue, this event is thought to contribute both beneficially by inducing the release of anti-inflammatory cytokines and growth factors, and negatively by increasing the lesion through a sustained release of proinflammatory cytokines and free radicals [29].

Within the process of the ischemic cascade, three points are identified that could classify as strategic to restore neuroprotection (ionic imbalance, excitotoxicity, and inflammation); nonetheless, most neuroprotective drugs act in many of the phases of the ischemic cascade, which is why they cannot be classified into a single step of neuroprotection.

## 3. Current stroke management in the clinical setting: the first step after the stroke

Early diagnosis of stroke is a predictor for better clinical outcomes [30]; therefore, its confirmation is a pressing matter for the treatment to begin as soon as possible from the recognition of symptoms onset [31]. Currently, different strategies for acute ischemic stroke are being used in the clinical setting and are part of the AHA/ASA clinical practice guidelines [32].

The differential diagnosis for stroke includes transient ischemic attacks, seizure, syncope, migraine, and brain tumors [33]. To establish a correct and timely diagnosis and to determine the best course of action, the clinician must rely on laboratory testing [34] (blood glucose is usually high, total cholesterol, LDL, HDL, AST, CPK-MB), and although the gold standard for diagnosis is a cerebral angiography, clinicians try to avoid it by choosing different methods such as imaging testing, including the first-line non-contrast CT scans, CT angiography, MRI, and MRI angiography [32, 35, 36]. In the earliest stages of acute stroke, CT scans are less useful for ischemic stroke diagnosis but can rule out hemorrhagic stroke [36]. Other clinical tests such as EKG, EEG, and the National Institutes of Health Stroke Scale (NIHSS) help establish differential diagnosis and treatment plan [35].

Specific and timely reperfusion treatment is essential to determine the course of the clinical outcome and to improve survival. Once the ischemic etiology has been established, and the patient is stable, treatment should start promptly. Currently, two major therapeutic strategies are being used to treat cerebral ischemia to allow for recanalization and reperfusion. The treatment of choice will depend on time to treatment and etiology of the injury; these therapies are thrombolysis using pharmacological agents and mechanical thrombectomy [35, 37–39].

At present and still after decades, the FDA only approves the use of recombinant tissue plasminogen activator (rTPA), also known as alteplase, as the sole pharmacological option for recanalization [35, 39]. Alteplase initiates local fibrinolysis when administered intravenously by hydrolyzing the peptide bond in plasminogen to form plasmin [40]. The standard IV dosage is 0.9 mg/kg for 60 min, with a 10% bolus over 1 min within 4.5 h of AIS onset [31].

Although alteplase is the only drug available for thrombolysis, most stroke sufferers do not receive this drug as treatment. There usually is a delay in recognition of the symptoms and the time window in which rTPA must be administered is from 3 to 4.5 h from onset of symptoms, and benefits diminish over time [39, 41], which is why the new AHA/ASA guidelines recommend not waiting for clinical improvement before administration [32]. Also, not all patients are eligible, since candidates must be ≤80 years of age, without diabetes or stroke history, with an NIHSS score ≤ 25, not currently taking oral anticoagulation, and without radiologic evidence of ischemic injury involving more than one-third of the MCA territory [42].

Complications that are associated with its use are limited: BBB integrity alterations, and hemorrhagic transformation, granting that other studies have shown it to be well tolerated by patients using warfarin or other anticoagulants [38], in controversy with the new AHA/ASA guidelines that suggest it should not be administered if the patient received heparin 24 h before [32, 35, 43]. Other drugs are also available, such as aspirin, which must be delivered within 24–48 h after stroke onset. Although the guidelines emphasize that it should not be used to replace mechanical thrombectomy or IV alteplase, aspirin continues to be the choice for secondary prophylaxis [32, 44], even when the 2018 guidelines find no benefit from its use for the treatment of an ongoing AIS [32].

Furthermore, the FDA approves of endovascular treatments, which are reported to have a time window of up to 8 hours from the onset of symptoms [38].

For patients with large vessel occlusion, less responsive to rTPA, intra-arterial therapy is recommended, since it leads to higher recanalization rates by being able to infuse the drug directly into the occluded area or the clot itself [35, 45]. About 10% of patients with AIS fall into this category, but only a few centers can perform endovascular procedures in proper conditions [46].

Also, endovascular mechanical thrombectomy using contact aspiration (CA) [47], which has been described before [48], and stent retrievers (SR), especially those of new generations [49], for clot rupturing and aspiration has shown significant benefits in large vessel occlusion [50] regarding clinical outcomes and lower complication rates [49]. Notwithstanding, CA alone, without the use of a SR, is associated with a greater need for rescue treatment, and thus, worse outcomes [51]; the SR might also increase the risk for hemorrhagic transformation and neurological deficit [52].

Increased costs of endovascular treatments, as well as their complexity and need for trained personnel, cause patients to have less access to them. Therefore, exploring new pharmacological therapies should be continued.

## 4. First neuroprotective pharmacological and non-pharmacological treatments

In the search to find new alternatives of neuroprotective agents, a great variety of molecules have been explored that affect one or several strategic points of the pathophysiology, and that promise good results; some are mentioned below.

During the onset of AIS, glucose and oxygen concentrations decrease, and this promotes the activation of adenosine monophosphate-activated protein kinase (AMPK). This process upregulates cellular pathways that control energy metabolism through catabolic pathways such as glycolysis and lipid oxidation to increase adenosine triphosphate (ATP) production and decrease its consumption through the inhibition of gluconeogenesis. Observations have been made regarding the fact that the activation of this enzyme for short periods increases neural survival, but its activation for extended periods will lead to cell death through apoptosis, necrosis, and autophagy [53], which is why several drugs that modulate AMPK activation have been tested recently in search for beneficial effects.

To mention some, metformin has been widely studied for cerebral ischemia since it possesses pleiotropic activity and modulates AMPK activation [54]. In 2016, Zhang et al. administered 7 mg/kg of metformin intraperitoneally to C57BL/6 mice for 7 days, before middle cerebral artery occlusion (MCAO). After MCAO, the authors observed that it induced neuroprotection by reducing infarct size, through lower AMPK, results that were not observed if administered for short periods of 1–3 days before MCAO, or after the occlusion; also, these benefits were not found in the case of reperfusion [55]. Also, the neuroprotective effect of metformin was observed in a global ischemia model in rats; after administration, apoptosis decreased, and mitochondrial biogenesis was induced [56]. Other experiments have demonstrated that metformin has the potential to improve memory and learning through the increase in brain-derived neurotrophic factor (BDNF) and p7056k protein [57]. On the other hand, it has also been implicated in the reduction of IL-6, IL-1β, TNF-α, and adhesion molecule levels, as well as a decrease in neutrophil infiltration [58]. Considering these results, it is crucial to clarify how this modulation is carried out since there is some controversy about the mechanism (**Table 1**).

Atorvastatin is a statin that has pleiotropic effects, since it allows angiogenesis and synaptogenesis, increases blood flow, blunts atherosclerotic plaque formation, and provides neuroprotection in cerebral ischemia model [59] by reducing aquaporin 4 expression (AQP4) [60], thus, preventing cerebral edema and the increase of infarct size. This statin has also been reported to attenuate cognitive deficit [61] through caspase 3 inhibition and avoiding neural death in the CA1 region of the hippocampus.

There is also a great variety of neuroprotective drugs or molecules that act closer by modulating inflammation, through the promotion of an anti-inflammatory microglial phenotype activation; only the most representative will be mentioned below.

DRα1 recombinant protein linked to the MOG peptide has demonstrated the ability to decrease macrophage migration and monocyte activation through its binding to CD74, which translates to a reduction in infarct size [62]. It has also been shown that it reduces proinflammatory cytokine expression, such as IL-1β, I-17, TNF-α, and INF-ϒ, as well as lowers T lymphocyte infiltration and promotes a polarization toward an M2 phenotype macrophage activation [63].

Cop-1 or glatiramer acetate is a copolymer formed by four amino acids (L-alanine, L-lysine, L-glutamic, and L-tyrosine) that has shown to exert neuroprotective effects by being able to reduce infarct size and improve neurological deficit [64]. Cop-1 increases the expression of IL-10, BDNF, Insulin-like growth factor-1 (IGF-1), and neurotrophin (NT-3) in the choroid plexus [65], and the cortex, which stimulates greater neurogenesis [66]. Mangin et al. and their study group obtained similar results; they reported that Cop-1 is capable of reducing COX-2, CD32, TNF-α, and IL-1β, as well as inducing greater neurogenesis and thus, reducing memory loss in mice with cerebral ischemia [67].

On the other hand, food strategies have also been proposed; for example, diet-induced ketosis has demonstrated its neuroprotective effects. Xu et al. observed, in 2017, that the ketogenic diet induced a reduction in infarct size through the overexpression of transcription factors HIF-1α, pAKT, and AMPK [68]; in 2018 Stefanovic, beneficial effects of administering exogenous β-hydroxybutyrate intraperitoneally were also observed in a model of cerebral ischemia induced by endothelin-1 in rats. He reported that the ischemic penumbra cells had a diminished glucose uptake, which translated into less ROS production, astrogliosis, and neuronal death [69]. Ketone bodies or ketosis is worth further exploration since clinical

| Drug | Mechanism | Observed effect | Authors |
|---|---|---|---|
| Metformin | ↓ AMPK<br>↓ Apoptosis | ↓ Infarct size<br>↓ Neurological deficit | Deng et al. [55] |
| | ↑ AMPK<br>↓ Apoptosis | ↓ Infarct size<br>↓ Neurological deficit | Ashabi et al. [56] |
| | ↓ AMPK<br>↑ BDNF<br>↑ P70S6K | ↑ Memory<br>↑ Learning | Ghadernezhad et al. [57] |
| | ↓ AMPK<br>↓ NFkβ<br>↓ IL-6<br>↓ IL-1β<br>↓ TNF-α<br>↓ ICAM<br>↓ Neutrophils | ↑ Protection of blood-brain barrier | Liu et al. [58] |
| Atorvastatin | ↓ Aquaporin AQP4 | ↓ Infarct size<br>↓ Neurological deficit<br>↓ Edema | Cheng et al. [60] |
| | ↓ pJNK3<br>◆ Caspase 3 | ↑ CA1 neurons of the hippocampus | Shao et al. [61] |
| Ketosis | ↑ HIF-α<br>↑ AMPK<br>↑ pAKT | ↓ Infarct size<br>↑ Neural survival | Xu et al. [68] |
| | ↓ ROS<br>↓ Astrogliosis | ↑ Neural survival | Bazzigaluppi et al. [69] |
| DHA | ↓● Macrophages<br>↓● Microglia<br>↓ Leukocyte infiltration<br>↓ TNF-α<br>↓ IL-6<br>↓ IL-1β | ↓ Infarct size<br>↓ Edema<br>↑ Protection of blood-brain barrier | Chang et al. [70] |
| | ↓ Macrophages<br>Neutrophils<br>T lymphocytes<br>B lymphocytes<br>Infiltration<br>■ Polarization of macrophages to M2 | ↓ Infarct size<br>↓ Neurological deficit | Cai et al. [71] |
| | ↑ Neurogenesis | ↓ Infarct size<br>↓ Neurological deficit | Belayev et al. [72] |

| Drug | Mechanism | Observed effect | Authors |
|---|---|---|---|
| DRα-1MOG35-55 | ↓ Macrophages migration<br>↓● Monocytes | ↓ Infarct size | Benedek et al. [62] |
| | ↓ TNF-α<br>↓ IL-17<br>↓ IL-1β<br>↓ INF-ϒ<br>↓ T lymphocytes<br>↓ Infiltration | ↓ Infarct size<br>↑ Motor functions | Wang et al. [63] |
| Cop-1 | Immunomodulation | ↓ Infarct size<br>↓ Neurological deficit | Ibarra et al. [64] |
| | ↑ IL-10<br>↑ BDNF<br>↑ IGF-1<br>↑ NT-3 | ↓ Neurological deficit | Cruz et al. [65]. |
| | ↑ Neurogenesis<br>↑ NT-3 | ↓ Neurological deficit | Cruz et al. [66] |
| | ↓ COX2<br>↓ Cd32<br>↓ TNF-α<br>↓ IL-1β | ↓ Infarct size<br>↓ Neurological deficit<br>↓ Edema<br>■ Memory | Mangin et al. [67] |

◆, *regulation* ; ●, *activation.*

**Table 1.**
*Main neuroprotective agents in ischemia.*

trials in Alzheimer's patients with mild cognitive decline have shown improvements in verbal memory after being treated with a ketogenic diet [73].

Dietary administration with docosahexaenoic acid (DHA) has also proven to have anti-inflammatory and neuroprotective effects in cerebral ischemia through the reduction of proinflammatory cytokine expression, such as TNF-α, IL-1β and IL-6; even, a decrease in macrophage and microglial activation and a decrease in leukocyte infiltration to the lesion site [70]. Similar observations were made by Cai et al. who noted that macrophage, neutrophil, and T and B lymphocyte infiltration was significantly decreased, besides stimulating an anti-inflammatory macrophage (M2) activation [71]; DHA is also capable of inducing neurogenesis and angiogenesis [72], which makes it a promising molecule for future experimental research.

## 5. Neurorestoration

Many of the cytokines and growth factors that result from immunomodulation processes are directly involved in neurorestoration processes, the latter understood as the set of strategies that seek to reconstruct the affected neural circuits through neuroplasticity or neurogenesis [74].

Neurotrophins are a group of proteins that are involved in the maintenance and survival of the central nervous system [75]; this includes BDNF, NT-3, NT-4, NT-5, nerve growth factor (NGF), and IGF-1. Neurotrophins interact with two types of receptors, Trk (tyrosine kinase receptors) and the p75 receptor that belongs to the TNFR receptor family, implicated in apoptosis processes.

Among the most studied neurotrophins are BDNF and NT-3; BDNF is produced by almost all brain cells and is known to participate in processes of proliferation, survival, and neuronal differentiation. Its receptors are widely distributed [76] and activate critical signaling pathways such as PLCγ, PI3K, and ERK, which ultimately lead to phosphorylation and activation of the transcription factor CREB that mediates the expression of genes that are essential for the survival and differentiation of neurons [77]. NT-3 has also been involved in the processes of cell proliferation and differentiation through the notch pathway [78], as well as participating in processes of memory and learning [76].

Experiments have shown that the increase of neurotrophic factors in the ischemia model is commonly related to a better functional or memory recovery and that it is usually associated with neurogenesis or neuroplasticity—as in the case of metformin, which showed an increase in BDNF expression and that induced a more significant recovery of memory and learning [57]. Also, Cop-1 was able to induce the increase of BDNF, IGF-1, and NT-3; which correlated with the increase in neurogenesis [65]; and the experiments of Luan et al. showed that patients with cerebral ischemia who presented higher levels of NGF obtained a better functional recovery at 3 months after the ischemia [79].

Stem cell transplantation has also been linked to better neurological recovery; although clinical trials have not reported the expected results [80], basic research using stem cells has shown an increase in neurological rehabilitation and suggested mechanisms include the overexpression of BDNF and IGF-1 [81, 82], as well as immunomodulatory cytokines like IL-10, which together induce a polarization toward an anti-inflammatory M2 microglial phenotype [83].

In recent years, there has been an increase in the interest of studying how the external environment has a direct effect on the structure and neuronal function, that is, on neuroplasticity [84], and that is why researchers keep studying what kind of external characteristics (specifically physical and social activity) can increase these factors and thereby obtain more significant benefits.

In 2017, Chen et al. explored whether a specific type of environment stimulated the production of BDNF in rats with cerebral ischemia, and what they observed was that physical stimulation increases the expression of neurotrophic factors more than social stimulation and obtains a higher neurological recovery [85]. Mang, on the other hand, observed that the increase in BDNF after an ischemic event is determined by the type of aerobic exercise and the val66met variant of the BDNF gene [86].

The effects on NT-3 have also been evaluated, and the results have been very similar; there is an increase in its levels with physical stimulation after the ischemic event and a more significant functional recovery [87]. Other proteins have also been associated with neuronal plasticity through axonal growth, such as the growth-associated protein 43 (GAP-43), which has been observed to increase when rats with cerebral ischemia undergo fastigial electrostimulation [88].

Electrical stimulation directly into the fastigial nucleus (FNS) has proven to be beneficial in a model of MCAO [89]. The mechanism through which FNS has shown to improve walking balance and neurological scores is due to the activation of the PKA/cAMP pathway, suppressing the expression of Rho-Kinase, and through the overexpression of GAP-43 protein [89].

In this sense, experiments continue to be designed to establish the efficacy of training types and times to modulate inflammation, the production of neurotrophins, and the impact on patient mobility, as in the proposal developed by Scalzo et al. [89] that gives rise to the continued development of a well-founded physical therapy for patients with cerebral ischemia.

## 6. Physical therapy as a coadjuvant to neural restoration through stimulation of neural plasticity

Post-stroke physical rehabilitation (PR) is of utmost importance as a non-pharmacological strategy for neuroprotection and neurorestoration but, most significantly, should be aimed at restoring and regaining motor impairment during the chronic period [90], and to promote the functional autonomy of the patient [4]. Recovery of body function assessment depends on whether the patients can perform everyday activities on their own and is measurable by several different scales such as UE-FM score for the upper extremity, and the Barthel Index for Activities for Daily Living scale [4].

Functional and cognitive deficit severity is related to tissue integrity [91], and it is not clear whether recovery results from biological processes or physical rehabilitation [91, 92]. Some clinical parameters that can be observed at the bedside, such as early finger extension and shoulder abduction, can act as predictors of long-term (over 6 months) recovery after stroke [93]. Spontaneous recovery of upper and lower limbs occurs depending on the type, location, and severity of the lesion, in approximately 60–70% of cases [93] during the first 2–6 months [4, 94], period after which most people believe they have achieved maximal recovery and stop with either physical or pharmacological therapy [4, 95]. Interventions should be designed according to the stage of neurological recovery the patient is in, with the consideration that early chronicity is not a contraindication for continuing rehabilitation [4].

Physical rehabilitation must start early, if possible, during the first week post-stroke [96], because there is an intensification in neuroplasticity during the early stages [91], employing different mechanisms such as the axon regeneration [88], and the higher expression of growth-promoting genes, such as GAP-43. This lesion-induced plasticity that happens during the first days post-stroke [90, 97, 98] reportedly lasts around 6 months after stroke [4, 91, 95, 97]. Also, therapy must continue after such a period, to take advantage of behavior-induced plasticity [95], which is still possible after 1 year of having had the stroke [4].

PR has also been proven to elicit neuroprotection and neurorestoration in other neurological disease models, such as Parkinson's, through the upregulation of BDNF and GDNF and prevention of inflammatory response [99]. The following therapies are currently under study for neurorestorative purposes during the post-stroke chronic period:

Environmental enrichment focuses on inducing adaptation to different environments, including toys and complex tasks, to improve functional outcomes [97]. Also, this type of therapy has shown to enhance angiogenesis by increasing CD31 and VEGF [97]. Furthermore, environmental enrichment upregulates BDNF secretion, and other neurotrophic factors [85, 90].

Wang et al. found improvements in spatial learning and memory, number of synapses, and an increase in the expression of synaptogenesis markers. GAP-43, a protein involved in neural plasticity through axonal growth, is upregulated during the first 28 days after stroke in mice exposed to environmental enrichment. Likewise, other markers involved in synaptogenesis like SYN and PSD-95 achieve better concentrations in the brains of mice treated with environmental enrichment [97].

Functional electrical therapy has been used alongside other types of electrical stimulation to induce repetitive muscular contraction to mobilize certain joints [6]. Somatosensory stimulation might enhance neurorehabilitation after stroke through the stimulation of corticomotoneuronal excitability [6]. It has been proposed that this type of therapy increases muscle strength, reduces spasticity, and facilitates voluntary movements, among other motor benefits [6].

Guided self-rehabilitation (GSR) is a method in which the intensity of training can be increased inside the home environment. While combined with conventional rehabilitation, it has proven to be efficacious in engaging the patients in their recovery through a contract between the patient and the therapist, allowing for an increased sense of responsibility and motivation for the patients, who are required to register their progress in a diary [100]. Although not many physical therapists accept such an approach [100], positive changes have been observed after 1 year of GSR and conventional rehabilitation in ultrasound measuring of the soleus' and medial gastrocnemius' thickness and fascicle length, as well as clinical improvement, observed in soleus extensibility and ambulation speed [101] in chronic stroke patients.

Constraint-induced therapy requires constraining the non-affected limb for 90% of the waking hours, forcing the patient to use the paretic limb, inducing the increase of use-dependent plasticity, although this therapy is not practical for most of the population [6].

Videogame- or virtual reality-based (VRb) therapies have been under study for upper extremity functional recovery in acute and subacute or chronic patients [91, 96, 99, 102]; the rationale for such approaches is that they promote motor learning and repetitive, intense movements, and in the specific case of virtual reality, the patient is exposed to interactive visual, auditive, and proprioceptive feedback [91, 102]. Different videogame and VRb therapies have reported improvements in fine dexterity, grip strength [96], and grasp force [99] in upper extremities, and, activities of daily living [91] and cognition [102] in young and elderly patients after several weeks of rehabilitation. Better results have been observed when combined with conventional therapy, although it is still not known whether it enhances or speeds up recovery [91].

## 7. Final remarks and future directions

In addition to continuing the search for pharmacological agents that allow the neuroprotection and neurorestoration of tissue affected by cerebral ischemia, the development of physical therapy and diet modification offers new horizons that have shown satisfactory results in the clinical setting in short times. However, it has not yet been possible to establish a protocolized treatment that can be added to the health care guidelines; so it is important to continue exploring all possible strategies to improve the quality of life of people who have suffered a cerebral infarction and that of their caregivers.

## Author details

María Yolanda Cruz Martínez[1], Karla Alejandra Cantú Saldaña[1,2] and José Juan Antonio Ibarra Arias[1*]

1 Facultad de Ciencias de la Salud, Centro de Investigación en Ciencias de la Salud (CICSA), Universidad Anáhuac México Norte, Estado de Mexico, Mexico

2 Tecnologico de Monterrey, Escuela de Medicina y Ciencias de la Salud, Monterrey, Nuevo León, México

*Address all correspondence to: jose.ibarra@anahuac.mx

## References

[1] WHO. The Top Ten Causes of Death. Fact Sheet. World Health Organization. Available from: https://www.who.int/en/news-room/fact-sheets/detail/the-top-10-causes-of-death [Accessed: 14 June 2018]

[2] IHME. Global Deaths Rate per 100k, Stroke. G. H. D. Exchange and (GHDx), editor. 2017

[3] Johnson W, Onuma O, Owolabi M, Sachdev S. Stroke: A global response is needed. Bulletin of the World Health Organization. 2016;**94**(9):634-634A

[4] Rubio Ballester B et al. A critical time window for recovery extends beyond one-year post-stroke. Journal of Neurophysiology. 1 July 2019;**122**(1):350-357. DOI: 10.1152/jn.00762.2018

[5] Silva SM, Corrêa FI, Faria CDCdM, Buchalla CM, Silva PF d C, Corrêa JCF. Evaluation of post-stroke functionality based on the international classification of functioning, disability, and health: A proposal for use of assessment tools. Journal of Physical Therapy Science. 2015;**27**(6):1665-1670. DOI: 10.1589/jpts.27.1665

[6] Balasubramanian S. Motor Impairments Following Stroke [Internet]. Unpublished; 2015. DOI: 10.13140/RG.2.1.3349.6804

[7] RTI. Cardiovascular Disease Costs will Exceed $1 Trillion by 2035. Available from: https://www.rti.org/news/cardiovascular-disease-costs-will-exceed-1-trillion-2035 [Accessed: 14 June 2019]

[8] Wahlgren N, Ahmed N. Neuroprotection in cerebral ischaemia: Facts and fancies—The need for new approaches. Cerebrovascular Diseases (Basel, Switzerland). 2004;**17**:153-166

[9] Meschia JF, Brott T. Ischaemic stroke. European Journal of Neurology. 2018;**25**(1):35-40. DOI: 10.1111/ene.13409

[10] Lo EH, Dalkara T, Moskowitz M. Neurological diseases: Mechanisms, challenges and opportunities in stroke. Nature Reviews Neuroscience. 2003;**4**(5):399-415

[11] Obel LF et al. Brain glycogen-new perspectives on its metabolic function and regulation at the subcellular level. Frontiers in Neuroenergetics. 2012;**4**:3. DOI: 10.3389/fnene.2012.00003

[12] Xing C, Arai K, Lo EH, Hommel M. Pathophysiologic cascades in ischemic stroke. International Journal of Stroke. 2012;7(5):378-385. DOI: 10.1111/j.1747-4949.2012.00839.x

[13] Song M, Yu SP. Ionic regulation of cell volume changes and cell death after ischemic stroke. Translational Stroke Research. 2014;**5**(1):17-27. DOI: 10.1007/s12975-013-0314-x

[14] Curcio M, Salazar IL, Mele M, Canzoniero LM, Duarte CB. Calpains and neuronal damage in the ischemic brain: The swiss knife in synaptic injury. Progress in Neurobiology. 2016;**143**:1-35. DOI: 10.1016/j.pneurobio.2016.06.001

[15] Lee BI, Lee DJ, Cho KJ, Kim GW. Early nuclear translocation of endonuclease G and subsequent DNA fragmentation after transient focal cerebral ischemia in mice. Neuroscience Letters. 2005;**386**(1):23-27. DOI: 10.1016/j.neulet.2005.05.058

[16] Coultrap SJ, Vest RS, Ashpole NM, Hudmon A, Bayer KU. CaMKII in cerebral ischemia. Acta Pharmaceutica Sinica B. 2011;**32**(7):861-872. DOI: 10.1038/aps.2011.68

[17] Muralikrishna Adibhatla R, Hatcher JF. Phospholipase A2, reactive

oxygen species, and lipid peroxidation in cerebral ischemia. Free Radical Biology and Medicine. 2006;**40**(3): 376-387. DOI: 10.1016/j.freeradbiomed.2005.08.044

[18] Lai TW, Zhang S, Wang YT. Excitotoxicity and stroke: Identifying novel targets for neuroprotection. Progress in Neurobiology. 2014;**115**: 157-188. DOI: 10.1016/j.pneurobio.2013.11.006

[19] Duchen MR. Roles of mitochondria in health and disease. Diabetes. 2004;**53** (Suppl. 1):S96-S102. DOI: 10.2337/diabetes.53.2007.s96

[20] Granger N, Kvietys P. Reperfusion injury and reactive oxygen species: The evolution of a concept. Redox Biology. 2015;**6**:524-551

[21] Rama R, Rodríguez J. Excitotoxicity and Oxidative Stress in Acute Stroke. 2016. DOI: 10.5772/64991

[22] Allen CL, Bayraktutan U. Oxidative stress and its role in the pathogenesis of ischaemic stroke. International Journal of Stroke. 2009;**4**(6):461-470. DOI: 10.1111/j.1747-4949.2009.00387.x

[23] Sugawara T et al. Neuronal death/survival signaling pathways in cerebral ischemia. NeuroRX. 2004;**1**(1):17-25. DOI: 10.1602/neurorx.1.1.17

[24] Saito A et al. Oxidative stress and neuronal death/survival signaling in cerebral ischemia. Molecular Neurobiology. 2005;**31**(1–3):105-116. DOI: 10.1385/mn:31:1-3:105

[25] Vidale S, Consoli A, Arnaboldi M, Consoli D. Postischemic inflammation in acute stroke. Journal of Clinical Neurology (Seoul, Korea). 2017;**13**(1): 1-9. DOI: 10.3988/jcn.2017.13.1.1

[26] Kim JY, Kawabori M, Yenari MA. Innate inflammatory responses in stroke: Mechanisms and potential therapeutic targets. Current Medicinal Chemistry. 2014;**21**(18):2076-2097

[27] Kim E, Cho S. Microglia and monocyte-derived macrophages in stroke. Neurotherapeutics. 2016;**13**(4): 702-718. DOI: 10.1007/s13311-016-0463-1

[28] Khoshnam SE, Winlow W, Farzaneh M, Farbood Y, Moghaddam HF. Pathogenic mechanisms following ischemic stroke. Neurological Sciences. 2017;**38**(7): 1167-1186. DOI: 10.1007/s10072-017-2938-1

[29] Selvaraj UM, Stowe AM. Long-term T cell responses in the brain after an ischemic stroke. Discovery Medicine. 2017;**24**(134):323-333

[30] Fransen PSS et al. Time to reperfusion and treatment effect for acute ischemic stroke: A randomized clinical trial time to reperfusion and treatment effect for acute ischemic stroke time to reperfusion and treatment effect for acute ischemic stroke. JAMA Neurology. 2016;**73**(2): 190-196. DOI: 10.1001/jamaneurol.2015.3886

[31] Powers William J et al. Guidelines for the early management of patients with acute ischemic stroke: 2019 update to the 2018 guidelines for the early Management of Acute Ischemic Stroke: A guideline for healthcare professionals from the American Heart Association/American Stroke Association. Stroke. 2019;**50**(12):e344-e418. DOI: 10.1161/STR.0000000000000211

[32] Powers William J et al. 2018 guidelines for the early management of patients with acute ischemic stroke: A guideline for healthcare professionals from the American Heart Association/American Stroke Association. Stroke. 2018;**49**(3):e46-e99. DOI: 10.1161/STR.0000000000000158

[33] Gibson LM, Whiteley W. The differential diagnosis of suspected stroke: A systematic review. The journal of the Royal College of Physicians of Edinburgh. 2013;**43**(2):114-118. DOI: 10.4997/jrcpe.2013.205

[34] Lipton SA, Samuels MA. Diagnosis of stroke by CPK isoenzymes. Annals of Neurology. 1982;**11**(4):434-435. DOI: 10.1002/ana.410110421

[35] Khaja AM. Diagnosis and management of ischemic stroke. In: Toth PP, Cannon CP, editors. Comprehensive Cardiovascular Medicine in the Primary Care Setting. Cham: Springer International Publishing; 2019. pp. 349-363

[36] Salmela MB et al. ACR appropriateness criteria((R)) cerebrovascular disease. Journal of the American College of Radiology. 2017;**14** (5s):S34-s61. DOI: 10.1016/j.jacr.2017.01.051

[37] Saver JL et al. Time to treatment with endovascular thrombectomy and outcomes from ischemic stroke: A meta-analysis endovascular thrombectomy and outcomes in ischemic stroke endovascular thrombectomy and outcomes in ischemic stroke. JAMA. 2016;**316**(12):1279-1289. DOI: 10.1001/jama.2016.13647

[38] Jovin TG et al. Thrombectomy within 8 hours after symptom onset in ischemic stroke. The New England Journal of Medicine. 2015;**372**: 2296-2306. DOI: 10.1056/NEJMoa1503780

[39] Campbell BC, Donnan GA, Davis SM. Vessel occlusion, penumbra, and reperfusion—Translating theory to practice. Frontiers in Neurology. 2014;**5**: 194. DOI: 10.3389/fneur.2014.00194

[40] Bansal S, Sangha KS, Khatri P. Drug treatment of acute ischemic stroke. American Journal of Cardiovascular Drugs: Drugs, Devices, and Other Interventions. 2013;**13**(1):57-69. DOI: 10.1007/s40256-013-0007-6

[41] Cheng NT, Kim AS. Intravenous thrombolysis for acute ischemic stroke within 3 hours versus between 3 and 4.5 hours of symptom onset. The Neurohospitalist. 2015;**5**(3):101-109. DOI: 10.1177/1941874415583116

[42] Mendez AA et al. Update in the early management and reperfusion strategies of patients with acute ischemic stroke. Critical Care Research and Practice. 2018;**2018**:9168731. DOI: 10.1155/2018/9168731

[43] Horsch AD et al. Relation between reperfusion and hemorrhagic transformation in acute ischemic stroke. Neuroradiology. 2015;**57**(12):1219-1225. DOI: 10.1007/s00234-015-1577-6

[44] Smith Wade S et al. Mechanical thrombectomy for acute ischemic stroke. Stroke. 2008;**39**(4):1205-1212. DOI: 10.1161/STROKEAHA.107.497115

[45] Alonso de Leciñana M et al. Endovascular treatment in acute ischaemic stroke. A stroke care plan for the region of Madrid. Neurologia. 2013; **28**(7):425-434. DOI: 10.1016/j.nrl.2012.12.009

[46] Furlan AJ. Endovascular therapy for stroke—It's about time. New England Journal of Medicine. 2015;**372**(24): 2347-2349. DOI: 10.1056/NEJMe1503217

[47] Boulanger M et al. First-line contact aspiration vs stent-retriever thrombectomy in acute ischemic stroke patients with large-artery occlusion in the anterior circulation: Systematic review and meta-analysis. Interventional Neuroradiology. 2019; **25**(3):244-253. DOI: 10.1177/1591019918821074

[48] Turk AS et al. Initial clinical experience with the ADAPT technique:

A direct aspiration first pass technique for stroke thrombectomy. Journal of Neurointerventional Surgery. 2014; **6**(3):231-237. DOI: 10.1136/neurintsurg-2013-010713

[49] Broussalis E, Trinka E, Hitzl W, Wallner A, Chroust V, Killer-Oberpfalzer M. Comparison of stent-retriever devices versus the merci retriever for endovascular treatment of acute stroke. American Journal of Neuroradiology. 2013;**34**(2):366. DOI: 10.3174/ajnr.A3195

[50] Mokin M et al. Endovascular treatment of acute ischemic stroke: The end or just the beginning? Neurosurgical Focus. 2014;**36**(1):E5. DOI: 10.3171/2013.10.FOCUS13374

[51] Kang D-H et al. Need for rescue treatment and its implication: Stent retriever versus contact aspiration thrombectomy. Journal of NeuroInterventional Surgery. 2019;**11**: 979-983. DOI: 10.1136/neurintsurg-2018-014696

[52] Coutinho JM et al. Combined intravenous thrombolysis and thromectomy vs. thrombectomy alone for acute ischemic stroke. A pooled analysis of the SWIFT and STAR studies. JAMA Neurology. 1 March 2017; **74**(3):268-274. DOI: 10.1001/jamaneurol.2016.5374

[53] Manwani B, McCullough LD. Function of the master energy regulator adenosine monophosphate-activated protein kinase in stroke. Journal of Neuroscience Research. 2013;**91**(8): 1018-1029. DOI: 10.1002/jnr.23207

[54] Arbelaez-Quintero I, Palacios M. To use or not to use metformin in cerebral ischemia: A review of the application of metformin in stroke rodents. Stroke Research and Treatment. 2017;**2017**: 9756429. DOI: 10.1155/2017/9756429

[55] Deng T et al. Pre-stroke metformin treatment is neuroprotective involving AMPK reduction. Neurochemical Research. 2016;**41**(10):2719-2727. DOI: 10.1007/s11064-016-1988-8

[56] Ashabi G, Khodagholi F, Khalaj L, Goudarzvand M, Nasiri M. Activation of AMP-activated protein kinase by metformin protects against global cerebral ischemia in male rats: Interference of AMPK/PGC-1alpha pathway. Metabolic Brain Disease. 2014; **29**(1):47-58. DOI: 10.1007/s11011-013-9475-2

[57] Ghadernezhad N, Khalaj L, Pazoki-Toroudi H, Mirmasoumi M, Ashabi G. Metformin pretreatment enhanced learning and memory in cerebral forebrain ischaemia: The role of the AMPK/BDNF/P70SK signalling pathway. Pharmaceutical Biology. 2016; **54**(10):2211-2219. DOI: 10.3109/13880209.2016.1150306

[58] Liu Y et al. Metformin attenuates blood-brain barrier disruption in mice following middle cerebral artery occlusion. Journal of Neuroinflammation. 2014;**11**:177. DOI: 10.1186/s12974-014-0177-4

[59] Sabogal AM, Arango CA, Cardona GP, Cespedes AE. Atorvastatin protects GABAergic and dopaminergic neurons in the nigrostriatal system in an experimental rat model of transient focal cerebral ischemia. Biomedica. 2014;**34**(2):207-217. DOI: 10.1590/s0120-41572014000200007

[60] Cheng ZJ, Dai TM, Shen YY, He JL, Li J, Tu JL. Atorvastatin pretreatment attenuates ischemic brain edema by suppressing aquaporin 4. Journal of Stroke & Cerebrovascular Diseases. 2018;**27**(11):3247-3255. DOI: 10.1016/j.jstrokecerebrovasdis.2018.07.011

[61] Shao S et al. Atorvastatin attenuates ischemia/reperfusion-induced hippocampal neurons injury via Akt-nNOS-JNK signaling pathway. Cellular and Molecular Neurobiology. 2017;

**37**(4):753-762. DOI: 10.1007/s10571-016-0412-x

[62] Benedek G et al. A novel HLA-DRalpha1-MOG-35-55 construct treats experimental stroke. Metabolic Brain Disease. 2014;**29**(1):37-45. DOI: 10.1007/s11011-013-9440-0

[63] Wang J, Ye Q, Xu J, et al. DRα1-MOG-35-55 reduces permanent ischemic brain injury. Translational Stroke Research. 2017;**8**(3):284-293. DOI: 10.1007/s12975-016-0514-2

[64] Ibarra A, Avendaño H, Cruz Y. Copolymer-1 (Cop-1) improves neurological recoveryafter middle cerebral artery occlusion in rats. Neuroscience Letters. 2007;**425**:110-113

[65] Cruz Y et al. Release of interleukin-10 and neurotrophic factors in the choroid plexus: Possible inductors of neurogenesis following copolymer-1 immunization after cerebral ischemia. Neural Regeneration Research. 2018; **13**(10):1743-1752. DOI: 10.4103/1673-5374.238615

[66] Cruz Y, Lorea J, Mestre H, Kim-Lee JH, Herrera J, Mellado R, et al. Copolymer-1 promotes neurogenesis and improves functional recovery after acute ischemic stroke in rats. PLoS ONE. 2015;**10**(3):e0121854. DOI: 10.1371/journal.pone.0121854

[67] Mangin G, Poittevin M, Charriaut-Marlangue C, Giannesini C, Merkoulova-Rainon T, Kubis N. Glatiramer acetate reduces infarct volume in diabetic mice with cerebral ischemia and prevents long-term memory loss. Brain, Behavior, and Immunity. 3 April 2019;**80**:315-327. DOI: 10.1016/j.bbi.2019.04.009

[68] Xu K et al. Diet-induced ketosis protects against focal cerebral ischemia in mouse. Advances in Experimental Medicine and Biology. 2017;**977**:205-213. DOI: 10.1007/978-3-319-55231-6_28

[69] Bazzigaluppi P et al. IMAGING the effects of beta-hydroxybutyrate on Peri-infarct neurovascular function and metabolism. Stroke. 2018;**49**(9): 2173-2181. DOI: 10.1161/strokeaha.118.020586

[70] Chang CY et al. Docosahexaenoic acid reduces cellular inflammatory response following permanent focal cerebral ischemia in rats. Journal of Nutritional Biochemistry. 2013;**24**(12): 2127-2137. DOI: 10.1016/j.jnutbio.2013.08.004

[71] Cai W et al. Post-stroke DHA treatment protects against acute ischemic brain injury by skewing macrophage polarity toward the M2 phenotype. Translational Stroke Research. 2018;**9**(6):669-680. DOI: 10.1007/s12975-018-0662-7

[72] Belayev L et al. Docosanoids promote neurogenesis and angiogenesis, blood-brain barrier integrity, penumbra protection, and neurobehavioral recovery after experimental ischemic stroke. Molecular Neurobiology. 2018; **55**(8):7090-7106. DOI: 10.1007/s12035-018-1136-3

[73] Krikorian R, Shidler MD, Dangelo K, Couch SC, Benoit SC, Clegg DJ. Dietary ketosis enhances memory in mild cognitive impairment. Neurobiology of Aging. 2012;**33**(2):425.e19-425.e4.25E27. DOI: 10.1016/j.neurobiolaging.2010.10.006

[74] Kidd PM. Integrated brain restoration after ischemic stroke—Medical management, risk factors, nutrients, and other interventions for managing inflammation and enhancing brain plasticity. Alternative Medicine Review. 2009;**14**(1):14-35

[75] Song M, Martinowich K, Lee FS. BDNF at the synapse: Why location matters. Molecular Psychiatry. 2017; **22**(10):1370-1375

[76] Vilar M, Mira H. Regulation of neurogenesis by neurotrophins during adulthood: Expected and unexpected roles. Frontiers in Neuroscience. 2016; **10**(26):1-9

[77] Cunha C, Brambilla R, Thomas KL. A simple role for BDNF in learning and memory? Frontiers in Molecular Neuroscience. 2010;**3**:1. DOI: 10.3389/neuro.02.001.2010

[78] Yan YH et al. Neurotrophin-3 promotes proliferation and cholinergic neuronal differentiation of bone marrow-derived neural stem cells via notch signaling pathway. Life Sciences. 2016;**166**:131-138. DOI: 10.1016/j.lfs.2016.10.004

[79] Luan X et al. High serum nerve growth factor concentrations are associated with good functional outcome at 3months following acute ischemic stroke. Clinica Chimica Acta. 2019;**488**:20-24. DOI: 10.1016/j.cca.2018.10.030

[80] Moniche F et al. Intra-arterial bone marrow mononuclear cells in ischemic stroke: A pilot clinical trial. Stroke. 2012; **43**(8):2242-2244. DOI: 10.1161/STROKEAHA.112.659409

[81] Xiang J et al. Bone marrow mesenchymal stem cells-conditioned medium enhances vascular remodeling after stroke in type 2 diabetic rats. Neuroscience Letters. 2017;**644**:62-66. DOI: 10.1016/j.neulet.2017.02.040

[82] Hsuan YC, Lin CH, Chang CP, Lin MT. Mesenchymal stem cell-based treatments for stroke, neural trauma, and heat stroke. Brain and Behavior. 2016;**6**(10):e00526. DOI: 10.1002/brb3.526

[83] Yang B et al. Multipotent adult progenitor cells enhance recovery after stroke by modulating the immune response from the spleen. Stem Cells. May 2017;**35**(5):1290-1302. DOI: 10.1002/stem.2600

[84] Castren E, Antila H. Neuronal plasticity and neurotrophic factors in drug responses. Molecular Psychiatry. 2017;**22**(8):1085-1095. DOI: 10.1038/mp.2017.61

[85] Chen X, Zhang X, Liao W, Wan Q. Effect of physical and social components of enriched environment on astrocytes proliferation in rats after cerebral ischemia/reperfusion injury. Neurochemical Research. 2017;**42**(5): 1308-1316. DOI: 10.1007/s11064-016-2172-x

[86] Mang CS, Campbell KL, Ross CJD, Boyd LA. Promoting neuroplasticity for motor rehabilitation after stroke: Considering the effects of aerobic exercise and genetic variation on brain-derived neurotrophic factor. Physical Therapy. 2013;**93**(12):1707-1716. DOI: 10.2522/ptj.20130053

[87] Chung JY, Kim MW, Im W, Hwang IK, Bang MS, Kim M. Expression of Neurotrophin-3 and trkC following focal cerebral ischemia in adult rat brain with treadmill exercise. BioMed Research International. 2017;**2017**: 9248542. DOI: 10.1155/2017/9248542

[88] Wang A-r, Hu M-z, Zhang Z-l, Zhao Z-y, Li Y-b, Liu B. Fastigial nucleus electrostimulation promotes axonal regeneration after experimental stroke via cAMP/PKA pathway. Neuroscience Letters. 2019;**699**:177-183. DOI: 10.1016/j.neulet.2019.02.016

[89] Oliveira DMG et al. Aerobic training efficacy in inflammation, Neurotrophins, and function in chronic stroke persons: A randomized controlled trial protocol. Journal of Stroke & Cerebrovascular Diseases. 2019;**28**(2): 418-424. DOI: 10.1016/j.jstrokecerebrovasdis.2018.10.016

[90] Corbett D, Nguemeni C, Gomez-Smith M. How can you mend a broken brain?—Neurorestorative approaches to stroke recovery. Cerebrovascular

Diseases. 2014;**38**(4):233-239. DOI: 10.1159/000368887

[91] Ho TH et al. Impact of virtual reality-based rehabilitation on functional outcomes in patients with acute stroke: A retrospective case-matched study. Journal of Neurology. 2019;**266**(3):589-597. DOI: 10.1007/s00415-018-09171-2

[92] Jeffers MS, Karthikeyan S, Corbett D. Does stroke rehabilitation really matter? Part A: Proportional stroke recovery in the rat. Neurorehabilitation and Neural Repair. 2018;**32**(1):3-6. DOI: 10.1177/1545968317751210

[93] Nijland RH, van Wegen EE, Harmeling-van der Wel BC, Kwakkel G. Presence of finger extension and shoulder abduction within 72 hours after stroke predicts functional recovery: Early prediction of functional outcome after stroke: The EPOS cohort study. Stroke. Apr 2010;**41**(4):745-750. DOI: 10.1161/strokeaha.109.572065

[94] Smith M-C, Byblow Winston D, Barber PA, Stinear Cathy M. Proportional recovery from lower limb motor impairment after stroke. Stroke. 2017;**48**(5):1400-1403. DOI: 10.1161/STROKEAHA.116.016478

[95] Gracies J-M et al. Guided self-rehabilitation contract vs conventional therapy in chronic stroke-induced hemiparesis: NEURORESTORE, a multicenter randomized controlled trial. BMC Neurology. 2019;**19**(1):39. DOI: 10.1186/s12883-019-1257-y

[96] Vanbellingen T, Filius SJ, Nyffeler T, van Wegen EEH. Usability of videogame-based dexterity training in the early rehabilitation phase of stroke patients: A pilot study. Frontiers in Neurology. 2017;**8**:654. DOI: 10.3389/fneur.2017.00654

[97] Wang C-J, Wu Y, Zhang Q, Yu K-W, Wang Y-Y. An enriched environment promotes synaptic plasticity and cognitive recovery after permanent middle cerebral artery occlusion in mice. Neural Regeneration Research. 2019;**14**(3):462-469. DOI: 10.4103/1673-5374.245470

[98] Carmichael ST, Archibeque I, Luke L, Nolan T, Momiy J, Li S. Growth-associated gene expression after stroke: Evidence for a growth-promoting region in peri-infarct cortex. Experimental Neurology. 2005;**193**(2):291-311. DOI: 10.1016/j.expneurol.2005.01.004

[99] Iosa M et al. Leap motion controlled videogame-based therapy for rehabilitation of elderly patients with subacute stroke: A feasibility pilot study. Topics in Stroke Rehabilitation. 2015;**22**(4):306-316. DOI: 10.1179/1074935714z.0000000036

[100] Marsal C, Gracies J-M, Dean C, Mesure S, Bayle N. Beliefs of rehabilitation professionals towards guided self-rehabilitation contracts for post stroke hemiparesis. Topics in Stroke Rehabilitation. 2017;**24**(8):608-613. DOI: 10.1080/10749357.2017.1373501

[101] Pradines M et al. Ultrasound structural changes in triceps surae after a 1-year daily self-stretch program: A prospective randomized controlled trial in chronic hemiparesis. Neurorehabilitation and Neural Repair. 2019;**33**(4):245-259. DOI: 10.1177/1545968319829455

[102] Lee K-H. Effects of a virtual reality-based exercise program on functional recovery in stroke patients: Part 1. Journal of Physical Therapy Science. 2015;**27**(6):1637-1640. DOI: 10.1589/jpts.27.1637

Chapter 17

# Rehabilitation Strategies and Key Related Mechanisms Involved in Stroke Recovery

*Hideki Nakano*

## Abstract

Poststroke rehabilitation requires a thorough understanding of the neural mechanisms underlying motor function recovery. This chapter outlines these mechanisms and also discusses the corresponding rehabilitation strategies based on the functional characteristics of the brain. The main topics we discuss are as follows: Although ipsilateral brain region activity is inhibited when using the limbs under normal conditions, it is thought that a decrease in this inhibition and the subsequent increased ipsilateral brain area activity post-injury promote recovery in the damaged contralateral neural network. For optimal poststroke motor function recovery, it is important to normalize the resulting imbalance in brain activity. Therefore, increased corticomotor excitation in the injured hemisphere or decreased excitation in the non-injured hemisphere must be promoted. Rehabilitation strategies include reducing non-paretic limb somatosensory input to decrease excitation in the non-injured hemisphere, increasing paretic limb somatosensory input to increase excitation in the injured hemisphere, increasing excitation in the injured hemisphere through movement training of the paretic hand and anesthesia of the paretic upper arm, increasing excitation in the injured hemisphere, or reducing excitation in the non-injured hemisphere. Considering the functional characteristics of the primary motor area, during the early stages after stroke, it is important to increase the somatosensory input to the paralyzed side and combine mental practices using motor imagery.

**Keywords:** neurorehabilitation, stroke, brain injury, neural plasticity, functional recovery, motor imagery, mental practice

## 1. Introduction

Stroke is a central nervous system condition that is prevalent worldwide. According to a report from the World Health Organization [1], approximately 15 million people experience a stroke each year globally, and stroke is the third leading cause of death after heart disease and cancer. As impairment of motor function after a stroke drastically impedes activities of daily living (ADL) and reduces the quality of life [2], the development of effective rehabilitation methods, which encourage the recovery of motor function in patients who have sustained a stroke, is an important task.

Although the 2014 Cochrane Stroke Systematic Review reported several rehabilitation methods demonstrating moderate results in the recovery of upper limb motor function after a stroke, a highly effective method is yet to be established [3]. Understanding the neural mechanisms underlying motor function recovery after brain injury is indispensable for the development of highly effective poststroke rehabilitation strategies. Therefore, in this chapter we will outline these mechanisms and introduce strategies based on these mechanisms as well as on the functional characteristics of the brain.

## 2. Brain reorganization after brain injury

The brain is a highly plastic organ with the ability to reorganize as a result of learning or injury. In cases of injury in the motor cortex or corticospinal tract, the recovery of motor function is taken care of by the surviving brain regions. Dancause [4] has reported on cortical reorganization accompanying injury in the primary motor cortex. Neurons in the hand area of the primary motor cortex receive input from the fingers as well as the wrist/forearm, and signals are sent from the hand area of the primary motor cortex to the corresponding ipsilateral premotor area. If the hand area of the primary motor cortex is injured, elimination of the inhibitory neurons in the primary motor cortex leads to an increase in the input to the hand area from the wrist/forearm. This results in an enlargement of the wrist/forearm area and shrinking of the hand area of the ipsilateral premotor area. However, as inhibitory neurons at the non-injured side are eliminated, the hand area of the premotor area and the primary motor cortex at the non-injured side also enlarge. Subsequently, reorganization leading to functional recovery occurs through learning and practice. The hand area of the primary motor cortex continues to enlarge as networks are stimulated or adjacent areas are inhibited through changes in synaptic receptor density or the creation of new synapses due to neuroplasticity. Neural networks are also reorganized through the formation of new connections between neurons and axonal sprouting. Thus, brain areas in both the injured and non-injured hemispheres are involved in the functional repair process accompanying recovery after brain injury.

Premotor area activity is also important for the recovery of motor function after a brain injury. Apart from being responsible for certain functions of the motor network, the premotor area is also involved in the integration of sensory and cognitive information in the course of goal-oriented behavior (actions carried out with a clearly established goal or aim, such as ADL). It receives sensory information from the parietal lobe and cognitive information from the dorsolateral prefrontal cortex and the supplementary motor cortex, which are then integrated and sent to the primary motor cortex. This information is also sent directly to the spinal cord via the corticospinal tract. These neural network connections are highly susceptible to plastic changes resulting from injury, learning, training, or therapy. Kantak et al. [5] discuss the reorganization of the premotor area involved in promoting motor function recovery after a brain injury. Reorganization of the premotor area on the injured/non-injured sides in the context of motor function recovery is influenced by the extent and site of the damage. For example, in cases of localized damage to the primary motor cortex or corticospinal tract, patients experience mild functional impairment. In this event, the premotor area on the injured side assists in the recovery of motor function, simultaneously increasing direct input to the corticospinal tract and to the remaining area of the primary motor cortex on the injured side. In cases of extensive damage to the primary motor cortex or corticospinal tract, patients exhibit severe functional impairment. In contrast to cases of localized injury, in these cases, the premotor area on the non-injured side increases input to the surviving sensorimotor area of the injured side. Thus, the premotor areas of the injured and non-injured sides are involved in reorganization contributing to motor function recovery post-brain injury by way of two different strategies.

It is known that reorganization of the brain after an injury changes over time along with recovery of motor function. Nishimura et al. [6] caused injury to the corticospinal tracts of monkeys and then carried out rehabilitation to examine the changes in brain activity during the initial phase (1 month) and the stable phase (3 months) of motor function recovery. The study confirmed activity in both the contralateral and ipsilateral primary motor cortices during the initial recovery phase, during which the pinching motion success rate was 80%. Meanwhile, when the success rate reached 100% for the same motion during the stable recovery phase, ipsilateral primary motor cortex activity decreased, while contralateral activity increased and the contralateral area expanded. Based on this study, although the activity of ipsilateral brain regions is inhibited when using the hands or feet under normal situations, it is thought that a decrease in this inhibition and the subsequent activity in the ipsilateral brain areas post-injury promote recovery in the damaged contralateral neural network. Furthermore, it can be concluded that when the injured neural network has recovered substantially, either through repair of the original network or the mobilization of an adjacent network, the ipsilateral brain area returns to a state of inhibition similar to that observed before the injury.

Similarly, the abovementioned phenomenon can be observed in the process of motor function recovery in stroke patients. Using functional magnetic resonance imaging (fMRI), Ward et al. [7] explored the correlation between stroke patient motor outcomes (motor function evaluations) 3 months after the onset and brain activity when performing a visually induced motor task with the paretic hand,. The results demonstrated that the number of motor-related brain areas utilized during the motor task was higher in patients with a poor outcome, while patients with a favorable outcome utilized fewer of these areas—a pattern of brain activity close to that of healthy individuals. Further, a negative correlation between motor outcome and the activity of task-related brain areas, such as the supplementary motor area, cingulate motor area, premotor cortex, posterior parietal cortex, and cerebellum, was shown. This negative correlation was confirmed for both the non-injured and injured primary motor cortices. Thus, it was understood that when performing motions with the paretic hand, the worse a patient's poststroke motor function, the more bilateral their brain activity. In a similar study, Rehme et al. [8] used fMRI to investigate longitudinal changes in motor network activity during the recovery of motor function in the initial phase after stroke onset. The authors measured the motor function recovery score and brain activity during movement of the non-paretic and paretic hands in stroke patients 2, 5, and 10 days after onset. The results demonstrated activity of the bilateral primary motor cortex, dorsal and ventral premotor area, and supplementary motor cortex during movement of the paretic hand in stroke patients (**Figure 1B**). Further, when the results were compared by level of motor function impairment, patients with mild impairment showed activity resembling that of healthy individuals at 2, 5, and 10 days, whereas patients with severe impairment showed increased bilateral activity over time (**Figure 1C**). As this bilateral activity demonstrated a positive correlation with motor function recovery (**Figure 1D**), it is thought to reflect neural restructuring in the initial phase after a stroke.

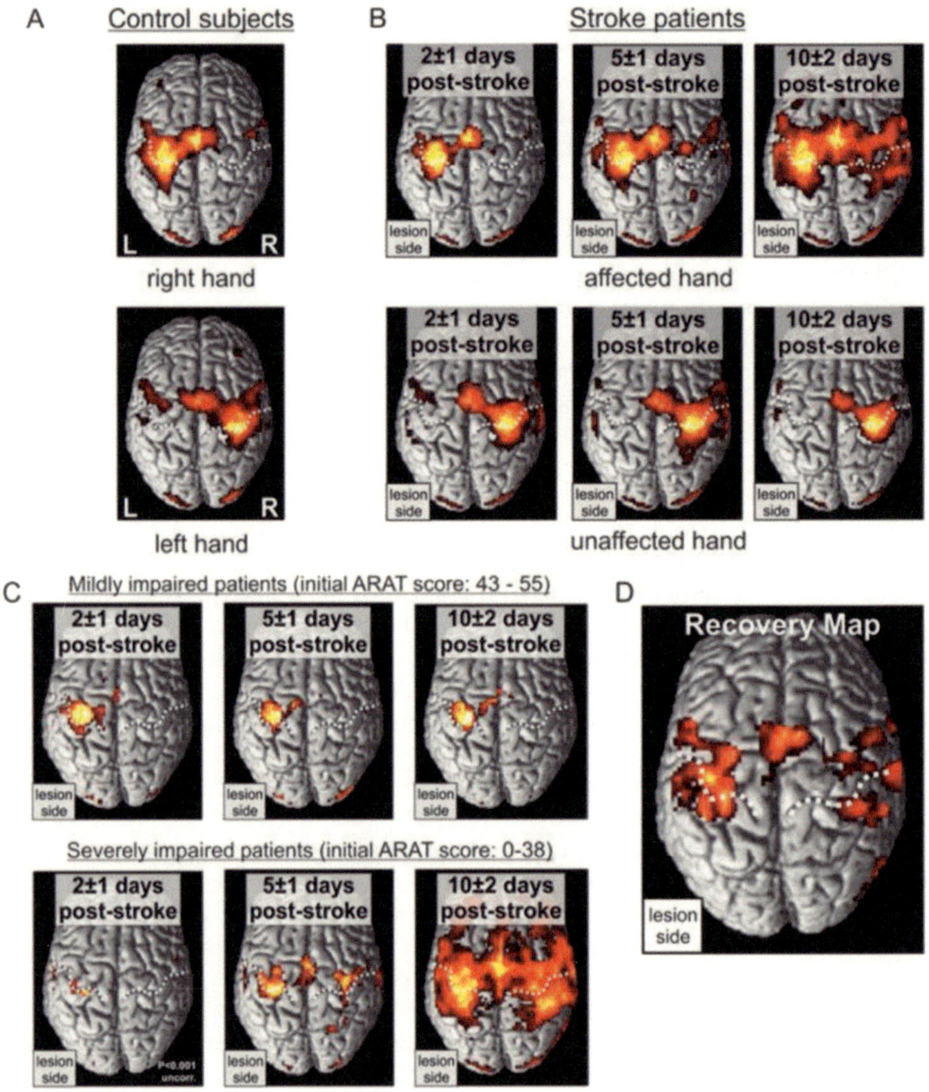


**Figure 1.**
*Longitudinal changes in motor network activity in the initial phase after stroke onset [8]. (A) Brain activity during right/left hand movement in healthy adults. (B) Brain activity during non-paretic/paretic hand movement in stroke patients (2, 5, and 10 days after onset). Bilateral activation is expanded for the paretic hand. (C) Brain activity during paretic hand movement for mild and severe stroke patients (2, 5, and 10 days after onset). In patients with mild functional impairment, only the contralateral hemisphere is active, whereas the activity in both hemispheres expands for severe patients. (D) Map of brain regions involved in favorable motor function recovery.*

## 3. Interhemispheric inhibition imbalance after brain injury

Interhemispheric inhibition refers to the phenomenon in which activation of one side of the cerebrum inhibits the activity of neurons in the opposite side of the brain [9]. In humans, sensory information from the right half of the body is normally conveyed to the neocortex of the left hemisphere, while sensory information from the left half of the body is conveyed to the neocortex of the right hemisphere. The left and right neocortices are connected via the corpus callosum. The inhibition of information exchange between the left and right hemispheres allows humans to move the bilateral upper and lower limbs dexterously. Recent research has revealed the mechanism of this neural network of interhemispheric inhibition. Palmer et al.

[10] explored neuronal activity in the left and right brain of conscious rats with foot stimulation in order to observe nerve activity in a more natural setting. This study revealed the following series of events: when information is conveyed to one side of the neocortex, excitatory information is conveyed to the other side via the corpus callosum, activating the inhibitory nerve cells that exist on its surface and releasing gamma aminobutyric acid (GABA)—an inhibitory neurotransmitter—within the brain. GABA binds to $GABA_B$ receptors on the dendrites of pyramidal neurons within layer V of the neocortex, thereby inhibiting nerve activity.

However, this interhemispheric inhibition between the left and right brain becomes imbalanced after a brain injury, leading to various dysfunctions. Grefkes et al. [11] investigated the functional intrahemispheric and interhemispheric connections of motor-related areas during voluntary hand movement in healthy individuals and stroke patients using fMRI. Interhemispheric inhibition functioned normally as described above for healthy individuals; it was found that in the resting condition, the left and right brain inhibited one another, while motor-related areas within each hemisphere stimulated one another (**Figure 2A**). It was further found that when healthy individuals moved the right hand, inhibition from the right hemisphere to the left hemisphere ceased, and inhibition from the left hemisphere to the right hemisphere was activated (**Figure 2B**). However, in contrast to healthy individuals, when stroke patients moved the paretic right hand, the right hemisphere (non-injured primary motor cortex) was found to inhibit the left hemisphere (injured primary motor cortex) (**Figure 2C**), such that the stronger the inhibition, the lower the motor performance in the paretic hand (**Figure 2D**). Use-dependent plasticity (use-dependent reorganization) is involved in this imbalance in interhemispheric inhibition in stroke patients [12]. Stroke causes paresis of the upper and lower limbs resulting in reduced motor function. As such, stroke patients commonly disuse the paretic limbs while overusing the non-paretic limbs. This poststroke disuse of the paretic and overuse of the non-paretic limbs—in other words, imbalance in the frequency of use for paretic vs. non-paretic limbs—is believed to influence the balance of the left and right cerebrum.

How does the disuse of the paretic limbs and overuse of the non-paretic limbs influence the left and right cerebrum in reality? Avanzino et al. [13] established an environment resembling that of a hemiplegic patient to explore the effect of restraining one-sided upper limb use in healthy individuals on interhemispheric balance using transcranial magnetic stimulation (TMS). To examine cortical changes due to abnormal unequal use of the hands, two experimental groups were compared: a group in which one hand (right) was fixed in place but the loose hand (left) could be moved freely and a group in which use of the left hand was also restricted. Note that the upper limbs were restrained for a period of 10 min. Despite the short restraint period, disuse of the right upper limb was found to decrease excitation in the left primary motor cortex and reduce interhemispheric inhibition from the left hemisphere to the right for both groups. Further, the group that not only disused the right upper limb but also overused the left upper limb showed increased excitatory activity in the primary motor cortex of the right hemisphere and increased interhemispheric inhibition from the right hemisphere to the left. Thus, it was revealed that disuse of one upper limb and overuse of the other—that is, imbalance in usage frequency between both upper limbs—causes imbalance between the cerebral hemispheres.

The hypothesis regarding the imbalance in interhemispheric inhibition post-brain injury is called the abnormal interhemispheric inhibition hypothesis [14, 15]. It states that in cases of subcortical brain injury, an abnormal inhibitory effect arises from the non-injured hemisphere, in which there is increased excitation, to the injured hemisphere. There are two conceivable strategies for

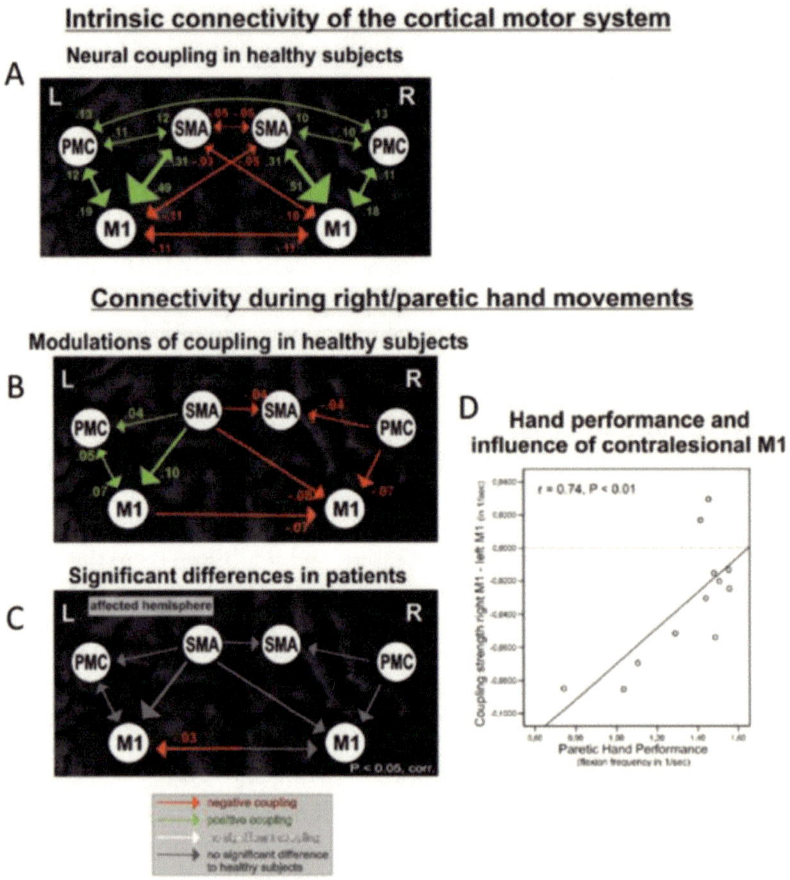


**Figure 2.**
*Differences in cortical connectivity between healthy adults and stroke patients [11]. Green arrows represent excitation and red arrows represent inhibition. (A) Intra-/interhemispheric functional connectivity in healthy adults at rest. (B) Intra-/interhemispheric functional connectivity in healthy adults during voluntary movement of the right hand. (C) Intra-/interhemispheric functional connectivity in stroke patients during voluntary movement of the paretic hand (right hand). (D) Correlation between interhemispheric inhibition of the primary motor cortex and motor performance for the paretic hand (right hand) in stroke patients. The stronger the inhibition from the non-injured hemisphere to the injured hemisphere, the more the paretic hand motor performance was reduced.*

treatment interventions corresponding to this hypothesis: increasing corticomotor excitation in the injured hemisphere or decreasing excitation in the non-injured hemisphere. Approaches for these strategies are known as hypothesis-driven approaches (**Figure 3**) [16]. Specifically, proposed methods include (1) reducing non-paretic limb somatosensory input in order to decrease excitation of the non-injured hemisphere, (2) increasing paretic limb somatosensory input in order to increase excitation of the injured hemisphere, (3) increasing excitation in the injured hemisphere through a combination of movement training of the paretic hand and anesthesia of the paretic upper arm, (4) directly increasing excitation in the injured hemisphere, or (5) directly reducing excitation in the non-injured hemisphere. With regard to procedures to directly manipulate excitation in one hemisphere, as in methods (4) and (5), effects can be exerted through the use of noninvasive brain stimulation methods such as transcranial direct current stimulation (tDCS) or repetitive transcranial magnetic stimulation (rTMS). These methods of stimulation bring about changes that are similar to long-term potentiation or long-term depression, resulting in increased or reduced excitation,

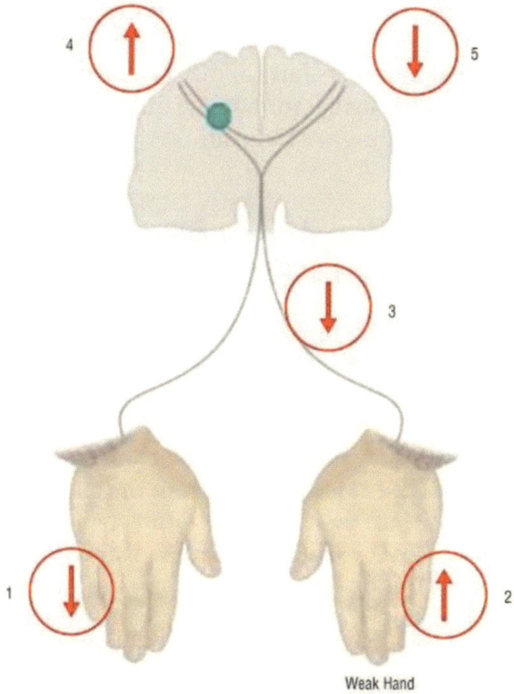


**Figure 3.**
*Approach based on the abnormal interhemispheric inhibition hypothesis (hypothesis-driven approach) [16]. (1) Reducing non-paretic limb somatosensory input in order to decrease excitation in the non-injured hemisphere. (2) Increasing paretic limb somatosensory input in order to increase excitation in the injured hemisphere. (3) Increasing excitation in the injured hemisphere through a combination of movement training of the paretic hand and anesthesia of the paretic upper arm. (4) Directly increasing excitation in the injured hemisphere. (5) Directly reducing excitation in the non-injured hemisphere.*

respectively, at the stimulation site. Regarding the efficacy of these methods, Hsu et al. [17] performed a meta-analysis that showed that rTMS was effective in motor function recovery in stroke patients. It was also reported in the 2011 Cochrane Review [18] that tDCS improved ADL function poststroke. At present, it has been established that the effects of rTMS and tDCS work on cortical neuromodulation and do not cause direct recovery from paresis. In other words, these methods are used for preconditioning to create a more plastic state in the brain or to stabilize the activity of the cerebral cortex. It is thought that these effects can be demonstrated with a combination of motor therapy, which is based on the process of motor learning. Constraint-induced movement therapy (CI therapy), established by Wolf et al. [19] and Taub et al. [20], is representative methods (1) and (2). In CI therapy, the non-paretic upper limb is first restrained in a sling or with a mitten to create a situation in which the patient is forced to use the paretic upper limb. Voluntary movement is then induced on the paretic side with intensive tasks of incremental difficulty levels leading to improvement in motor function. Regarding the results of this method, the 2009 Cochrane Review [21] confirmed the short-term effects on the recovery of motor function in stroke patients directly after CI therapy intervention. A meta-analysis by Langhorne et al. [22] about the effects of various rehabilitation methods on upper limb paresis in stroke patients also found that CI therapy had better intervention effects than other methods and that there was little variation among such effects. In addition, recent studies have used randomized comparative experiments to study the effects of behavioral strategies for the utilization of function acquired through CI therapy in daily life (transfer package) [23, 24], as well as research examining the effects of motor therapy, which combines CI therapy with the abovementioned rTMS and tDCS [25, 26]. In this way, it is essential that motor therapy in the rehabilitation of stroke patients be developed with sufficient consideration to the imbalance in interhemispheric inhibition between the left and right cerebrum.

## 4. Rehabilitation strategies based on the functional characteristics of the brain and advances in clinical practice guidelines

Research by Geyer et al. [27] showed that the human primary motor cortex consists of two different regions: the anterior portion (IVa area) and the posterior portion (IVp area). These two regions differ in cell structure and receptor density. The IVa area is located in the anterior (rostral) portion of the primary motor cortex. This area is phylogenetically ancient and is thus referred to as the old primary motor cortex (Old M1). Outputs from the Old M1 control physical movement via the corticospinal tract and spinal interneurons. Meanwhile, the IVp area is found in the posterior (caudal) portion of the primary motor cortex and, being a newer section of the motor cortex compared to the IVa, is known as the New M1. New M1 includes cortical motoneurons, which synapse directly with spinal motoneurons. These synaptic connections are not mediated by spinal interneurons and are involved in the execution of extremely masterful and complex movements [28].

In light of the neural network functional disparity between the IVa and IVp areas of the primary motor cortex, Sharma et al. [29] proposed the somatosensory feedback for the paretic limb as one factor influencing the recovery of motor function after stroke (**Figure 4A**). The authors suggested that increased neural activity in the IVp area due to somatosensory input is involved in the recovery of motor function. Loubinoux et al. [30] investigated brain areas involved in motor function recovery for stroke patients using fMRI. They found that stroke patients with high neural activity in the IVp area had favorable motor function recovery in the hand and that neural activity in the IVp area predicted motor performance 1 year later. This suggests that early poststroke stimulation of neural activity in the IVp area of the injured hemisphere is critical for rehabilitation. As described above, the IVa and IVp areas are structurally disparate, but they are also functionally different with respect to afferent somatosensory information processing. Strick et al. [31] investigated differences in neural activity in the rostral (IVa) and caudal (IVp) areas of the primary motor cortex in monkeys using inputs from different sensory modalities. Their study found that the rostral primary motor cortex has plentiful cells that respond to the characteristic sensory input of muscles and joints, while the caudal area has an abundance of cells responding to cutaneous sensation input. Thus, it was suggested that providing cutaneous sensation to the paretic limb was important for increasing excitation in the IVp area. It was further found that neural activity in this IVp area was influenced by actively drawing attention. Binkofski et al. [32] examined the effect that directing attention to behavior had on neural activity in the IVa and IVp areas of the human primary motor cortex using fMRI. The authors found that the neural activity in the IVp area was affected by drawing attention to behavior, but this effect was not present in the IVa area. This suggested that apart from providing simple sensory stimulation, directing participants' active attention would also be beneficial for increasing neural activity in the IVp area. To summarize, for poststroke motor function recovery, it is considered important to increase the neural activity of the IVp area by providing somatosensory input to the paretic limb while capturing the patient's active attention.

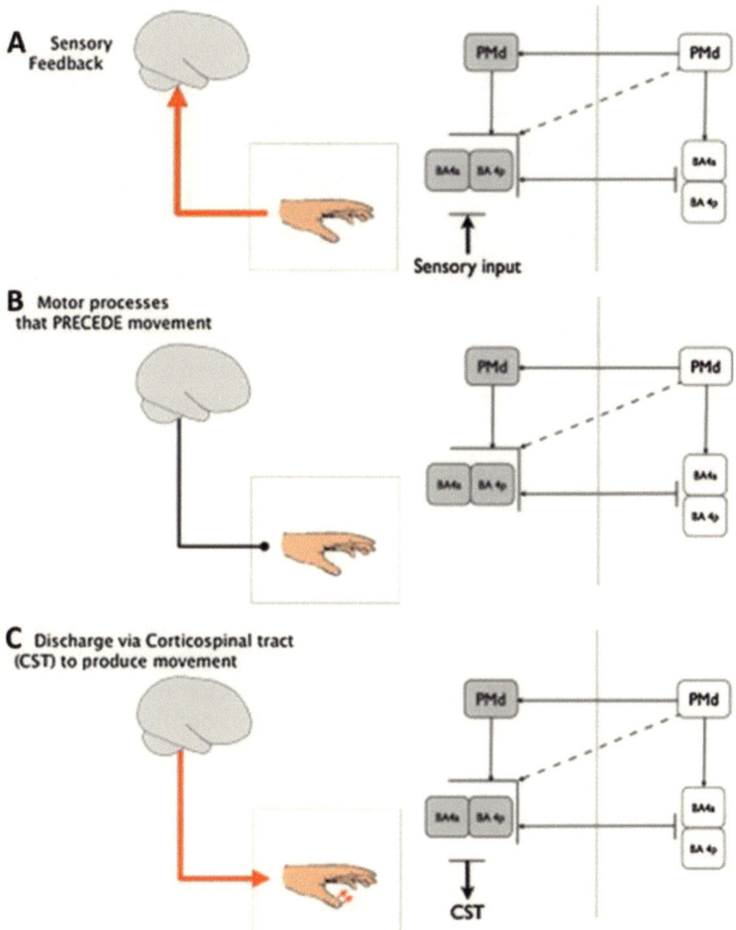


**Figure 4.**
*Three factors influencing motor function recovery after a stroke and the corresponding neural networks [29]. The injured hemisphere is shown in gray and the non-injured hemisphere in white. (A) Somatosensory feedback: This network can be accessed through somatosensory input such as peripheral nerve stimulation. (B) Processes preceding movement such as a movement plan: This network can be accessed through motor imagery or action observation. (C) Discharge via the corticospinal tract to produce movement: This network is involved in physical movement but predominantly through the combination of the other two (A and B).*

Sharma et al. [29] proposed, as a second factor involved in poststroke recovery of motor function, activities preceding movement (**Figure 4B**). We know that the IVp area is excited in the same way by both the abovementioned somatosensory input and mental representations, such as motor imagery and preceding movement. Using fMRI and healthy adults, Sharma et al. [33] conducted a study of neural activity in the primary motor cortex (IVa and IVp areas) while the subjects imagined movement. The results demonstrated that the relative involvement of imagining movement was larger in the IVp area than that in the IVa area. Sharma et al. [34] then explored the relationship between neural activity in the primary motor cortex (IVa and IVp areas) in stroke patients, while imagining movement and motor performance using fMRI. The authors found that, while imagining movement of the paretic hand, the neural activity in the injured side of the IVp area of stroke patients was positively correlated with motor performance. These studies suggest that the neural activity of the IVp area, when imagining movement, can be used as a tool to predict motor function in stroke patients and, further, that intervention with tasks involving motor imagery may increase excitation in the IVp area.

A third factor influencing recovery of motor function after stroke suggested by Sharma et al. [29] is discharge via the corticospinal tract to produce movement (**Figure 4C**). This network is involved in all physical movement but predominantly through the combination of the other two. That is, this neural network for producing movement is predominantly utilized via the mutual involvement of the neural network based on somatosensory feedback and the neural network preceding movement. As a specific example, Nilsen et al. [35] and López et al. [36] conducted a systematic review and found that combining mental practice and the use of motor imagery with physical movement improved intervention effects. Further, a Cochrane Review [37] also reported that mental practice interventions combined with motor therapy, including physical movement, were more effective than mental practice alone. We also reported that neurofeedback-based motor imagery training combined with physical movement contributed to improving upper extremity function in stroke patients [38]. These findings indicate that somatosensory feedback accompanying physical movement promotes the effects of motor imagery interventions. In other words, the neural network preceding movement and that for somatosensory feedback may work together to enhance motor performance.

To summarize, the factors influencing motor function recovery accompanying the reorganization of the IVp area after a stroke are (1) somatosensory feedback to the paretic side; (2) movement-preceding activities, which utilize motor imagery and action observation; and (3) discharge via the corticospinal tract to produce movement. As (3) is ultimately effective through the combination of the neural networks involved in (1) and (2), information processing combined with somatosensory input to the paretic limb should take priority in motor therapy for hemiparetic stroke patients exhibiting motor paresis. Next, treatment should precede mental practice interventions utilizing motor imagery induction, based on estimations from that information processing and from motor practice producing movement through an exercise program based on those movement-preceding activities. This step-by-step intervention strategy is considered vital.

Nevertheless, according to the Guidelines for the Management of Stroke [39], the following therapies are recommended for rehabilitation for upper limb dysfunction—for patients with mild paralysis, a therapy that suppresses the non-paralyzed upper limb and forces the use of the paralyzed upper limb in life is highly recommended (grade A). For moderate paralytic muscles (such as wrist and finger extensors), electrical stimulation is recommended (grade B). For patients with mild to moderate paralysis, training should be performed with repetition of certain movements (reach movement of the upper limb on the paralyzed side, goal-oriented movement, repetitive movement of both upper limbs, mirror therapy, repetitive facilitation exercise, etc.) is recommended (grade B). rTMS and tDCS may be considered, but care must be taken in patient selection and safety (grade C1).

Moreover, the following therapies are recommended for rehabilitation for gait disorders—increasing the amount of limb training associated with walking or of walking itself is strongly recommended to improve walking ability (grade A). For stroke hemiplegic patients with equinovarus feet, it is recommended to use short leg braces to improve walking (grade B). Botulinum therapy and intramuscular nerve block to the tibial nerve or the lower leg muscle using 5% phenol is recommended when the spastic equinovarus foot hinders walking and ADL (grade B). Tendon transfer may be considered for patients presenting with spastic equinus and abnormal gait (grade C1). Biofeedback using electromyogram and joint angle is also recommended to improve walking (grade B). Functional electrical stimulation is recommended for chronic stroke patients with drooping foot, but the duration of treatment effect is short (grade B). Treadmill training is recommended because it improves walking speed and endurance in ambulatory stroke patients (grade B).

Walking training using a walking assist robot is recommended for those who cannot walk within 3 months of onset (grade B).

Furthermore, the following therapies are recommended for rehabilitation in cases of movement disorders and ADL. For stroke sequelae, active rehabilitation from the early stage is strongly recommended to promote the recovery of dysfunction and disability (grade A). It is strongly recommended to increase the amount and frequency of training early after onset to promote more effective recovery of disability in patients (grade A). For lower limb function and ADL, repeated task training is recommended (grade B).

Based on the above guidelines, it is necessary to consider three points: (1) dose dependency, (2) task dependency, and (3) neuroplasticity, in order to promote effective functional recovery in stroke rehabilitation.

In clinical practice, it is important to perform optimal rehabilitation for stroke patients while keeping the functional characteristics of the brain and the existing guidelines in mind.

## 5. Final remarks

In this chapter, we outlined the neural mechanisms underlying motor function recovery after stroke-related brain injury. We have also outlined the corresponding rehabilitation strategies based on the functional characteristics of the brain and advances in clinical practice guidelines. We discussed how, considering the functional characteristics of the primary motor area, it is important during the early stages after stroke to increase the somatosensory input to the paralyzed side and combine mental practices using motor imagery. The existing guidelines highlighted the importance of dose dependency, task dependency, and neuroplasticity, in promoting effective functional recovery in stroke rehabilitation. Understanding the rehabilitation strategies and key related mechanisms involved in stroke recovery is indispensable for the development of highly effective poststroke rehabilitation.

## 6. Future directions

Previous studies have shown that the recovery of motor function after stroke is acutely related to the functional replacement of damaged neuronal circuits and the interhemispheric imbalance model. Therefore, it is important to promote neuroplasticity related to motor function recovery in rehabilitation. In addition to the use of evidence-based clinical practice guidelines, rehabilitation strategies that take into account the functional characteristics of the brain may maximize the recovery of motor function in stroke patients. In the future, it is expected that improved intervention strategies will be widely applied in the clinical setting by accumulating knowledge about the pathology of relevant cases and brain areas.

## Conflict of interest

The authors declare no conflict of interest.

## Author details

Hideki Nakano
Neurorehabilitation Laboratory, Graduate School of Health Sciences, Kyoto Tachibana University, Kyoto, Japan

*Address all correspondence to: nakano-h@tachibana-u.ac.jp

## References

[1] World Health Organization. The Atlas of Heart Disease and Stroke [Internet]. Available from: http://www.who.int/cardiovascular_diseases/resources/atlas/en/ [Accessed: 14 December 2019]

[2] Kim K, Kim YM, Kim EK. Correlation between the activities of daily living of stroke patients in a community setting and their quality of life. Journal of Physical Therapy Science. 2014;**26**:417-419. DOI: 10.1589/jpts.26.417

[3] Pollock A, Farmer SE, Brady MC, Langhorne P, Mead GE, Mehrholz J, et al. Interventions for improving upper limb function after stroke. Cochrane Database of Systematic Reviews. 2014;**11**:CD010820. DOI: 10.1002/14651858.CD010820.pub2

[4] Dancause N. Vicarious function of remote cortex following stroke: Recent evidence from human and animal studies. The Neuroscientist. 2006;**12**:489-499. DOI: 10.1177/1073858406292782

[5] Kantak SS, Stinear JW, Buch ER, Cohen LG. Rewiring the brain: Potential role of the premotor cortex in motor control, learning, and recovery of function following brain injury. Neurorehabilitation and Neural Repair. 2012;**26**:282-292. DOI: 10.1177/1545968311420845

[6] Nishimura Y, Onoe H, Morichika Y, Perfiliev S, Tsukada H, Isa T. Time-dependent central compensatory mechanisms of finger dexterity after spinal cord injury. Science. 2007;**318**:1150-1155. DOI: 10.1126/science.1147243

[7] Ward NS, Brown MM, Thompson AJ, Frackowiak RS. Neural correlates of outcome after stroke: A cross-sectional fMRI study. Brain. 2003;**126**:1430-1448. DOI: 10.1093/brain/awg145

[8] Rehme AK, Fink GR, von Cramon DY, Grefkes C. The role of the contralesional motor cortex for motor recovery in the early days after stroke assessed with longitudinal FMRI. Cerebral Cortex. 2011;**21**:756-768. DOI: 10.1093/cercor/bhq140

[9] Asanuma H, Okuda O. Effects of transcallosal volleys on pyramidal tract cell activity of cat. Journal of Neurophysiology. 1962;**25**:198-208. DOI: 10.1152/jn.1962.25.2.198

[10] Palmer LM, Schulz JM, Murphy SC, Ledergerber D, Murayama M, Larkum ME. The cellular basis of GABA(B)-mediated interhemispheric inhibition. Science. 2012;**335**:989-993. DOI: 10.1126/science.1217276

[11] Grefkes C, Nowak DA, Eickhoff SB, Dafotakis M, Küst J, Karbe H, et al. Cortical connectivity after subcortical stroke assessed with functional magnetic resonance imaging. Annals of Neurology. 2008;**63**:236-246. DOI: 10.1002/ana.21228

[12] Mark VW, Taub E, Morris DM. Neuroplasticity and constraint-induced movement therapy. Europa Medicophysica. 2006;**42**:269-284. DOI: 10.33425/2639-944X.1037

[13] Avanzino L, Bassolino M, Pozzo T, Bove M. Use-dependent hemispheric balance. The Journal of Neuroscience. 2011;**31**:3423-3428. DOI: 10.1523/JNEUROSCI.4893-10.2011

[14] Nowak DA, Grefkes C, Ameli M, Fink GR. Interhemispheric competition after stroke: Brain stimulation to enhance recovery of function of the affected hand. Neurorehabilitation and Neural Repair. 2009;**23**:641-656. DOI: 10.1177/1545968309336661

[15] Hummel FC, Cohen LG. Non-invasive brain stimulation: A new

strategy to improve neurorehabilitation after stroke? Lancet Neurology. 2006;**5**:708-712. DOI: 10.1016/S1474-4422(06)70525-7

[16] Ward NS, Cohen LG. Mechanisms underlying recovery of motor function after stroke. Archives of Neurology. 2004;**61**:1844-1848. DOI: 10.1001/archneur.61.12.1844

[17] Hsu WY, Cheng CH, Liao KK, Lee IH, Lin YY. Effects of repetitive transcranial magnetic stimulation on motor functions in patients with stroke: A meta-analysis. Stroke. 2012;**43**:1849-1857. DOI: 10.1161/STROKEAHA.111.649756

[18] Elsner B, Kugler J, Pohl M, Mehrholz J. Transcranial direct current stimulation (tDCS) for improving function and activities of daily living in patients after stroke. Cochrane Database of Systematic Reviews. 2013;**11**:CD009645. DOI: 10.1002/14651858.CD009645.pub2

[19] Wolf SL, Lecraw DE, Barton LA, Jann BB. Forced use of hemiplegic upper extremities to reverse the effect of learned nonuse among chronic stroke and head-injured patients. Experimental Neurology. 1989;**104**:125-132. DOI: 10.1016/s0014-4886(89)80005-6

[20] Taub E, Miller NE, Novack TA, Cook EW 3rd, Fleming WC, Nepomuceno CS, et al. Technique to improve chronic motor deficit after stroke. Archives of Physical Medicine and Rehabilitation. 1993;**74**:347-354

[21] Sirtori V, Corbetta D, Moja L, Gatti R. Constraint-induced movement therapy for upper extremities in stroke patients. Cochrane Database of Systematic Reviews. 2009;**4**:CD004433. DOI: 10.1002/14651858.CD004433.pub2

[22] Langhorne P, Coupar F, Pollock A. Motor recovery after stroke: A systematic review. Lancet Neurology. 2009;**8**:741-754. DOI: 10.1016/S1474-4422(09)70150-4

[23] Takebayashi T, Koyama T, Amano S, Hanada K, Tabusadani M, Hosomi M, et al. A 6-month follow-up after constraint-induced movement therapy with and without transfer package for patients with hemiparesis after stroke: A pilot quasi-randomized controlled trial. Clinical Rehabilitation. 2013;**27**:418-426. DOI: 10.1177/0269215512460779

[24] Taub E, Uswatte G, Mark VW, Morris DM, Barman J, Bowman MH, et al. Method for enhancing real-world use of a more affected arm in chronic stroke: Transfer package of constraint-induced movement therapy. Stroke. 2013;**44**:1383-1388. DOI: 10.1161/STROKEAHA.111.000559

[25] Gillick BT, Krach LE, Feyma T, Rich TL, Moberg K, Thomas W, et al. Primed low-frequency repetitive transcranial magnetic stimulation and constraint-induced movement therapy in pediatric hemiparesis: A randomized controlled trial. Developmental Medicine and Child Neurology. 2014;**56**:44-52. DOI: 10.1111/dmcn.12243

[26] Bolognini N, Vallar G, Casati C, Latif LA, El-Nazer R, Williams J, et al. Neurophysiological and behavioral effects of tDCS combined with constraint-induced movement therapy in poststroke patients. Neurorehabilitation and Neural Repair. 2011;**25**:819-829. DOI: 10.1177/1545968311411056

[27] Geyer S, Ledberg A, Schleicher A, Kinomura S, Schormann T, Bürgel U, et al. Two different areas within the primary motor cortex of man. Nature. 1996;**382**:805-807. DOI: 10.1038/382805a0

[28] Rathelot JA, Strick PL. Subdivisions of primary motor cortex based on

cortico-motoneuronal cells. Proceedings of the National Academy of Sciences of the United States of America. 2009;**106**:918-923. DOI: 10.1073/pnas.0808362106

[29] Sharma N, Cohen LG. Recovery of motor function after stroke. Developmental Psychobiology. 2012;**54**:254-262. DOI: 10.1002/dev.20508

[30] Loubinoux I, Dechaumont-Palacin S, Castel-Lacanal E, De Boissezon X, Marque P, Pariente J, et al. Prognostic value of FMRI in recovery of hand function in subcortical stroke patients. Cerebral Cortex. 2007;**17**:2980-2987. DOI: 10.1093/cercor/bhm023

[31] Strick PL, Preston JB. Sorting of somatosensory afferent information in primate motor cortex. Brain Research. 1978;**156**:364-368. DOI: 10.1016/0006-8993(78)90520-6

[32] Binkofski F, Fink GR, Geyer S, Buccino G, Gruber O, Shah NJ, et al. Neural activity in human primary motor cortex areas 4a and 4p is modulated differentially by attention to action. Journal of Neurophysiology. 2002;**88**:514-519. DOI: 10.1152/jn.2002.88.1.514

[33] Sharma N, Jones PS, Carpenter TA, Baron JC. Mapping the involvement of BA 4a and 4p during motor imagery. NeuroImage. 2008;**41**:92-99. DOI: 10.1016/j.neuroimage.2008.02.009

[34] Sharma N, Simmons LH, Jones PS, Day DJ, Carpenter TA, Pomeroy VM, et al. Motor imagery after subcortical stroke: A functional magnetic resonance imaging study. Stroke. 2009;**40**:1315-1324. DOI: 10.1161/STROKEAHA.108.525766

[35] Nilsen DM, Gillen G, Gordon AM. Use of mental practice to improve upper-limb recovery after stroke: A systematic review. The American Journal of Occupational Therapy. 2010;**64**:695-708. DOI: 10.5014/ajot.2010.09034

[36] López ND, Monge Pereira E, Centeno EJ, Miangolarra Page JC. Motor imagery as a complementary technique for functional recovery after stroke: A systematic review. Topics in Stroke Rehabilitation. 2019;**26**:576-587. DOI: 10.1080/10749357.2019.1640000

[37] Barclay-Goddard RE, Stevenson TJ, Poluha W, Thalman L. Mental practice for treating upper extremity deficits in individuals with hemiparesis after stroke. Cochrane Database of Systematic Reviews. 2011;**5**:CD005950. DOI: 10.1002/14651858.CD005950.pub4

[38] Nakano H, Kodama T, Murata S, Nakamoto T, Fujihara T, Ito Y. Effect of auditory neurofeedback training on upper extremity function and motor imagery ability in a stroke patient: A single case study. International Journal of Clinical Trials. 2018;**3**:126. DOI: 10.15344/2456-8007/2018/126

[39] The Japan Stroke Society. Japanese Guidelines for the Management of Stroke 2015. 3rd ed. Tokyo: Kyowa Kikaku; 2019. pp. 286-294

Chapter 18

# Supporting Survivors of Stroke in Low Resource Settings

*Farayi Kaseke, Tecla Mlambo, Aimee Stewart, Lovemore Gwanzura and James Hakim*

## Abstract

Stroke occurs suddenly and has major impact on both the survivor and their caregiver. A third of stroke victims usually die from its direct effects or complications. The survivors usually have functional deficits resulting in the need for caregiver support. The caregivers may have inadequate knowledge of how to care for their affected relatives. The result is high caregiver burden and complications among the survivors. Once a person has stroke, it becomes important that their caregivers and their needs are determined so that they get the necessary support from the health professionals. Education of both the stroke survivors and the caregivers, and follow-up to determine if their needs are being met may be the support required. This is important in low resource settings where the survivors and caregivers may not always afford to go to stroke clinics for support visits and follow-up. Furthermore, stroke will result in reduced quality of life, poor functional outcomes, and poor community reintegration, which are important areas in life. Caregivers who look after the survivor for long periods may suffer burnout and have poor quality of life. Educating both the stroke survivor and their caregiver may result in better quality of life and survival rate.

**Keywords:** survivors of stroke, caregivers of stroke, low resource settings, outcomes of stroke, caregiver training

## 1. Introduction

Stroke is a common neurological problem and one of the leading causes of death in developing countries of the world [1]. It is one of the most disabling diseases and has great emotional impact on both the survivors of stroke and their relatives [2]. Stroke can affect virtually all human functions and unlike other disabling conditions, the onset is sudden, leaving the survivor and family unprepared to deal with the consequences which can be clinical, social and economic [3]. In most developing countries, people affected by stroke present late to hospital and even then, are only kept in hospital for a short period until they are medically stable. They are then discharged home while still functionally dependent to the care of relatives who lack knowledge on what to do hence the need to be trained [3–5]. There are no institutions where they can get community support and the few that are available are beyond the reach of many. This puts the burden of care at home on the relatives. This is the case in Zimbabwe, Rwanda, Tanzania and South Africa [5, 6]. The chapter therefore gives information on supporting informal caregivers in order to improve functional outcomes among survivors of stroke and quality of life among both the survivors and caregivers [7].

It also gives an overview of the extent and consequences of the stroke problem in low resource settings, length of hospital stay and the implications on stroke survivors and their caregivers, and the impact of stroke in terms of mortality and morbidity. Furthermore, the chapter looks at the rehabilitation of stroke patients, the impact of stroke on caregivers, and how patient and caregiver training can improve outcomes for both the patient and caregiver in low resource settings. In addition, it highlights the reason why supporting survivors of stroke and their caregivers are important in these settings considering that there are no consistent hospital-based services to support them. Finally, it outlines how a training programme for stroke patients and their caregivers can be developed using Kern's six step model [8].

## 2. Epidemiology of stroke

Projected figures indicate that stroke is reaching epidemic proportions due to increased non-communicable diseases and HIV, and will be the number one killer by 2020 [9–11]. According to the Centre for Disease Control and Prevention, the incidence of stroke has increased by 100% in middle-to-low-income countries since 2002 [10, 12]. Although this increase is related to the increasing burden of cardiovascular risk factors and the ageing population, infectious causes of stroke are also thought to contribute. According to the World Health Organisation, 15 million people suffer from a stroke worldwide each year, and of these, 5 million die, 5 million fully recover and another 5 million are permanently disabled and need assistance with activities of daily living [13]. Low- and middle-income countries have 70% of strokes and 87% of both stroke-related deaths and disability-adjusted life years [14, 15] consequently making stroke the major cause of disability in Sub-Saharan Africa [16].

The incidence of stroke varies by race and country [17]. In SSA, most cases of stroke occur in relatively young people (mean age < 60 years in most studies), some 10–15 years younger than patients with stroke in developed countries [11, 17–21]. Earlier, Feigin and colleagues had found the mean ages for men and women to be 70 and 75 years respectively [22]. In Chile, the mean age was reported to be 66.4 years [23]; while it was found it to be less than 50 years for sub Saharan Africa [24]. This was in line with findings in Malawi where the mean age was 54.2 ± 16.9 years [11]. A Gambian study found the mean age to be 58 years (10–15 years) younger than patients in developed countries [25]; as is the case with Brazil where the mean age was 64.1 years [26]. In Ghana the mean age of stroke patients is 63.68 years and the male to female ratio is 1:0.96 [27]. In Sudan the mean age was found to be 56.61 [28]. However in Zimbabwe there were more females than male [5, 20, 29].

It is hoped that improved post stroke care, through caregiver support and training would reduce morbidity and mortality among stroke survivors and improve caregiver outcomes in low income countries. Information on causes and prevention of subsequent strokes may be important to give during caregiver support so as to empower them and improve compliance with medications.

## 3. Length of hospital stay (LOS)

Generally, LOS in African hospitals and other developing countries is short and range from 2 to 30 days [20, 30–37]. Shorter LOS may be indicative of fewer rehabilitation sessions and reduced impact on stroke survivor outcomes [6]. In 2012, 6 ± 4 days were reported in South Africa [32]. This was however lower than the 14 days previously reported for public hospitals in the same country in 2002 [34]. Other authors reported up to 30 days of hospital stay in South Africa [37]. LOS has a bearing on the state at which patients are discharged in terms of function. This may mean that the stroke survivor will still need care, and within 2 days, caregivers may not have been trained on care or even have met rehabilitation personnel to get information about their sick relative.

There are other reasons too. In most instances, survivors of stroke and their relatives cannot afford long LOS as this means higher hospital bills [33–35]. Hospitals also need beds for other ill patients so once patient is stable, they are discharged home to the care of relatives more likely due to pressure for beds as survivors of stroke do not pay in the public hospitals in many developing countries [36, 38, 39]. Furthermore, most patients would have presented late to hospital due to several factors and the stroke would have progressed, and condition worsened [5, 40]. This is not unique to African countries as this was also the case in Jordan where 32% of the population was not covered by any health and social insurance, and also spent less time in hospital [41]. Short hospital stay also means that patients are discharged before they are fully functional [39, 42]. This may be an indication that patients are kept in hospital until they are medically stable but not for rehabilitation [6]. As in the Zimbabwean setting, there may be no community services available to cater for the stroke survivors and their caregivers in most instances. Even in developed countries, it was found that caregivers lack knowledge on how to care for their relatives with stroke and are not trained to care [42].

Survivors do better with an organised, multidisciplinary approach to treatment in which they and the caregivers are a part, hence the need to offer support to caregivers [7, 43]. The ideal management of stroke involves several aspects although these are not uniform in different countries. These include rapid response systems to stroke where patients are seen within 3 hours and proper diagnosis is made which includes Computerised Tomography (CT) scans and Magnetic Resonance Imaging (MRI). Patients are also put in Stroke units for transition of care and given thrombolysis. Once stable they start rehabilitation treatment before being discharged home or to institutions. However, well-organised stroke services are virtually absent in the government sector in most developing countries [44]. For example, in Zimbabwe, current stroke management is hospital-based because most of the hospitals are acute care facilities and are not designed to provide rehabilitation in the wards beyond patient's discharge from the acute ward. From experience, rapid response is not available as most patients are not able to present to hospital on time after stroke. Most survivors also cannot afford the diagnostic procedures hence physicians depend on clinical symptoms for diagnosis. This is also compounded by a high staff turn-over making it difficult for patients to get consistent care. Challenges may then occur with coordination, availability of health care professionals and finances [34, 45].

The short length of stay in most hospitals in developing countries, (on average, up to 2 weeks) may be too short considering the time required to restore function post stroke. After the survivors of stroke are stable in terms of blood pressure, they are discharged back into the community usually with a disability, to the care of their family who have to offer physical, emotional and psychological support. This is indicative of a situation where survivors are discharged home to families who may not be fully prepared to cope with the changes that have occurred in the stroke survivors. This scenario has been going on for a long time even in middle income countries like South Africa [32, 34, 46, 47]. It is therefore necessary to involve caregivers in the pre-discharge planning of stroke survivors as failure to do so may result in unsatisfactory care-giving as a result of higher caregiver burden and poor quality of life for both the stroke survivor and the caregiver.

It is not clear if during the hospitalisation period the rehabilitation personnel in developing countries meet with the caregivers of people who have survived a stroke to discuss ongoing progress and pre-discharge plans. Maybe this could facilitate caregivers' access to information on stroke and its consequences, prevention and management options.

In Zimbabwe, management of survivors of stroke involves acute care in hospitals and not much of the rapid response and thrombolytic therapy in government hospitals. Even in private hospitals the costs of thrombolytic therapies are prohibitive. Most survivors cannot afford the CT scans and MRIs either. Once survivors are medically stable the rehabilitation professionals intervene whilst patients are still admitted. However, rehabilitation systems to support survivors of stroke have also not been fully developed. This means that hospital management of survivors of stroke is also deficient. Survivors are then discharged home with very minimal preparation and not notwithstanding the challenges of bringing them back for review. There are also no call centres in communities to assist, hence no support systems for caregivers in communities.

## 4. Outcome of stroke

Few studies have been done on the outcomes of stroke in Sub Saharan Africa (SSA) [11, 32, 48]. Initial stroke severity and in-hospital complications were found to be determinants of 28-day case fatality in Mozambique [48]; while in South Africa the case fatality was found to be associated with poor functional ability but not with age [32]. An important outcome post stroke is function which will be discussed in the next section. In Malawi mild stroke and the male gender were associated with favourable outcomes and being HIV positive did not worsen the outcomes of stroke [11]. In Zimbabwe, a 25% in hospital case fatality rate was reported [20]. Some of the patients who died had pneumonia, most probably from aspiration [20].

As mentioned before, a third of all patients with stroke will fully recover, a third will live with some disabilities and the other third will die [13]. Those who survive stroke and are disabled will require some form of care [7, 13, 49, 50]. Several factors affect prognosis post stroke. Some of these include demographic characteristics, type of stroke, severity and immediate and long-term post stroke care [51]. Factors that may contribute to a good prognosis after stroke are youth, mild deficit, speedy resolution of symptoms, no loss of consciousness, independent sitting balance, no cognitive impairment or urinary incontinence [52]. Medical complications are frequent among individuals who have had a stroke, increasing the length of hospitalisation as well as the costs of care. These complications are a major cause of death in the acute and sub-acute stroke phases [53]. Some events, such as cardiac abnormalities, dysphagia and pneumonia, are often apparent early after stroke onset whereas others, such as bed sores, venous thrombosis, and falls, can occur after several days [54, 55]. Potential cardiac complications such as atrial fibrillation and myocardial infarction are also common after stroke [54].

Neurological recovery in stroke occurs mainly within 1–3 months post stroke, whilst functional recovery occurs more fully at 4–6 months [56]. According to Doğan et al., 10% of stroke patients recover spontaneously within the first month, and 80% of patients are candidates for rehabilitation while the last 10% do not respond to treatment [57]. This is however different from the 2007 WHO report [13]. The neurological recovery of stroke often improves significantly within 3 weeks and function may continue to improve up to 18 months [46].

### 4.1 Mortality among people who suffer from stroke

Two-thirds of stroke deaths occur in people living in developing countries and 40% of those with stroke aged less than 70 years [58]. The Inter-stroke phase 1 study 2007–2009 reported that 5.7 million deaths in 2005 were due to stroke and the number is projected to rise to 7.8 million by 2030 and 87% of these will be in low or middle in-come countries. Similar findings were reported when it was estimated that approximately 80% of all deaths by stroke occur in developing countries [59]. However, age adjusted stroke mortality in adults in SSA seemed to be like developed countries [60]. This they attributed to lack of accuracy of longitudinal data collection in different regions.

In Africa, stroke accounts for 0.9–4% of hospital admissions and 2.8–4.5% of total deaths [61]. This is in line with findings elsewhere where it was reported that mortality due to stroke in low- and middle-income countries was the 5th leading cause of death in adults aged 15–59 years [62]. The same study found stroke to be the 7th leading cause of death in SSA with HIV/AIDS at the top. According to UNAIDS, HIV related deaths made up 16% in South Africa, 17% in Nigeria and 6% in Zimbabwe of total death [63]. This makes the need to support survivors of stroke more important so as to reduce mortality in communities.

This high stroke case fatality in Africa was found to be related to limited healthcare facilities and uncontrolled risk factors such as hypertension and diabetes which conditions and resultant death can be prevented [64]. Higher values have been found from community studies where deaths due to stroke contribute 5–10% of deaths in Tanzania [65]. Other studies in Africa have reported between 20 and 45% case fatality rates between admission and one-year post stroke [31, 32]. Stroke has been projected to be the 3rd leading cause of death in low income countries by 2030. Therefore, there is need for vigilance in prevention and care of patients with stroke as previously mentioned.

In South Africa based on an 11-disability adjusted number of life years lost per 1000 of the population, stroke was declared a catastrophic illness as the prevalence of stroke in South Africa was reported to be 3000/100,000 people [66], much higher than the 500/100,000 people living with strokes in developed countries [67]. It may be safe to conclude that Sub-Saharan Africa has relatively low stroke incidence and prevalence but has high mortality rates [17]. This is may be attributed to high prevalence of smoking and other risk factors for stroke. Factors associated with mortality include severity of stroke, being a woman, haemorrhagic stroke, low level of consciousness upon admission and failing a swallow test, irreversible coma, stroke recurrence and other secondary infections and pressure sores, increased age, diabetes mellitus and stroke subtypes as independent predictors of 30-day case fatalities. Similarly, the relative risk of death from stroke was found to be higher for females in Ghana [68].

Ischaemic stroke patients with a National Institutes of Health Stroke Scale (NIHSS) score of less than 10 have a 60–70% chance of a favourable outcome at 1 year compared with only a 4–16% chance if the score is more than 20 [53]. However, ischaemic strokes have better prognosis, but less functional prognosis compared to haemorrhagic strokes [69]. Upon follow up, 23% of patients with ischaemic stroke had died while 65% of the survivors were functionally independent at 1 year [69]. Meanwhile, among the patients with haemorrhagic strokes, 62% had died, and among the survivors, 68% were functionally independent at 1 year. Among those with subarachnoid haemorrhage, 48% were dead and 76% of the survivors were functionally independent. The differences in mortality during the acute phase between the two types of strokes are said to be due to the fact that haemorrhagic strokes are more severe at onset than ischaemic strokes. This results in increased pressure in the brain with mass shifting of brain which may be the reason for increased fatality. Later, as resolution occurs, swelling and pressure reduce with resultant reduction in mortality. Function is also better in Haemorrhagic strokes because there is less brain damage and once swelling and pressure have resolved, function is restored [70]. In Zimbabwe, not all patients with stroke can afford CT scans for diagnostic purposes, hence comparison is difficult. This also makes it difficult for typing the strokes although this is an important aspect of this study.

### 4.2 Functional outcomes in stroke

Poor functional recovery is associated with bowel and urinary incontinence, long time between stroke onset and hospital admission, more severe hemiparesis, visuospatial deficits and lower FIM scores [71, 72]. Functional recovery after stroke is also closely related to age, aetiology and severity of neurological deficit, nature of lesion and localization including integrity of collateral blood supply [52, 71]. The authors also reported that factors such as patient's education, motivation and socio-economic level may be important in recovery. Psychosocial and cognitive impairments and other neurological and sociodemographic factors have been seen to affect the functional recovery of stroke survivors [73].

Functional prognosis is better among the patients with haemorrhagic stroke in the long term compared to patients with ischaemic stroke even when someone is caring for them [74–81]. This is however different from findings that report worse functional outcomes among haemorrhagic strokes [82]. In line with the study by Bamford et al. [69], Kelly et al., had comparable results when they used the Functional Independence Measure (FIM) and found that among 1064 patients with stroke, 871 had ischaemic stroke and these had better functional abilities at admission compared to those with haemorrhagic stroke [81]. However, at follow up, the patients with haemorrhagic stroke had better recovery in comparison to those with ischaemic stroke. However, the treatment they received was not standardised. Unfortunately there are not many studies where comparison of functional outcomes was done after training in Africa. In South Africa poor functional outcomes were found to be associated with female gender, and more severe stroke and poor physical condition when patients were followed up at 6 weeks, 6 months and 1 year [32]. This was also the case later in Malawi [31]. Stroke has both psychosocial and physical impact upon both the survivors of stroke and their caregivers and it is important to discuss this area. These are aspects that affect quality of life.

### 4.3 Participation

Participation restriction means that survivors are unable to take part in areas of life such as usual roles and hobbies. They are the challenges individuals would have 'in involvement in life situations' [83]. Achieving independent ambulation within the community post stroke is not easy [84]. This has an impact on community reintegration post stroke as the survivors may not be able to take part in their former activities and may become isolated [85]. It is therefore important to assess stroke survivor's participation post stroke to get a complete picture of caregiver burden [86]. The relationship between participation and the environment was also highlighted elsewhere where the authors reported that perceptions of danger in the environment may make survivors increase speed for safety as seen when crossing roads [87]. In some cases, fear and the terrain may not be conducive for mobility. This is because there may be stones around and the terrain may be hilly thus reducing wheelchair mobility [6, 87]. Rehabilitation professionals may face difficulties in trying to equip stroke survivors with the skills for community mobilisation in different terrains. Further, survivors may not be able to manoeuvre wheelchairs given for mobilisation as the environment plays a role in the outcome of rehabilitation and the patient's recovery after stroke as it may act as a barrier [6, 87, 88]. This is more so because the objects, their position and orientation in the environment drives the motor pattern in an action as survivors try to move about [6].

Inability to ambulate within the community by survivors of stroke directly affects their community participation [87]. Reduced ambulation leads to poor accessibility of community facilities and this in turn causes poor social integration of survivors of stroke [89]. Once the survivors cannot access facilities, integration into community becomes poor, leading to non-compliance with medications [85]. This is further compounded by the fact that about 66% of community dwelling survivors of stroke will need help with at least one activity of daily living (ADL) [90]. Availability of support from family, acquaintances, peers, colleagues, neighbours and personal care providers are facilitators to activity participation but these are not always available as they have other roles to play [91]. The impact of stroke on ADLs, emotions, cognition, and participation in social activities therefore significantly compromises survivor well-being and inevitably alters their and caregiver's quality of life [67]. However, stroke survivors generally function better in activities of daily living than they do in social activities [92]. This is because stroke survivors are dependent on their caregivers for single and multiple tasks for up to one-year post stroke thus further compromising social integration [91]. Unfortunately, this need for help may cause dependency as they may continue to play the sick role.

## 5. Rehabilitation and caregiving of stroke survivors

The occurrence of stroke is devastating and overwhelming for both the survivor who becomes disabled suddenly and the family who are not prepared for the changes brought about in their lives when managing the multiple problems of a patient post stroke [7]. This is because they may face financial worries and are not prepared for the long care-giving hours and emotional stress which are predominant factors in increasing caregiver stress when one is caring for stroke survivors [93]. Caregivers should therefore be involved early on in the rehabilitation phase so that they understand and deal with the problems and prepare for after discharge life. The quality of rehabilitation, timing of treatment and amount of time spent in hospital have a bearing on the functional outcomes of the patients [6, 94–96]. Success of rehabilitation is also determined by emotional and physical challenges that the patient faces post stroke [97]. It is therefore important to identify barriers to an efficient rehabilitation service [6, 98, 99]. This is because availability of resources will affect the standard of stroke rehabilitation that patients receive [6, 100]. Effective rehabilitation initiated early after stroke can help enhance the recovery process and minimise functional disability which in turn improves quality of life of both the patient and the caregiver [42, 43, 97, 101–103]. Caregivers need to be well prepared for the emotional and physical challenges that the survivor faces as they may become barriers to care or even have a bearing on caregiver burden.

Moreover, organised respite care services that are available in developed countries may not be available in Zimbabwe to help with care of stroke survivors. This means that caregivers who have to look after survivors for long periods of time in most cases have no respite support. Disability benefits or allowances and voluntary support services to assist people living with disabilities and their caregivers may not be available as is the case in Zimbabwe [104, 105]; yet the caregiver's role in the health delivery system and support of stroke survivors is important. The global prevailing economic meltdown may also affect development of community services in most developing countries. This is despite home-based rehabilitation being considered an important complementary component of health-care to address stroke related disability as advocated by WHO in the case of HIV/AIDS. In South Africa, Hale et al. noted that stroke care leaves the caregiver who has no knowledge of what is going on in a predicament of what to do as information provided may not meet all their needs [33]. This results in increased caregiver strain as they may be the only source of rehabilitation available to the survivors of stroke as most cannot afford formal services due to poverty [34, 98]. There is therefore a missing link between hospital rehabilitation and survivors of stroke and their caregivers post discharge within the community.

The large numbers of people affected by stroke may also mean that the caregiver burden will increase and quality of life among many people will be affected. It is therefore important that caregivers of stroke survivors receive adequate caregiver support. When caregivers do not receive support, they may become strained resulting in inadequate support to survivors that will affect their quality of life. It is hoped that equipping caregivers by training them to look after stroke survivors may hopefully improve their outcomes and those of stroke survivors they care for. This is because elsewhere it has also been previously reported that disability affects quality of life and functional independence among survivors of stroke and increases burden of care among the caregivers [7].

## 6. Community management of stroke

Post stroke, many stroke survivors want to return to the roles they had prior to the stroke and integrate into their communities [46, 106]. However, the specific support systems required in helping stroke survivors and their caregivers remain unclear as the onset of stroke is sudden and patients and relatives are ill prepared to deal with the subsequent disability [7, 93, 107]. Survivors of stroke are primarily rehabilitated as inpatients and are then discharged home once it is felt that the person and their primary caregivers can cope [108]. In most low-income countries community support for stroke survivors and their families remains fragmented and poorly coordinated [6, 42, 101, 107]. In rural areas this problem is further compounded by physical geographical surroundings which are not conducive for mobility in any form [109, 110]. This results in patients receiving minimal therapeutic interventions to assist with recovery due to lack of access to rehabilitation services. In addition, this further strengthens the need for home-based rehabilitation [111, 112]. Due to low numbers of rehabilitation personnel and inaccessibility of communities, family caregivers are important among survivors of stroke.

After experiencing a stroke, 60–74% of survivors need caregivers to take care of them since some recover with physical and cognitive limitations [7, 90, 113]. This is usually provided by informal caregivers [114]; who are mainly women [38, 115]; and may be children, spouses or other relatives of the stroke survivors [116, 117]. Due to shortage of resources in low resourced countries, support of caregivers to enable them to offer home rehabilitation may be the option of choice. Many caregivers end up suffering from emotional, physical and psychological burnout due to the burden of caring for stroke relatives over a long period [7, 116]. They are also left with little time for their own responsibilities. Financial constraints may limit visits to hospitals to get support and distances to health centres may be prohibitive [32]. The fate of stroke victims has been documented elsewhere where many die or live with morbidities [13, 32, 93]. The challenges that caregivers face require that they get support from the health professionals to carry out the caregiving duties.

Earlier on, the importance of caregivers as part of the community support for survivors of stroke was highlighted [118]. Their involvement may help reduce stroke recurrence and complications associated with stroke, improve function and physical health as well as community reintegration [42, 47, 107, 119]. Caregiver involvement may reduce disability and depression [120] which can occur due to increased caregiver burden [114, 121]; and improve quality of life [122]; among survivors of stroke. Women, younger caregivers and caregivers with poor physical health are at a higher risk of suffering caregiver burden [123]. Caregiver support programmes should focus on self-efficacy, social support and coping strategies among these caregivers. Financial constraints are the chief causes of burden in caring for stroke survivors post discharge and could be minimised by educating caregivers on basic stroke management principles to reduce the economic burden when accessing rehabilitation services [32].

After suffering a stroke, stroke survivors and relatives are faced with physical, emotional and mental problems and health care providers should educate them about basic care before the patient is discharged to adequately prepare for life at home [124, 125]. As previously mentioned, after experiencing a stroke, 66–78% of survivors world-wide need caregivers to help with activities of daily living since some recover with physical and cognitive limitations [7, 66, 67, 113]. Caring for a stroke survivor is a complex, stressful, life changing experience for both the survivors and their family caregivers especially when one had not prepared for it [7, 117].

Caring for a stroke survivor requires both informal and formal caregivers. While formal caregivers are trained, the informal caregivers are not, and are also not paid for the services they offer yet play an important role in the survival of patient with stroke after discharge [38, 126, 127]. Most caregivers are therefore put into a carer role without any idea of what to do with the resultant increase in caregiver burden and poor quality of life [38, 42, 47, 100, 108]. As previously discussed, this lack of training can overwhelm caregivers who are ill prepared to care for someone with these limitations [7, 38, 42, 128–130]. The caregivers and survivors of stroke rarely receive information on the nature of stroke, its cause, management and prognosis [131]. In support of this finding other authors also noted that the specific caregiver needs were information on causes of stroke, stroke progression, prevention of recurrence, practical care, emotional care and guidelines on use of medicines as needed by people who have survived a stroke [42, 132, 133]. This further complicates their lives as their duties will also involve administration of drugs, assisting with rehabilitation exercises and performing medical procedures for which they are not trained [90, 134]. Assisting with rehabilitation exercises make them play an important role in rehabilitation [127].

Stroke is also associated with many complications such as falls, pressure sores, urinary tract infections, chest infections and caregivers must deal with these too [135]. The amount of time needed to look after an individual varies depending on several factors which may include severity of the stroke and relationship of caregiver to stroke survivor [136, 137]. Caregivers were found to complain of long hours of caregiving which in turn leads to increased caregiver strain and reduced sleep [138]. Caregiver strain also increases over time [139, 140]. Length of care is determined by the severity of the stroke where the more severely affected stroke survivors need constant care thus more strain in the caregivers [141, 142]. In contrast, another in their study found no difference in strain between those who had looked after a survivor of stroke over a long time compared to those who had cared over a short period [123]. This is because the authors found that other factors such as cognitive, emotional and behavioural changes in the survivor have a negative influence on caregiver strain. On the other hand, high confidence knowledge about efficacy, high satisfaction with social support and frequent use of coping strategy confronting all had a positive influence [123]. They therefore concluded that caregiver support programs should include education about self-efficacy, stimulation of the use of the coping strategy confronting and training in mobilising social support in a way that is satisfactory to caregivers. Furthermore, support programs should be offered both to caregivers who recently started to take care of a survivor and to caregivers who have been taking care of a patient for a longer time [123].

The mean age of caregivers ranged from 36 to 70 years [100, 142]. The most common informal caregivers are spouses and adult children or other relatives most of whom are poor [100, 116, 121, 143, 144]. Most of the caregivers are females [32, 100, 123, 142, 145]. In most cases there is no one else to carry out the caregiving task [146]. Female caregivers usually encounter more caregiving demands than male caregivers [147, 148]. This is because the female caregivers spend more time doing care giving tasks and other multiple family responsibilities [147, 149]. They are also the cornerstone for development and implementation of community care policies [141]. Further to this it was also found that 93% of men were cared for by women (their spouse in 73% of cases), while 55% of women were cared for by men [100]. Governments should make sure that poor people are educated on reduction of chronic diseases [150]. This is because they will end up caring for their sick relatives.

An attractive option is the use of formal caregivers, but they are expensive and for low resources settings like SSA, where accessibility to health settings is difficult [6, 109]. Home rehabilitation using informal caregivers is therefore the option of choice and if they receive support, may provide alternative cost-effective care compared to usual care [36, 151]. However, caregivers may end up giving up their jobs to care for the stroke survivor full time, give up their houses to stay with the stroke survivor and give up some social activities like going out with friends and going to church [38, 116, 138]. As discussed before, caregivers have not been made an integral part of the health care system [118], yet are responsible for the improvement of quality of life and survival of stroke survivors post discharge and suffer burnout themselves [38, 122].

In most SSA countries, most of the caregivers are informal [36]. Due to the high HIV burden the occurrence of stroke in HIV positive patients causes a dual burden of care [10, 31, 32]. Lack of support systems in poor countries also pose challenges as most of those affected are poor and cannot afford outside support [6, 44]. It was further noted that caregivers in developing countries are usually family not educated about care and face challenges in dealing with patients' problems [32]. At the same time, they are expected to help lower the risk of stroke recurrence, reduce stroke related complications, improve function and subsequently improve community integration [42, 46, 47]. There is need to address the perceived needs of caregivers of stroke survivors to improve quality of life and reduce caregiver burden which may arise from long term caregiving. Caregiver training may be the best choice as these are available and will not need payment.

## 7. Training of caregivers of survivors of stroke

To help support survivors of stroke, stroke rehabilitation services should address caregiver issues and include practical training in nursing skills and counselling sessions, which will help in reducing the caregiver burden and improve stroke survivor recovery. Survivors of stroke spend most of their time with caregivers who therefore need to be trained and educated on how to take care of the survivor and on what to expect [42].

In high income countries, caregiver training consisting of basic skills of moving and handling, facilitation of activities of daily living and simple nursing tasks have been seen to reduce caregiver burden and improve quality of life [42, 101]; and was cost-effective [101]. Trained caregivers were also followed up over time in South Africa, and the structured caregiver training positively impacted on survivors' quality of life post discharge [98]. They recommended an exploration of different caregiver education programs to determine those that would produce the best outcomes in patients and caregivers so that they can be adopted regionally and internationally [98]. That education of caregivers reduce the burden of care and was also later reported in other studies on home-based care in HIV [32, 152]. The authors reported that those who received support from a nurse or community care worker had a lower caregiver burden and had more than twice the odds of wanting to care for another person living with HIV in the future [152]. Any training or educational program should start during the acute phase of rehabilitation to prepare patients and caregivers for the trajectory of problems they may face during the recovery period [153].

Education may benefit both the survivors of stroke and caregivers by preventing stroke. Education is defined as 'a planned experience that uses a combination of methods such as teaching, counselling and behaviour modification techniques to influence knowledge and behaviour' [154]. Various interventions have been developed and evaluated with the intention of supporting informal caregivers. However, there are conflicting reports on their effectiveness and even for those with positive outcomes, only modest effects are reported [155, 156]. Caregiver training is a non-pharmacological intervention to reduce the burden on informal caregivers and facilitate patient recovery after stroke [131, 157].

Caregivers should receive information regarding stroke survivor handling, positioning and how to communicate with the stroke survivor [42, 101, 158]. These findings were supported by authors who reported that caregivers' training programs should mainly be focused on practical demonstrations on physical activities which they do whilst performing their roles to reduce physical strains among caregivers [158, 159].

Education should be given to family caregivers as this will benefit the community as they may relay the information to others for sustainability and improve quality of life of stroke survivors [42, 132]. They should be educated on how to look after the stroke survivor to prevent complications as well as recurrence [64, 160]. Training should cover self-efficacy and enable coping strategies like how to mobilise social support and also help the stroke survivor [123]. Training caregivers will also reduce adverse outcomes [145] However, the long-term impact of training on caregivers is not known in that they may end up thinking that the training is a qualification.

In Africa, about two thirds of caregivers of stroke survivors in rural areas receive no basic stroke education before discharge due to scarcity of rehabilitation services [6, 161]. On a positive note, educating the public and health care providers about prevention of stroke, warning signs and symptoms of the disease has been found to be useful when treating patients with hypertension [64, 162]. Lack of training is associated with high mortality among stroke survivors and severe forms of disabilities which could be minimised if training is done prior to discharge [161, 163]. Comparing the effects of training on the outcomes of caregivers and stroke survivors may highlight the importance of this aspect of care.

The training should not be generic, but tailor made or individually adapted for clients and include written information for caregivers given during the training session together with pictorial charts [156, 157, 164–166]. Stroke survivors should also be educated about their condition, treatment, prognosis and what they may need to do or not do and about hypertension as their knowledge was found to be suboptimal [64, 154, 160]. This finding strengthened findings from South Africa, which reported that 79% of hypertension and 64% of strokes said they did not know about the risk of stroke [167]. Development of a caregiver training programme that can be adapted to individual needs is important as any caregiver may receive this mode of support.

Any assistive devices used during training should be offered to them to take home to prevent regression of the stroke survivors' condition and difficulties in execution of the exercise programs [168]. Any training involving stroke survivors should be done after the acute phase, when they are less overwhelmed and able to comprehend the information [158, 169]. It is also important for stroke survivors and caregivers to be educated about the importance of incorporating the survivor back into the family [170]; although in some instances it may not result in improved perceived health status [171]. This is because education may improve carers' knowledge about stroke and its consequences but may fail to provide positive solutions to their problems hence lack of improvement in perceived health status [171]. It is therefore important for health workers to disseminate the training to other staff for sustenance of the training programme [172]. Training after the acute phase may be a challenge in situations where beds are required for other patients. In that case the caregivers may only receive training and later survivors of stroke may be included once they are ready.

## 8. Patient and caregiver outcomes after training

Several studies were carried out to determine effect of training on the outcomes of survivors of stroke and their caregivers. Most of the studies compared intervention and control groups. Most studies that found better outcomes in the intervention group were from developed countries and looked at functional status of patients and physical/emotional health of family caregivers, quality of life, caregiver optimism, task difficulties and use of intervention [42, 101, 173–176]. In some instances, 89% of the control group was functionally independent at 3 months compared to 93% in the intervention group. At 6 months, this was 86 and 89% respectively. Similarly, Foster and colleagues found a significant difference in two of the satisfaction questions on satisfaction with hospital services [177].

The differences found between the intervention and control group were largely attributed to extended training time and longer call durations in the intervention group [175]. Effects of the intervention can persist over a long-term period as the intervention can sustain home care by reducing institutionalisation and mortality as well as improve clinical outcomes for caregivers [173, 175]. On the other hand, some findings showed no difference in outcomes between the control and intervention groups and in other cases are contrasting [42, 175, 177, 178]. These authors found no statistically significant difference between groups in functional Barthel Index score or functional independence at 6 months among patients. They did not give caregiver outcomes. No significant differences in patient activities of daily living or functioning or in caregiver emotional distress, anxiety, depression and strain were also reported [177]. On the other hand, the intervention group had more patients referred for depression in one study [178]; although stroke recurrence was similar in both groups. It was therefore concluded that there was no evidence of a clinically significant benefit of the intervention to both patients and caregivers [177]. However it is important to consider the differences in this study with those that found positive results.

Studies that involved caregivers only were carried out in other places [176, 178]. One study in the rural areas in the United States found that all caregivers were satisfied with the intervention and were willing and able to use the intervention [178]. The intervention helped the caregivers make informed decisions about health care needs of stroke survivors thus reducing stress. This was further supported when the caregiver training program was found to have a positive impact on the functional status, post stroke depression and caregivers' knowledge and practices [179].

Caregivers were trained alone or in some instances together with the stroke survivor [42]. In other instances, both the caregivers and patients were trained [101, 176]. However different findings were reported in that some found the intervention to improve quality of life in both caregivers and patients [42] On the other hand, improvement in quality of life among the caregivers was found but not in the other outcomes [101]. No significant differences in survivors' activities of daily living or functioning or in caregiver emotional distress, anxiety, depression and strain were found in other studies [177]. On the other hand, in South Africa, improvement in quality of life, mobility and reduction in caregiver burden were found in the intervention group [98]. When training caregivers it is important to take into account other factors that may confound the outcomes such as culture and level of education.

All the results point towards a trend for caregiver targeted interventions having some value, but there is need for further research to confirm this and improve generalizability [155]. A caregiver training programme in low resource settings may be of value to offer support to stroke survivors and caregivers.

## 9. Developing a caregiver training programme

Education of caregivers is important [32, 42, 47, 101, 158]. However any developed training programme should be repeatable [8]. To come up with a training programme that is relevant, objective and feasible, it is important to consider the cultural and socio-economic context in which it will be used. The Kern model of curriculum development for medical education a six-step approach that links health needs to the education process was used to develop a caregiver training programme. The process does not usually proceed in sequence but is rather an interactive and dynamic one and can be adapted for low resource settings. According to Kern et al., the curriculum development is based on the following six steps [8]:

Step 1. Problem identification and general needs assessment

This begins with identification and analysis of health care needs. A general analysis of the current approach to address the identified needs is done. The difference between the ideal approach and the current approach represents a general needs assessment. This helps identify the gaps that exist in the care of stroke survivors. There is need to assess how other countries are dealing with training issues and compare outcomes of the stroke survivors and those in one's country. In most cases key informant interviews are carried out and other training programmes are assessed for adaptability. The observed gaps help in coming up with a targeted needs analysis.

Step 2. Targeted needs analysis

This involves assessing the needs of the targeted group of caregivers and stroke survivors which may be different from their needs in general. A triangulation of methodologies is used to come up with their needs and challenges that they face. This should be done among those that are likely to have faced challenges, meaning that they have experienced the challenges for a certain length of time.

### 9.1 Syllabus

Based on the findings from the targeted needs assessment, the syllabus for the training programme includes information on the condition and presentation of stroke, physical changes, causes, complications and risk factors, and related

| Topic | Notes to assist with topic development |
|---|---|
| The disease stroke | What is stroke? What are the causes of stroke? How does stroke present? How is the diagnosis made? What is the prognosis? |
| Identifying stroke | Use appropriate evaluation procedures to assess psychological and physical state of patients. Accurate identification of the patient's immediate and potential problems |
| Problems that patients face | These range from sudden change in body image, immobility, dependence on others for activities of daily living and care and personality changes. Also includes fears of loss of self-care and income and insecurities |
| Problems that caregivers face | Sudden changes from being thrust into caregiver role. Patient dependent on caregiver |
| Complications and prevention of stroke | Changes in motor and sensory problems. Secondary issues from immobility in cardio-respiratory and muscular skeletal systems. Issues with urinary system, particularly incontinence |
| Progression time frames | Changes in status from flaccidity to spasticity, immobility to mobility and recovery of lost function. |
| Comorbidities | Additional diseases that may be found in stroke patients such as HIV and other potential infections |
| Infection control | Use of gloves and disinfectants to minimise exposure to HIV and other potential infections |
| Handling of stroke patients | Handling and training for positioning, preventing shoulder-hand syndrome and shoulder subluxations |
| Lifting and transfers | Different methods of lifting stroke patients. Use of one-man method as well as methods for patients who are completely dependent. Help with facilitation of mobility and transfers as well as correct application of lifting and transferring techniques for safety reasons. |
| Activities of daily living | Teach feeding, bathing, toileting and alternatives to assist with dressing and any other personal activities of daily living |
| Treatment | Devising a plan of care for treatment that includes an appropriate progression and post discharge program of management. Recognition of contraindications and precautions for treatment, delivery of effective treatment and progression based on regularly scheduled evaluation of the patient's progress. |
| Communication | Tailored to the needs of each individual with identification and referral to appropriate resource persons or sources within the hospital and community |
| Dealing with bereavement | Explain the different stages of bereavement from shock, anger, denial, depression, acceptance and that the cycle may repeat. |
| Role of different departments and of the community in patient care | Establishment of appropriate relationships with the patient and other caregivers and members of the health care team. |

**Table 1.**
*Notes to assist with topic development [166].*

diseases are also included. The syllabus also addresses the activity limitations, participation restrictions and treatment needs of the stroke survivors in a practical way. **Table 1** presents the notes to assist with topic development for training.

Step 3. Developing goals and objectives

After identifying the needs of caregivers and the stroke survivors, goals and objectives for the training programme are developed. The objectives may include cognitive (knowledge), affective (attitudinal) and psychomotor (skill and behaviour) for the caregivers and stroke survivors. Objectives help determine the content of the training programme, learning methods/educational strategies and communicate what the curriculum is about and provide the basis for evaluation.

Step 4. Developing educational strategies

Educational strategies are based on the objectives and the content of training programme. After the educational needs of caregivers and stroke survivors have been identified, it is decided on what has to be taught based on the needs and the methods of delivery that will be effective. The selected strategies are the ones most likely to achieve the educational objectives.

Step 5. Implementation

Implementation of the training programme includes getting buy-in from the people who will allow use of the training programme, and the identification of any barriers to the use of programme. Usually these are the health professionals who will do the training later on or even Directors of health who have to enforce the training of caregivers and stroke survivors. The programme is introduced and

| Resources | Outputs | Program outcomes | Impact |
|---|---|---|---|
| Caregivers of stroke survivors<br>Stroke survivors<br>Training materials<br>Places where training will be held<br>Support from communities of interest. | Number of CGs enrolled<br>Number of caregivers trained<br>Number of drop outs<br>Number of caregivers who develop competencies in looking after stroke survivors<br>Number of CGs who are satisfied with the training program<br>Number of CGs confident to look after SS after training | All caregivers of stroke survivors are knowledgeable, compassionate, dedicated in caring for stroke survivors.<br>Caregivers of stroke survivors demonstrate competencies in the following areas:<br>Explaining the causes and symptoms of stroke<br>Explaining how to handle and lift a patient with stroke<br>Can handle, lift, mobilise and help a stroke survivor to perform activities of daily living.<br>CGs have confidence and good attitude in dealing with problems of stroke<br>Stroke survivors have increased access to home based support. | Hospitals have optimal holistic health care that reduces the impact of stroke on caregivers and people who have survived a stroke. |

**Underlying Assumptions:**

- The caregiver training program is fully implemented with fidelity to written goals and objectives.
- Government policies and resources are supportive
- The total health care system is improved to support the work of caregivers

**Table 2.**
*Logic model for the training programme implementation [166].*

administered. Implementation is critical for success of programme as it converts a mental exercise into reality [8]. A logic model (**Table 2**) is used to help with the implementation process as exemplified below.

Step 6. Evaluation and feedback

In this phase the caregivers and stroke survivors as well as the training programme are evaluated. This may be either formative (at the beginning) or summative (at the end) [8]. Evaluation of the content and delivery of the programme to caregivers is important as it leads to its acceptance [42, 172]. Evaluation is also important for recognition of caregiver and stroke survivor needs during and after training leading to appropriate and timeous interventions which are perceived as beneficial by the caregivers and the survivors of stroke [180].

## 10. Conclusion

Stroke occurs suddenly and affects functional outcomes in stroke survivors and the quality of life of both the caregivers and the stroke survivors. Most of the survivors end up with disabilities and have to depend on caregivers to survive. Unfortunately, most of the caregivers are not knowledgeable about looking after stroke survivors and end up with high caregiver burden. This chapter explained how the caregivers can be assisted in supporting stroke survivors. It also outlined the steps that can be followed in developing a training programme that can be adapted for low resource settings, and for conditions that may also affect function and quality of life. This is because supporting survivors of stroke is best done through training their caregivers. The training programme should take into account the cultural issues surrounding the caregivers and the stroke survivors. It is worth noting that over and above training the caregivers, health departments should continue to offer support to the stroke survivors through provision of appropriate rehabilitation services so that they become functionally independent. The support and training should be ongoing.

## Author details

Farayi Kaseke, Tecla Mlambo*, Aimee Stewart, Lovemore Gwanzura and James Hakim
Department of Rehabilitation Harare, University of Zimbabwe College of Health Sciences, Zimbabwe

*Address all correspondence to: teclamlambo@hotmail.com

## References

[1] Gyagenda JO et al. Post-stroke depression among stroke survivors attending two hospitals in Kampala Uganda. African Health Sciences. 2015;**15**(4):1220-1231. DOI: 10.4314/ahs.v15i4.22

[2] Litton J, Lokesh S. A cross-sectional study of prevalence and determinants of depression among stroke patients. International Journal of Advances in Medicine. 2016;**3**(3):527-532. DOI: 10.18203/2349-3933.ijam20162213

[3] Ali MA, Chidi OV, Timothy AO. Demographic and clinical factors on depression among stroke patients. American Journal of Clinical Medicine Research. 2016;**4**(3):38-42

[4] Mlambo T, Amosun SL, Concha ME. Assessing the quality of occupational therapy records for stroke patients at one academic hospital in South Africa. South African Journal of Occupational Therapy. 2004;**34**(3):10-13

[5] Seremwe F, Kaseke F, Chikwanha TM, Chikwasha V. Factors associated with hospital arrival time after the onset of stroke symptoms: A cross-sectional study at two teaching hospitals in Harare, Zimbabwe. Malawi Medical Journal. 2017;**29**(2):171-176

[6] Rhoda A, Cunningham N, Azaria S, Urimebenshi G. Provision of inpatients rehabilitation and challenges experienced with participation post discharge: Quantitative and qualitative inquiry of African stroke patients. BMC Health Services Research. 2015;**15**:423

[7] Lutz BJ, Young ME. Rethinking intervention strategies in Stroke family care giving. Rehabilitation Nursing. 2010;**35**(4):152-160

[8] Kern DE, Thomas PA, Howard D, et al. Curriculum Development for Medical Education: A Six-Step Approach. Baltimore, MD: Johns Hopkins University Press; 2009

[9] Centres for Disease Control and Prevention. Stroke related deaths and disability. 2008. Available from: https://www.gov/mmwr/preview/mmwrhtml/su6001a21.htm?.Retrieved [Accessed: 3 April 2014]

[10] Benjamin Laura A, Bryer A, Emsley Hedley CA, Khoo S, Solomon T, Connor Myles D. HIV infection and stroke: Current perspectives and future directions. Lancet Neurology. 2012;**11**:878-890

[11] Heikinheimo T, Chimbayo D, Kumwenda JJ, Kampondeni S, Allain TJ. Stroke outcomes in Malawi, a country with high prevalence of HIV: Prospective follow –up study. PLoS One. 2012;**7**(3):e33765

[12] Strong K, Mathers C, Bonita R. Preventing stroke: Saving lives around the world. Lancet. 2007;**6**:182-187

[13] World Health Organisation. Future health: Projected deaths for selected causes to 2030. World Health Statistics. Chapter 3:12. Geneva: World Health Organization; 2007. Available from: https://www.who.int/whosis/whostat 2007-10 highlights.pdf. [Retrieved: 03/04/2014]

[14] Feigin VL, Rinkel GJ, Lawes CM, Alga A, Bennet DA, van Gijn J, et al. Risk factors for subarachnoid haemorrhage: An updated systematic review of epidemiological studies. Stroke. 2005;**36**(12):2773-2780

[15] Owolabi MO, Arulogun O, Melikam S, Adeoye AM, Akarolo-Antony S, et al. The burden of stroke in Africa: A glance at the present and a glimpse of the future.

Cardiovascular Journal of Africa. 2015;**26**:S27-S38

[16] Moran A, Forouzanfar M, Sampson U, Chugh S, Feigin V, Mensah G. The epidemiology of cardiovascular diseases in sub-Saharan Africa: The global burden of diseases, injuries and risk factors 2010 study. Progress in Cardiovascular Diseases. 2013;**56**(3):234-239

[17] Feigin VL, Forouzanfar MH, Krishnamurthi R, Mensah GA, Connor M, Bennet DA, et al. Global burden of stroke during 1990-2010: Findings fro the global burden of disease study 2010. Lancet. 2014;**383**:245-255

[18] Kengne AP, Anderson CS. The neglected burden of stroke in sub-Saharan Africa. International Journal of Stroke. 2006;**1**:180-190

[19] Urton ML, Kohla M, Davis J, Neill MR. Systematic review of treatment interventions for upper extremity hemiparesis following stroke. Occupational Therapy International. 2007;**14**(1):11-27

[20] Kaseke F, Stewart A, Gwanzura L, Hakim J, Chikwasha V. Clinical characteristics and outcomes of patients with stroke admitted to three tertiary hospitals in Zimbabwe: A retrospective one-year study. Malawi Medical Journal. 2017a;**29**(2):177-182. Non-Communicable Diseases Special Issue

[21] Mlambo T, Amosun SL, Concha M. Timing of occupational therapy services in the rehabilitation of stroke patients in an academic hospital in South Africa. South African Journal of Occupational Therapy. 2006;**36**(2):5-8

[22] Feigin VL, Lawes CMM, Bennet DA, Anderson CS. Stroke epidemiology: A review of population based studies of incidence, prevalence and case fatality in the 20th century. Lancet. 2003;**2**:43-53

[23] Lavados PM, Sacks C, Prina L, Escobar A, Tossi C, Araya F, et al. Incidence, case fatality rate, and prognosis of ischaemic stroke subtypes in a predominantly Hipsnaic-mestizo population in Iquique, Chile (PISCIS project): A community-based incidence study. Lancet Neurology. 2007;**6**:140-148

[24] Seedat YK. Meeting the challenges of hypertension in sub-Saharan Africa (editorial). Cardiovascular Journal of South Africa. 2006;**17**(2):47-48

[25] Walker RW, Rolfe M, Kelly PJ, George MO, James OFW. Mortality and recovery after stroke in the Gambia. Stroke. 2003;**34**:1604-1609

[26] Martins ANN, deFiqueiredo MM, Rocha Orlandil D, Fernandes MAF, Jeronimo SMB, Dourado ME. Frequency of stroke types at an emergency hospital in Natal Brazil. *Arquivos de Neuro-Psiquiatria*. 2007;**65**(4b):1139-1143

[27] Attah-Adjepong G. A retrospective descriptive study on cerebrovascular accidents at the Komfo Anokye Teaching Hospital (KATH) in Kumasi. A dissertation submitted to the school of Graduate studies. Kwame Nkrumah University of Science and Technology; 2008

[28] Iburahim S, Hussein A, Sidig A, Yasin F, Mohmad AB, Gadour O, et al. Stroke in women (Sudanese experience). American Journal of Scientific and Industrial Research. 2011;**2**(2):157-160

[29] Chimusoro FR, Mlambo T. Activities and participation domains considered important by outpatient stroke patients attending rehabilitation in Harare, Zimbabwe. Central African Journal of Medicine. 2013;**59**. Nos 9/12. RD/54/13:20

[30] Garbusinski JM, van Sande MAB, Bartholome EJ, et al. Stroke presentation and outcome in developing countries: A prospective study in the Gambia. Stroke. 2005;**36**:1388-1393

[31] Heikinheimo T, Chimbayo D. Quality of life after first ever stroke: An interview-based study from Blantyre, Malawi. Malawi Medical Journal. 2015;**27**(2):50-54

[32] Mudzi W, Stewart A, Musenge E. Case fatality of patients with stroke over a 12-month period post stroke. South African Medical Journal. 2012;**102**(9):765-767

[33] Hale LA, Eales CJ, Fritz VU. The Soweto stroke questionnaire. South African Journal of Physiotherapy. 1998;**54**(4):16-20

[34] Hale LA. The problems experienced by people with stroke living in Soweto, South Africa. PhD thesis. University of the Witwatersrand; 2002

[35] Whitehead M, Dahlgren G, Evans T. Equity and health sector reforms: Can low-income countries escape the medical poverty trap? The Lancet. 2001;**358**:833-836

[36] Thorogood M, Connor M, Tollman S, Hundt GL, Fowkes G, Marsh J. A cross-sectional study of vascular risk factors in a rural south African population: Data from the southern African stroke prevention initiative (SASPI). BMC Public Health. 2007;7:326. Available: http://www.biomedcentral.com/147-2458-7-326

[37] Green AR. The human face of health disparities. Public Health Reports. 2003;**118**:303-308

[38] Smith LN, Lawrence M, Kerr SM, Langhorne P, Lees KR. Informal caregivers' experiences of caring for stroke survivors. Journal of Advanced Nursing. 2004a;**46**(3):235-244

[39] Johansson L, Sundstrom G, Hassing LB. State provision down, offspring's up: The reversed substitution old-age acre in Sweden. Ageing and Society. 2003;**23**:269-280

[40] Ekeh B, Isamade E. Time of presentation of stroke patients in a tertiary hospital in Northern Nigeria, West Africa. Journal of Medical Investigations and Practice. 2014;**9**(1):1-4

[41] Suhimat T. Health services in Jordan. Jordan Times. 3 January. P7; 2001

[42] Kalra L, Evans A, Perez I, Melbourn A, Patel A, Knapp M, et al. Training carers of stroke patients: Randomised controlled trial. British Medical Journal. 2004;**328**(7448):1099

[43] Duncan PW, Zorowitz R, Bates B, Choi JY, Glasberg JJ, Graham GD, et al. Management of adult stroke rehabilitation care: A clinical practice guideline. AHA/ASA – Endorsed practice guidelines. Stroke. 2005;**36**:e100-e143

[44] Pandian JD. Stroke and thrombolysis in India. Neurology India. 2007;**55**:173

[45] Brainin M, Zorowitz RD. Advances in stroke: Recovery and rehabilitation. Stroke. 2013;**44**(2):311-313

[46] Han B, Haley WE. Family care giving for patients with stroke. Review and analysis. *Stroke*. 1999;**30**:1478-1485

[47] Hankey GJ. Informal caregiving for disabled stroke survivors. Editorial: Training the caregiver benefits the patient, caregiver and the community. British Medical Journal. 2004;**328**:1085-1086

[48] Gomes J, Damasceno A, Carrilho C, et al. The effects of season and temperature variation on hospital admissions for incident stroke events in Maputo, Mozambique. Journal of Stroke and Cerebrovascular Diseases. 2014;**23**(2):271-277. DOI: 10.1016/j.jstrokecerebrovasdis.2013.02.012

[49] Michael-Titus AT, Revest P, Shortland P. The Nervous System: Basic Science and Clinical Conditions, Stroke and Head Injury. 2nd ed. Chapter 11. Churchill Livingstone, London, UK: Elsevier; 2007

[50] Ogunmola JO, Oladosu OY. Patient outcome of admissions in the medical wards of a tertiary health Centre in a rural community of Ekiti state Nigeria. Annals of African Medicine. 2014;**13**(4):195-203

[51] Walker R, Whiting D, Nigel U, Mugusi F, Swai M, Aris E, et al. Stroke incidence in rural and urban Tanzania: A prospective, community –based study. Lancet Neurology. 2010;**9**:786-792

[52] Stokes M. Physical Management in Neurological Rehabilitation. 2nd ed. Edinburgh: Elsevier Limited; 2004

[53] Hong K et al. Impact of neurological and medical complications on 3-month outcomes in acute ischaemic stroke. European Journal of Neurology. 2008;**15**(12):2310

[54] Khaja AM, Grotta JC. Established treatments for acute ischaemic stroke. The Lancet Neurology. 2007;**369**:319-330

[55] Kumar V, Abbas AK, Fausto N, Mitchell R. Robbins' Basic Pathology. 8th ed. Philadelphia: Saunders; 2007

[56] Schaetcher JD. Motor rehabilitation and brain plasticity after hemiparetic stroke. Progress in Neurobiology. 2004;**73**:61-72

[57] Doğan A, Nakipoğlu GF, Aslan DM, Kaya ZA, Ozgirgin N. The rehabilitation results of hemiplegic patients. Turkish Journal of Medical Sciences. 2004;**34**:385-389

[58] Truelsen T, Piechowski-Jozwiak B, Bonita R, Mathers C, Bogousslavsky J, Boysen G. Stroke incidence and prevalence in Europe: A review of available data. European Journal of Neurology. 2006;**13**:581-598

[59] Connor MD, Walker R, Modi G, Warlow CP. Burden of stroke in black populations in sub Saharan Africa. The Lancet Neurology. 2007a;**6**:269-278

[60] Connor MD, Thorogood M, Modi G, Warlow CP. Burden of stroke in Sub Saharan Africa. *American Journal of Preventative Medicine*. 2007b;**33**(2):172-173. (Letters to the Editor)

[61] Njoku CH, Adujolu AB. Stroke in Sokoto Nigeria: A five year retrospective study. Annals of African Medicine. 2004;**3**(2):73-76

[62] Mathers CD, Lopez AD, Murray JL. The burden of disease and mortality by condition: Data, methods, and results for 2001. In: Lopez AD, editor. Global Burden of Disease and Risk Factors. Chapter 3. The International Bank for Reconstruction and Development/ The World Bank. New York: Oxford University Press; 2006

[63] UNAIDS. Regional statistics. Gapreport factsheet. Aavailable from: http://www.unaids.org/en/resources/ campaigns.2014gapreport [Accessed: 21 December 2014]

[64] Lemogoum D, Degaute JP, Bovet P. Stroke prevention, treatment and rehabilitation in sub-Saharan Africa. American Journal of Preventive Medicine. 2005;**29**:95-101. DOI: 10.1016/j.amepre.2005.07.025

[65] Walker RW, McLarty DG, Kitange HM, Whiting D, Masuki G, Mtasiwa DM, et al. Stroke mortality in urban and rural Tanzania. Adult morbidity and mortality project. Lancet. 2000;**355**:1684-1687

[66] Connor M, Bryer A. Stroke in South Africa. Chronic Disease of Lifestyle in South Africa. 2005;**1995-2005**:195-203

[67] Donnan GA, Fisher M, Macleod M, Davis SM. Stroke. Lancet. 2008;**371**:1612-1623

[68] Wiredu EK, Nyame PK. Stroke related mortality at Korle Bu teaching hospital, Accra, Ghana. East African Medical Journal. 2001;**78**:180-184

[69] Bamford J, Sanderock P, Dennis M, Burn J, Warlow C. A prospective study of acute cerebrovascular disease in the community: The Oxfordshire community stroke project –1981 –86. 2. Incidence, case fatality rates and overall outcome at one year of cerebral infarction, primary intracerebral and subarachnoid haemorrhage. Journal of Neurology, Neurosurgery, and Psychiatry. 1990;**53**(1):16-22

[70] AndersenKK,OlsenTS,DehlendorffC, Kammersgaard LP. Haemorrhagic and ischaemic strokes compared. Stroke severity, mortality and risk factors. Stroke. 2009;**40**(6):2068-2070

[71] Jongbloed L. Prediction of function after stroke: A critical review. Stroke. 1986;**17**(4):765-776

[72] Perna R, Temple J. Rehabilitation outcomes: Ischaemic versus haemorrhagic strokes. Behavioural Neurology. 2015;**2015**:891651. DOI: 10.1155/2015/891651

[73] Saxena S, Ng T, Yong D, Fong N, Kohn G. Functional outcomes in inpatient rehabilitative care of stroke patients: Predictive factors and the effect of therapy intensity. Quality in Primary Care. 2006;**14**:145-153

[74] Paolucci S, Antonucci G, Grasso MG, Bragoni M, Coiro P, de Agelis D, et al. Functional outcome of ischaemic and haemorrhagic stroke patients after in-patient rehabilitation. Stroke. 2003;**34**(12):2861-2865

[75] Caplan LR. Intracerebral haemorrhage. Lancet. 1992;**3391**: 656-658

[76] Labovitz DL, Allan A, Sacco RL. Prevalence and predictors of early seizure and status epilepticus after first stroke. Neurology. 2001;**57**:200-206

[77] Qureshi AI, Tuhrim S, Broderick JP, Batjer HH, Hondo H, Hanley DF. Spontaneous intracerebral haemorrhage. New England Journal of Medicine. 2001;**344**:1450-1460

[78] Vemeer SE, Koudstaal PJ, Oudkerk M, Hofman A, MMb B. Prevalence and risk factors of silent brain infarcts in the population-based Rottedan scan study. Stroke. 2002;**33**:21-25

[79] Wei JW, Heeley EL, Wang JG, Huang Y, Wong LKS, Li Z, et al. Comparison of recovery patterns and prognostic indicators for ischaemic and haemorrhagic stroke in China: The China quest (quality evaluation of stroke care and treatment) registry study. Stroke. 2010;**41**:1877-1883

[80] Van Asch CJ, Luitse MJ, Rinkel GJ, van der Tweel I, Algra A, Klijn CJ. Incidence, case fatality and functional outcome of intracerebral haemorrhage over time, according to age, sex and ethnic origin: a systematic review and meta analysis. Lancet Neurology. 2010;**9**:167-176

[81] Kelly PJ, Furie KL, Shafqat S, Rallis N, Chang Y, Stein J. Functional recovery following rehabilitation after haemorrhagic and ischaemic stroke. Archives of Physical Medicine and Rehabilitation. 2003;**84**:968-972

[82] Dennis MS. Outcome after brain haemorrhage. Cerebrovascular Diseases. 2003;**16**(Suppl 1):9-13

[83] World Health Organization. ICF: International Classification of Functioning, Disability and Health/ World Health Organization. Geneva: WHO; 2001. pp. 1-299

[84] Lord S, McPherson KM, McNaughton HK, Rochester L, WeatherallM.Howfeasibleistheattainment of community ambulation after stroke? A pilot randomised controlled trail to evaluate community-based physiotherapy in sub-acute stroke. Clinical Rehabilitation. 2008;**22**:215-225

[85] Hale LA, Eales CJ, Stewart A, Fritz VU. The problems experienced by black stroke patients in Soweto, South Africa. South African Journal of Physiotherapy. 1999;**55**(2):17-22

[86] Rochette A, Desrosiers J, Bravo G, St-Cyr Tribble D, Bourget A. Changes in participation level after spouse' first stroke and relationship to burden and depressive symptoms. Cerebrovascular Diseases. 2007;**24**:255-260

[87] Taylor D, Stretton CN, Mudge S, Garret N. Does clinic measured gait speed differ from gait speed measured in the community in people with stroke? Clinical Rehabilitation. 2006;**20**:436-444

[88] Carr J, Shepherd R. Neurological Rehabilitation: Optimising Motor Performance. 2nd ed. Edinburgh: Butterworth-Heinmann; 2010

[89] Belanger L, Bolduc M, Noel M. Relative importance of after effects, environment and socio-economic factors on the social integration of stroke victims. International Journal of Rehabilitation Research. 1988;**11**:251-260

[90] Connor MD, Thorogood M, Casserly B, Dobson C, Warlow CP (for the SASPI Project Team). Prevalence of stroke survivors in rural South Africa; results from the southern African stroke prevention initiative (SASPI) Agincourt field site. Stroke. 2004;**35**(3):627-632

[91] Mudzi W, Stewart A, Musenge E. Community participation of patients 12 months post stroke in Johannesburg, South Africa. African Journal of Primary Health Care & Family Medicine. 2013;**5**(1):426

[92] Schmidt SM, Herman LM, Koenig P, Leuze M, Monahan MK, Stubbers RW. Status of stroke patients: a community assessment. Archives of Physical Medicine and Rehabilitation. 1986;**67**(2):99-102

[93] Bhattacharjee M, Vairale J, Gawali KD. Factors affecting burden on caregivers of stroke survivors: Population-based study in Mumbai (India). Annals of Indian Academy of Neurology. 2012;**15**(2):113-119

[94] Paolucci S, Antonucci G, Grasso MG, Morelli D, Troisi E, Coiro P, et al. Early versus delayed In-patient stroke rehabilitation: A matched comparison conducted in Italy. Archives of Physical Medicine and Rehabilitation. 2000;**81**:695-700

[95] Maulden SA, Gassaway J, Horn SD, Smout RJ, DeJong G. Timing of initiation of rehabilitation after stroke. Archives of Physical Medicine Rehabilitation. 2005;**86**(Supervision 2): S34-S40

[96] Horn SD, DeJong G, Smout RJ, Gassaway J, James R, Conroy B. Stroke rehabilitation patients, practice, and outcomes: Is earlier and more aggressive therapy better. Archives of Physical Medicine Rehabilitation. 2005;**86**(Supervision 2):S34-S40

[97] Aprile I, Di Stasio E, Romitelli F, Lancellotti S, Caliandro P, Gilardi A, et al. Effects of rehabilitation on quality of life in patients with chronic stroke. Brain Injury. 2008;**22**(6): 451-456

[98] Mudzi W. Impact of caregiver education on stroke survivors and their caregivers. Phd thesis. University of Witwatersrand; 2010

[99] Chestnut TJ. Fatigue in stroke rehabilitation patients: A pilot study. Physiotherapy Research International. 2011;**16**:151-158

[100] Penido S, SanMartin V, Zaldibar B, Miranda M, Tejada P, Erazo P, et al. Quality of life of stroke patients and their caregivers. International Journal of Physical Medicine and Rehabilitation. 2017;**5**(1):386-392

[101] Patel A, Knapp M, Evans A, Perez I, Kalra L. Training care givers of stroke patients: Economic evaluation. British Medical Journal. 2004;**328**:1102

[102] Chouhan S, Kumar S. Comparing the effects of rhythmic auditory cueing and visual cueing in acute hemiparetic stroke. International Journal of Therapy and Rehabilitaion. 2012;**19**(6):344-351

[103] Carod-Artal FJ, Egido JA. Quality of life after stroke: The importance of a good functional recovery. Cerebrovascular Diseases. 2009;**27**(Suppl 1):204-214

[104] Mugumbate J, Nyoni C. Disability in Zimbabwe under the new constitution: Demands and gains of people with disabilities. Southern Peace Review Journal (Special Issue in association with the OSSREA Zimbabwe Chapter). 2013:180-199. Available from: https://www.academia.edu/7762774/ [Retrieved 12/02/2018]

[105] Government of Zimbabwe. Constitution of Zimbabwe. 2013. Available from: https://www.constituteproject.org>constitution>Zimbabwe_2013

[106] Parker CJ, Gladman JR, Drummond AE. The role if leisure in stroke rehabilitation. Disability and Rehabilitation. 1997;**19**:1-13

[107] Mayo NE, Wood-Dauphinee S, Ahmed S, et al. Disablement following stroke. Disability and Rehabilitation. 1999;**21**:258-268

[108] Hale LA. Community –based or home –based stroke rehabilitation: Confusion or common sense. New Zealand Journal of Physiotherapy. 2004;**32**(3):131-139

[109] Rhoda AJ. Limitations in activity and participation experienced by stroke patients: A qualitative inquiry. South African Journal of Physiotherapy. 2012;**68**(1):1-5

[110] Urimubenshi G, Rhoda A. Environmental barriers experienced by stroke patients in Musanze district in Rwanda: A descriptive qualitative study. African Health Sciences. 2011;**11**(3):398-406

[111] Khondowe O, Rhoda A, Mpofu R. Perceived needs of caregivers of stroke patients receiving out-patient physiotherapy treatment in Lusaka, Zambia. South African Journal of Physiotherapy. 2012;**68**(1):1-5

[112] Steihaug S. Addressing the organisation of home-based rehabilitation. International Journal of Physical Medicine and Rehabilitation. 2015;**3**:293

[113] Bakas T, Austin JK, Jessup SL, Williams LS, Oberst MT. Time and difficulty of tasks provide by family caregivers of stroke survivors. The Journal of Nursing Science. 2004b;**36**(2):95-106

[114] Dewey HM, Thrift AG, Mihalopoulos C, Carter R, Macdonell RAL, Mcneil JJ, et al. Informal care for stroke survivors. Results from the North Melbourne stroke incidence study (WEMESIS). Stroke. 2002;**33**:1028-1033

[115] Anderson R. The contribution of informal care to the management of stroke. International Journal of Disability Studies. 1988;**10**:107-112

[116] Anderson CS, Linto J, Stewart-Wynne EG. A population-based assessment of the impact and burden of caregiving for long-term stroke survivors. Stroke. 1995;**26**:843-849

[117] Draper B, Bowring G, Thompson C, et al. Stress in caregivers of aphasic stroke patients: A randomized controlled trial. Clinical Rehabilitation. 2007;**21**:122-130. DOI: 10.1177/0269215506071251

[118] Twigg J. Informal care of older people. In: Bernard M, Phillip L, editors. The Social Policy of Old Age. London: Centre for Policy of Ageing; 1998. pp. 128-141

[119] Glass TA, Matchar DB, Belyea M, Feussner JR. Impact of social support on outcome in first stroke. Stroke. 1993;**24**:64-70

[120] Carod-Artal J, Egido JA, Gonzalez JL, Varela de Seijas E. Quality of life among stroke survivors evaluated 1 year after stroke: Experience of a stroke unit. Stroke. 2000;**31**:2995-3000

[121] Bugge C, Alexander H, Hagen S. Stroke patients' informal caregivers. Patient, caregiver, and service factors that affect caregiver strain. Stroke. 1999;**30**:1517-1523

[122] Pomeroy V, Tallis R. Neurological rehabilitation: A science struggling to come of age. Physiotherapy Research International. 2002;**7**:76-89

[123] van den Heuvel ETP, de Witte LP, Schure LM, Sanderman R, Meyboom-de Jong B. Risk factors for burnout in caregivers of stroke patients, and possibilities for intervention. Clinical Rehabilitation. 2001;**15**:669-677

[124] Saunders R. Prevention and treatment of acute ischemic stroke. Nursing Older People. 2013;**25**(8):34-38

[125] Cameron JI, Naglie G, Silver FL, et al. Stroke family caregivers' support needs change across the care continuum: a qualitative study using the timing it right framework. Disability and Rehabilitation. 2013;**35**:315-324. DOI: 10.3109/09638288.2012.691937

[126] Ski C, O'Oconnell B. Stroke: The increasing complexity of carer needs. Journal of Neuroscience Nursing. 2007;**39**(3):172-179

[127] Low JT, Payne S, Roderick P. The impact of stroke on informal carers: A literature review. Social Science & Medicine. 1999;**49**:711-725

[128] Bakas T, Kroenke K, Plue LD, Perkins SM, Williams LS. Outcomes among family caregivers of aphasic versus nonaphasic stroke survivors. Rehabilitation Nursing. 2004b;**31**(1):33-42

[129] Berg A, Palomaki H, Lonnqvist J, Lehtihalmes M, Kaste M. Depression among caregivers of stroke survivors. Stroke. 2005;**36**:639-643

[130] Hickey JV, editor. The Clinical Practice of Neurological and Neurosurgical Nursing. 5th ed. New York/Philladelphia: JB Lippincott Company; 2001

[131] Smith J, Forster A, Young J. A randomized trial to evaluate an education programme for patients and carers after stroke. Clinical Rehabilitation. 2004b;**18**:726-736. DOI: 10.1191/0269215504cr790oa

[132] Gijn v, Dennis MS. Issues and answers in stroke care. The Lancet. 1998;**352**(Suppl. II):23-27

[133] Ang SY, Tin AS, Pavita G, Ng WM, Lee KE, Lim LH, et al. A qualitative study into stroke caregivers' educational needs –perspectives of caregivers and healthcare professionals. Proceedings of Singapore Healthcare. 2013;**22**(3):163-173

[134] Kaseke F, Gwanzura L, Hakim J, Chiwayo DF, Stewart A. Targeted needs analysis for people who have survived stroke and their caregivers in local communities in Zimbabwe. Central African Journal. 2017b;**63**(1/3):7-14

[135] Henderson C. Partial View. Dallas: Southern Methodist University Press; 1998

[136] Davenport R, Dennis M. Neurological emergencies: Acute stroke. Journal of Neurology and Psychiatry. 2000;**68**:277-288

[137] Pinquart M, Sorenson S. Associations of stressors and uplifts of caregiving with caregiver burden and depressive mood: a meta analysis. The Journals of Gerontology: Series B, Psychological Sciences and Social Sciences. 2003; **58**(2):112-128

[138] Gosman-Hedstrom G, Claesson L, Blomstrand C. Consequences of severity at onset for health-related quality of life (HRQL) and informal care: A 1-year follow-up in elderly stroke survivors. Archives of Gerontology and Geriatrics. 2008;**47**:79-81

[139] Jaffe J, Blackley B. Coping as a rural caregiver: The impact of health care reforms on rural women informal caregivers. Priaire Women's Health Centre of Excellence. (Online); 2000. Available at: www.pwhce.ca/copingRuralCaregiver.htm

[140] Blake H, Lincoln NB, Clarke DD. Caregiver strain in spouses of stroke patients. Clinical Rehabilitation. 2003;**17**:312-317

[141] Simon C, Kumar S, Kendrick T. Cohort study of informal cares of first time stroke survivors: Profile of health and social changes in the first year of caregiving. Social Science & Medicine. 2009;**69**:404-410

[142] Forsberg-Warleby G, Moller A, Blomstrand C. Spouses of first-ever stroke patients. Psychological well-being of spouses of stroke patients during the first year after stroke. Stroke. 2001;**32**:1646-1651

[143] Roopchand-Martin S, Creary-Yan S. Level of caregiver burden in Jamaican stroke caregivers and relationship between selected sociodemographic variables. West Indian Medical Journal. 2014;**63**(6):605-609

[144] Wade DT, Leigh-Smith J, Hewer RL. Effects of living with and looking after stroke survivors of a stroke. British Medical Journal. 1986;**293**:418-420

[145] Lin I, Fee HR, Wu H. Negative and positive caregiving experiences: A closer look at the intersection of gender and relationship. Family Relations. 2012;**61**:343-358

[146] McCullagh E, Brigstocke G, Donaldson N, Kalra L. Determinants of care giving burden and quality of life in caregivers of stroke patients. Stroke. 2005;**36**:2181-2186

[147] Jullamate P, de Azeredo Z, Rosenbrug E, Paul C, Subgranon R. Informal stroke rehabilitation: What are the main reasons of than caregivers? International Journal of Rehabilitation Research. 2007;**30**(4):315-320

[148] Choi-Kwon S, Kim H, Kwon SU, Kim JS. Factors affecting the burden on caregivers of stroke survivors in South Korea. Archives of Physical Medicine and Rehabilitation. 2005;**86**:1043-1048

[149] Hsiao C. Family demands, social support and caregiver burden in Taiwanese family caregivers living with mental illness. The role of family caregiver gender. Journal of Clinical Nursing. 2010;**19**:3494-3503

[150] Chiou C, Chen I, Wang H. The health status of family caregivers in Taiwan: An analysis of gender differences. International Journal of Geriatric Psychiatry. 2005;**20**:821-826

[151] Abegunde DO, Mathers CD, Adam T, Ortegon M, Strong K. The burden and costs of chronic disease in low income and middle income countries. The Lancet. 2007;**370**:1929-1938

[152] Singh D, Chaudoir SR, Escobar MC, Kalich man S. Stigma, burden, social support and willingness to care among carers of PLWHA in home-based care in South Africa. AIDS Care. 2011;**23**(7):839-845

[153] Flick CL. Stroke rehabilitation. Stroke outcome and psychosocial concequences. Archives of Physical Medicine and Rehabilitation. 1999;**80**:521-526

[154] Teng J, Mayo NE, Latimer E, Hanley J, Wood-Dauphinee S, Cote R, et al. Costs and caregiver consequences of early supported discharge for stroke patients. Stroke. 2003;**34**:528-536

[155] Schrieber L, Colley M. Patient education. Best Practice & Research. Clinical Rheumatology. 2004;**18**(4):465-476

[156] Margaret H, Anne F, Andy H, Anita P. A systematic review of the economic evidence for interventions for family carers of stroke patients. Clinical Rehabilitation. 2016;**30**(2):119-133

[157] Legg LA, Mahmood F, Weir CJ, Tierney J, Stott OJ, Smith LN, Langhorne P. Non-pharmacological interventions for caregivers of stroke survivors (Review). Cochrane Database System Review. 2011;**5**(10):CD008179. DOI: 10.1002/14651858.CD008179.pub2

[158] Pop-Busui R, Low PA, Waberski RAmas J, Courbon A, Roche F, Bethoux F, et al. Effects of training programmes and exercise in adult stroke patients: A literature review. Annales de Réadaptation et de Médecine Physique. 2007;**50**(6):438-444

[159] Forster A, Dickerson J, Young J, et al. A structured training programme for caregivers of inpatients after stroke (TRACS): a cluster randomised controlled trial and cost-effectiveness analysis. Lancet. 2013;**382**:2069-2076. DOI: 10.1016/S0140-6736(13)61603-7

[160] Akosile CO, Okoye EC, Adegoke BOA, Mbada CE, Marufu FA. Burden, health and quality of life of Nigerian stroke caregivers. Health Care Current Reviews. 2013;**1**:105. DOI: 10.4172/hccr.1000105

[161] Flaherty ML, Kleindorfer D, Kissela BM. Public stroke awareness and education. Seminars in Cerebrovascular Diseases and Stroke. 2004;**4**:130-133

[162] Wasserman S, de Villiers L, Bryer A. Stroke care in a rural African setting. International Journal of Stroke. 2009;**4**:151

[163] Poungvarin N. Stroke in the developing world. The Lancet. 1998;**352**(Suppl. III):19-22

[164] Klinedist NJ, Dubar SB, Clark PC. Stroke survivor and informal caregiver perceptions of poststroke depressive symptons. Journal of Neuroscience Nursing. 2012;**44**(2):72-81

[165] King RB, Hartke RJ, Denby F. Problem-solving early intervention: A pilot study of stroke caregivers. Rehabilitation Nursing. 2007;**32**:68-76

[166] Kaseke F, Challender A, Rapport MJ. Designing a curriculum to meet the needs of caregivers and patients who are living with stroke

in local communities in Zimbabwe. The Internet Journal of Allied Health Sciences and Practice. 2016;**14**(1):6

[167] Bogoshi G, Stewart A, Hale L, Fritz V. Knowledge of stroke risk factors amongst black diabetic, hypertensive and stroke patients. South African Journal of Physiotherapy. 2003;**59**(4):25-30

[168] Dermain S, Burridge J, Ellis-Hill C, Hughes A-M, Yardley L, Tedesco-Triccas L, et al. Assistive technologies after stroke: Self-management or fending for yourself? A focus group study. BMC Health Services Research. 2013;**13**:334. 1-12. http://www.biomedcentral.com/1472-6963/13/334

[169] Moreland JD, Depaul VG, Dehueck AL, Pagliuso SA, Yip DWC, Pollock BJ, et al. Needs assessment of individuals with stroke after discharge from hospital stratified by acute functional Independence measure score. Disability and Rehabilitation. 2009;**31**(26): 2185-2195

[170] Dorsey MK, Vaca KJ. The stroke patient and assessment of caregiver needs. Journal of Vascular Nursing. 1998;**16**(3):62-67

[171] Rodgers H, Atkinson C, Bond S, Suddes M, Dobson R, Curless R. Randomized controlled trial of a comprehensive stroke education program for patients and caregivers. Stroke. 1999;**30**:2585-2591

[172] Forster A, Dickerson J, Melbourn A, Steadman J, Wittink M, Young J, et al. The development and implementation of the structured training program for caregivers of inpatients after stroke (TRACS) intervention: The London stroke carers training course. Clinical Rehabilitation. 2015;**29**(3):211-212. DOI: 10.1177/0269215514543334

[173] Grasel E, Schmidt R, Biehler J, Schupp W. Long-term effects of the intensification of the transition between in-patient neurological rehabilitation and home care of stroke patients. Clinical Rehabilitation. 2006;**20**:577-583

[174] Mant J, Carter J, Wade DT, Winner S. Family support for stroke: A randomised controlled trial. Lancet. 2000;**356**:808-813

[175] Bakas T, Li Y, Habermann B, McLennon SM, Weaver MT. Developing a cost template for a nurse-led stroke caregiver intervention program. Clinical Nurse Specialist. 2011;**25**:41-46

[176] Pierce LL, Steiner V, Govoni AL, Hicks B, Cervantez Thompson TL, Friedemann ML. Internet-based support for rural caregivers of persons with stroke shows promise. Rehabilitation Nursing. 2004;**29**:95-99

[177] Forster A, Young J, Green J, Patterson C, Wanklyn P, Smith J, et al. Structured re-assessment system at 6 months after a disabling stroke: a randomised controlled trial with resource use and cost study. Age and Ageing. 2009;**38**:576-583

[178] Glass TA, Berkman LF, Hiltunen EF, Furie K, Glymour MM, Fay ME, et al. The families In recovery from stroke trial (FIRST): Primary study results. Psychosomatic Medicine. 2004;**66**:889-897

[179] Shebl Amany M, Abd Elhameed SH. Impact of informal caregivers training program on geriatric patients' functional status and post-stroke depression. IOSR Journal of Nursing and Health Science. 2014;**3**(4):45-53. e-ISSN: 2320-1959.p- ISSN: 2320-1940. Ver. I (Jul-Aug. 2014)

[180] Cameron JI, Gignac MAM. "Timing it right": A conceptual framework for addressing the support needs of family caregivers to stroke survivors from the hospital to the home. Patient Education and Counseling. 2008;**70**:308-314